Manual of
Pharmacologic Calculations
With Computer Programs
Second Edition

Ronald J. Tallarida   Rodney B. Murray

Manual of
Pharmacologic Calculations
With Computer Programs

Second Edition

With 28 Figures

Springer-Verlag
New York   Berlin   Heidelberg
London   Paris   Tokyo

Ronald J. Tallarida, Ph. D.
Professor of Pharmacology
Department of Pharmacology
Temple University School of Medicine
Philadelphia, PA 19140
USA

Rodney B. Murray, Ph. D.
Department of Pharmacology
Biosearch Inc.
Philadelphia, PA 19134
USA

Library of Congress Cataloging-in-Publication Data

Tallarida, Ronald J.
  Manual of pharmacologic calculations with
computer programs.

  Includes bibliographical references and
index.
  1. Pharmaceutical arithmetic—Computer
programs. I. Murray, Rodney B.   II. Title.
RS57.T22   1986   615'.1'0285425   86-13029
ISBN 0-387-96357-X

Typeset by Composition House Ltd., Salisbury, England.
Printed and bound by R. R. Donnelley & Sons, Harrisonburg, Virginia.
Printed in the United States of America.

9 8 7 6 5 4 3 2 1

ISBN 0-387-96357-X Springer-Verlag New York Berlin Heidelberg
ISBN 3-540-96357-X Springer-Verlag Berlin Heidelberg New York

Preface to the Second Edition

This book contains a collection of quantitative procedures in common use in pharmacology and related disciplines. It is intended for students and researchers in all fields who work with drugs. Many physicians, especially those concerned with clinical pharmacology, will also find much that is useful. The procedures included may be considered "core" since they are generally applicable to all classes of drugs. Some of the procedures deal with statistics and, hence, have even wider application.

In this new edition we have increased the number of procedures from 33 (in the first edition) to 48. Other procedures have been revised and expanded. Yet the basic philosophy of this new edition remains unchanged from the first. That is, the pharmacologic basis of each procedure is presented, along with the necessary formulas and one or more worked examples. An associated computer program is included for each procedure and its use is illustrated with the same worked example used in the text. The discussions of theory and the sample computations are brief and self-contained, so that all computations can be made with the aid of a pocket calculator and the statistical tables contained in Appendix A. Yet it is realized that the proliferation of lower-priced microcomputers is likely to mean that more and more readers will utilize a computer for most calculations. Accordingly, we have modified the format of the book to facilitate computer usage.

In contrast to the first edition, which was divided into Part I for text and calculation and Part II for computer screens and programs, this edition provides a different, more usable format in which the text of each procedure is immediately followed by the computer screens. These screens, generated by the master program (called PHARM/PCS), use the data from the text example and show the user how data are entered and results received. It is recommended that the text of a procedure and its worked example be read and understood, and, subsequently entered into the associated computer routine. In some cases results of the computer analysis will differ in the second or third decimal place from those given in the text example. The slight difference is due to roundoff that inevitably accompanies hand calculation. Instructions for using the computer program are given in an introductory chapter. The appendix contains a complete listing of the program that may be of value to experienced programmers who wish to modify parts for their own specialized use.

The computer program is vastly enhanced over that contained in the first edition. Provision is now made for saving and editing data files. Also the program diskette (available separately) contains many of the statistical tables, thereby obviating the need for many of the tables in Appendix A. The current program now generates neatly formatted reports which may be saved onto disk to merge with text files when preparing manuscripts that contain both text and tables.

The following procedures are new to this edition:

11. Relative Potency II: Statistical Analysis
28. Pharmacokinetics III: Volume of Distribution
29. Pharmacokinetics IV: Plasma Concentration-Time Data
30. Pharmacokinetics V: Renal Clearance
31. Pharmacokinetics VI: Renal Excretion Data Following Intravenous Administration
32. Pharmacokinetics VII: Multiple Dosing from Absorptive Site
34. Analysis of Variance II: Two-Way, Single Observation
35. Analysis of Variance III: Two-Way, with Replication
36. Newman–Keuls Test
37. Duncan Multiple Range Test
38. Least Significant Difference Test
41. Ratio of Means
43. Proportions: Confidence Limits
47. Litchfield and Wilcoxon II
48. Differential Equations

The authors are grateful to our many colleagues who have communicated with us and offered many valuable suggestions. Special thanks are due Joseph Aceto, and Professor Alan Cowan of Temple University, Professor Frank Porreca of the University of Arizona (Tucson) and Dr. William Schmidt of E.I. Du Pont Company.

Information regarding procurement of the computer disk is given after Appendix B or may be obtained by writing to the authors.

Ronald J. Tallarida
Rodney B. Murray

Preface to the First Edition

This book provides a collection of quantitative procedures in common use in pharmacology and related disciplines. The procedures we selected may be considered "core" since it is likely that all scientists who work with drugs will use these procedures at some time or another. By excluding very specialized topics, we managed to keep the size of the book small, thus making it handy for quick reference—a handbook in the true sense.

Since many scientists and students now have access to electronic computers, and since the advent of lower cost microcomputers is likely to increase computer availability even further, we also included a computer program for each procedure.* The user need not know computer programming since all necessary information needed to run the programs is included here.

The manual is divided into two parts. In the first, the pharmacologic basis for the calculation is briefly stated for each of the procedures (numbered 1 through 33). Then the appropriate equations (formulas) are given and an example of each calculation is provided. For each procedure, the discussion of theory and illustration of the calculation are brief and self-contained. With the tables in the Appendix and a pocket calculator, all of the calculations can be done without reference to any other source. It is recommended that the procedure and sample calculation be read and understood before going to the automated "magic" of the computer program in Part II. This will ensure an understanding of the theory, particularly the possible limitations of the theory to the data in question.

The computer programs (written in standard BASIC) in Part II are numbered corresponding to their Part I equivalent, prefixed with the code S (programs are

---

* All computer programs are available on cassette tape or disk. Information on their purchase may be obtained by writing the authors or by referring to the last page of this volume.

also called subroutines). For example, S5 is the program for performing the computations of Procedure 5, *Analysis of the regression line*. All that is necessary is that the desired programs be accurately typed into the computer. Preferably, they should be stored on a disk or tape for loading when they are to be used; the user then need only type RUN and the number of the desired procedure. The computer will ask for the data, which the user types in. The computer then gives the results of the analysis.

For each of the 33 programs in Part II, we give an example of the user's interaction with the computer. The use of the same data in the computer example and in the text example allows the user to relate the knowledge gained in Part I to the use of the computer. The user should actually enter the sample data for a particular program before trying other data, and the results should agree with that given in this book. Erroneous results would indicate that the program was typed in wrong. Details of the computer operation are given in the introduction to Part II.

The authors are grateful to our many friends and colleagues who helped in so many ways in the preparation of this work. We owe special thanks to Alan Cowan, Paul McGonigle, Frank Porreca, Robert Raffa, Mary Jane Robinson, Theresa Tallarida, and Mark Watson for their help with the proofreading and for several valuable suggestions.

Contents

Introduction

The procedures presented in this book are, either directly or indirectly, concerned with the quantitative identification and comparative evaluation of drug properties. These are key computational methods needed to analyze experiments that search for new drugs and in elucidating, in a rigorous way, metrics that characterize existing drugs. The term "pharmacometrics" might therefore describe the major content of this volume. Two main ideas underly most of the calculations: how much effect? and how much drug? These questions must be answered in any experimental design in which the evaluation of a new compound is to be made by comparing it to a different known compound.

The measurement of effect may be obvious, as in the determination of the drug-induced tension in an isolated muscle preparation, or it may be less obvious as, for example, in evaluating changes in animal behavior. It is essential that the student make a clear definition of effect. Following this, should one examine graded responses, or should a single biologic endpoint (quantal effect) be used in a sample of subjects to assess variability among the subjects? The former is discussed in Procedure 8 (and related Procedures 10–17), whereas the latter is given in Procedure 9, 46, and 47. In some cases a procedure may be applied to either graded or quantal data.

Besides the assessment of effect, several procedures are aimed at determining concentrations. Such calculations are straightforward when dosages are administered *in vitro*, where only dilutions of stock solutions are calculated (Procedure 1). These are more complicated when experiments are carried out in animals and pharmacokinetic considerations apply (Procedures 26–32). Many procedures deal entirely with statistics. These are obviously applicable to many analyses.

The student should in every case understand the pharmacologic basis of the calculation and illustrative examples, for these are guides to the analysis of one's own data. In many cases it may be desirable to plot data prior to entering these into the computer, especially when only portions of the data should be used, for example, in situations in which only steady-state data are wanted. Then the data are ready for entry into the computer and the speed and accuracy of the computer analysis is best utilized. Equal attention should be paid to becoming familiar with the operation of the programs.

Many procedures use linear regression for parts of the computation. The theory that underlies linear regression analysis is well known.* The independent variables $x_1, x_2, \ldots, x_n$, are assumed to be measured with negligible error, or might be controlled by the experimentor. The corresponding y values can inevitably be expected to vary but their distributions are normally distributed. Further, the variances in the population distributions of y values are assumed to be all the same, that is, independent of the x value. In many transformations of data to linear form (e.g., Scatchard plots, double-reciprocal plots, etc.) the assumptions underlying the use of linear regression may not strictly apply. In the case of dose–effect data, it is generally accepted that the use of log(dose) versus effect is preferable in applying linear regression for a variety of reasons. In other transformations, and the biomedical literature is rich with such examples, linear regression analysis gives results which are only approximate. Students are cautioned to understand the limitation of this analysis in such situations.

Computer Program (PHARM/PCS)

The program, PHARM/PCS, will carry out all of the 48 procedures presented in this book. The program will run with little or no modification on computers that use the Microsoft BASIC language. This part of the introduction provides just enough instruction to enable a user to enter data quickly and run each procedure as quickly as possible. Technical details about running PHARM/ PCS and the actual source code listing are found in Appendix B.

Program Listing vs. Diskette

It should be noted that the program listing in Appendix B is intended for experienced programmers who may wish to modify the program to their own specifications. Program remarks (REM statements) are found only in the printed listing and not in the diskette version of the program. The listing is, of necessity, a somewhat abbreviated version of PHARM/PCS. For example, the PHARM/PCS diskette contains help files and statistical tables required by most procedures. These tables are *not* contained in the listing. (See Appendix B for more detailed information and specifics on obtaining the PHARM/PCS diskette for your particular computer.)

* See, for example, Busby, R. C. and Tallarida, R. J. *J. Theor. Biol. 93*: 867–879, 1981.

Sample Screens and Reports

The text of each procedure is followed by sample computer screens generated by PHARM/PCS. These screens follow the text examples closely. The user may familiarize himself/herself with the operation of the program by following the examples illustrated in the sample screens and comparing these with the text example.

Menus

The sample screens show all the prompts given by the program as well as the responses required by the user to accomplish a given procedure. Responses by the user are shown underlined in the examples below and in the sample screens. PHARM/PCS is "menu" oriented. Selections from a menu are chosen by pressing the appropriate key as indicated by angle brackets, ⟨ ⟩. Menus and the general steps required to carry out most procedures are as follows:

Step 1. Choose procedure.

Select procedure, press ⟨?⟩ for help, or press ⟨ENTER⟩ (also called "RE-TURN") to see the "Table of Contents" screen.

Procedure: ⟨# #⟩, ⟨E⟩xit, ⟨?⟩, or ⟨ENTER⟩ for next screen? 10

Step 2. Enter data.

Select the source of the input data (i.e., keyboard entry or data file entry from disk).

Input: ⟨K⟩eyboard, ⟨D⟩isk, or ⟨E⟩xit this procedure? D

Step 3. Edit, list and/or save data.

Data can be viewed and/or edited. Also, files (data sets) saved during this step make it easy to submit the same data for further analysis at a later time. Of course, you will be given the opportunity to save data files again, after editing.

Data: ⟨E⟩dit, ⟨L⟩ist, ⟨S⟩ave, or ⟨ENTER⟩ to continue? E
Edit: ⟨C⟩hange, ⟨D⟩elete, ⟨I⟩nsert, ⟨L⟩ist, or ⟨R⟩ename? C

Step 4. Answer any procedure-specific prompts.

Some procedures allow one to view intermediate results, for example...

Do you want to show intermediate results ⟨Y/N⟩ ? Y

Step 5. Print, view, and/or save results.

A final report may be viewed on the screen, printed immediately or saved on disk for printing at a later time. This feature allows one to save the results of computation for inclusion in a word processing file. The user may then easily incorporate the results in a manuscript.

Report: ⟨P⟩rint, ⟨S⟩ave, or ⟨V⟩iew? <u>S</u>

Help Screens

It should be noted that "Help Screens" are available at any of the program menu choices by pressing ⟨?⟩. These are printed in Appendix B and display the additional options available at each of the menu selections shown above.

Keyboard Data Entry and Editing

Special attention should be paid to the sample screens of Procedure 2, "Mean, Standard Deviation and Confidence Limits," and Procedure 3, "Linear Regression I." Sample screens for these procedures illustrate the entry and editing of data from the keyboard, while most of the remaining sample screens use the data file (disk) method of data entry.

Data Types

Procedure 2 requires the entry of one or more groups of single variable data, called "Y" type data. Procedure 3 requires the entry of one or more groups of paired two-variable data, called "XY" type data. You will find that most procedures call on the computations that are performed in these two procedures; thus these are good examples to study.

In addition, a few procedures require entry of three variable or "XYZ" type data. Procedures requiring "Y," "XY," and "XYZ" data types lend themselves to creating data files. Finally, some procedures require only keyboard input in response to individual prompts, and thus cannot use data files at all.

Procedure 1

Dosage and Concentration: Drug Stock Solutions

A drug is to be dissolved in a saline solution in order to make a given volume of specified molarity. If the molarity is denoted by M, the molecular weight by W, and the desired volume by v (ml), then the amount (in grams) of drug is given by

$$G = \frac{MWv}{1000}. \tag{1.1}$$

Isotonic saline (0.009 g/ml) is added to make the volume v.

If the drug is in a concentrated stock solution, the volume of stock solution (in ml) is computed by dividing G by the concentration of stock solution. The concentration of stock solution, denoted by c, is usually expressed either in units of percent ($g/100$ ml) or in units of g/ml. Hence, the volume of stock needed will be determined by either of the formulas:

for c in units of g/ml

$$x_1 \text{ (ml of stock)} = \frac{MWv}{1000c} = \frac{G}{c} \tag{1.2}$$

for c in units of percent

$$x_2 \text{ (ml of stock)} = \frac{MWv}{10c} = \frac{100G}{c}. \tag{1.3}$$

If the concentration of the final solution is low the drug molecules will not seriously affect the osmolarity of the final solution. However, if the concentration of drug is appreciable and, in particular, if the drug is an electrolyte, the amount of NaCl should be determined in order that the final solution be isotonic with blood. It is necessary, therefore, to find the NaCl equivalent of the grams of drug. The NaCl equivalent of 1 g of drug is first computed. Since the molecular weight of NaCl is 58.5 and since it is 80% dissociated we get the NaCl equivalent of 1 g of drug, denoted by E:

$$E = \frac{58.5}{1.8} \frac{i}{W} = 32.5 \frac{i}{W}, \tag{1.4}$$

where i is the dissociation factor of the drug and W is its molecular weight. The dissociation factor for a drug is related to its number of ions and, in the absence of more specific information, may be obtained from Table 1.1.

Table 1.1
Dissociation Factors[a]

Substance	i
nonelectrolyte	1.0
2 ions	1.8
3 ions	2.6
4 ions	3.4
5 ions	4.2

[a] Stoklosa, M. J. *Pharmaceutical Calculations*, Lea and Febiger, Philadelphia, 1974.

Since $G (= MWv/1000)$ grams of drug are needed, the NaCl equivalent of this amount is EG. Now the NaCl alone that would be contained in an isotonic solution of volume v (ml) is $0.009v$. Hence, the amount of NaCl (in grams) that is needed is given by Q:

$$Q = 0.009v - EG. \qquad (1.5)$$

Water is added to bring the volume to v.

Example

It is desired to make 25 ml of a $10^{-2}\ M$ solution of phenylephrine hydrochloride. A 1% stock solution is to be used. The molecular weight is 204 and the drug dissociates into 2 ions. We have the following:

$$W = 204$$
$$v = 25\ \text{ml}$$
$$M = 0.01$$
$$c = 1\%$$
$$i = 1.8.$$

Equation (1.3) is used to compute the volume of stock solution:

$$x_2 = 0.01 \times 204 \times 25/10$$
$$= 5.1\ \text{ml}.$$

The NaCl equivalent of 1 g of drug is determined from Equation (1.4):

$$E = 32.5 \times 1.8/204$$
$$= 0.29$$

and the amount of NaCl needed for isotonicity is from Equation (1.5):

$$Q = 0.009 \times 25 - 0.29 \times 0.01 \times 204 \times 25/1000$$
$$= 0.21\ \text{g}.$$

Computer Screen

```
            < 1> Dosage & Concentration: Drug Stock Solutions
        Pharmacologic Calculation System - Version 4.0 - 03/10/86

Enter molecular weight of drug ? 204<ENTER>
Enter concentration of stock drug solution
(grams <ENTER> mls <ENTER> )? 1<ENTER>? 100<ENTER>
Enter desired molarity of drug sol'n ? 0.01<ENTER>
Enter volume of sol'n desired (mls) ? 25<ENTER>
Is the drug an electrolyte (Y/N) ? Y
Enter # of ions (2-5) ? 2

Molecular weight of drug          =  204
Conc. of stock drug solution      =  .01 grams/ml
Desired molarity of drug sol'n    =  .01
Total volume of desired sol'n     =  25 ml

Add 5.1 mls of drug stock and 210 milligrams of NaCl to
 19.9 mls of distilled water to give an isotonic solution.

Report: <P>rint, <S>ave, or <V>iew?
```

Computer Report

```
            < 1> Dosage & Concentration: Drug Stock Solutions
        Pharmacologic Calculation System - Version 4.0 - 03/10/86

Molecular weight of drug          =  204
Conc. of stock drug solution      =  .01 grams/ml
Desired molarity of drug sol'n    =  .01
Total volume of desired sol'n     =  25 ml

Add 5.1 mls of drug stock and 210 milligrams of NaCl to
 19.9 mls of distilled water to give an isotonic solution.
```

Procedure 2

Mean, Standard Deviation, and Confidence Limits

The arithmetic mean is the most commonly used number for describing a set of data from a population or a sample. For the n numbers $x_1, x_2, \ldots, x_n$, in a sample the arithmetic mean, denoted by $\bar{x}$, is given by

$$\bar{x} = \frac{x_1 + x_2 + \cdots + x_n}{n} = \frac{\sum_{i=1}^{n} x_i}{n}. \tag{2.1}$$

The formula for the mean of a population, denoted μ, is identical to equation (2.1), i.e., $\mu = (\sum_{i=1}^{N} x_i)/N$, where N is the number of items in the population.

The *standard deviation* of a sample of a population measures the dispersion of the set of data about the mean. For a sample having mean $\bar{x}$ the standard deviation s (or $\hat{s}$) is defined by either of the formulas

$$\hat{s} = \sqrt{\frac{\sum_{i=1}^{n} (x_i - \bar{x})^2}{n-1}} \tag{2.2}$$

or

$$s = \sqrt{\frac{\sum_{i=1}^{n} (x_i - \bar{x})^2}{n}}. \tag{2.3}$$

For a population having mean μ, the standard deviation σ is defined by

$$\sigma = \sqrt{\frac{\sum_{i=1}^{N} (x_i - \mu)^2}{N}}. \tag{2.4}$$

Although we measure the sample mean we are really interested in the population mean. For example, we might determine the tension produced in an isolated muscle by a constant drug concentration and make this determination in a sample of muscles. From these values we compute the sample mean $\bar{x}$ as in Equation (2.1). We ask then, to what extent is the sample mean an estimate of the population mean μ? For this purpose we need to specify a confidence level, such as 95% or 99%, and find the upper and lower confidence limits. The confidence limits depend upon the sample size n and the population standard deviation σ. In most research situations, we do not know σ. In such cases the sample standard deviation s (given by Equation 2.3) may be used provided n is sufficiently large, say $n > 30$. The confidence interval, that is, the interval between the confidence limits, is $\bar{x} \pm z \cdot s/\sqrt{n}$. The value of z is that corresponding to an area under the standard normal curve. If the required confidence (or probability) is 95%, then $z = 1.96$ (See Table A.1).

Thus, the 95% confidence limits for the population mean μ are

$$(95\%: n > 30) \qquad \bar{x} \pm 1.96s/\sqrt{n}. \tag{2.5}$$

For the 99% confidence interval the value of z is 2.58. Thus,

$$(99\%: n > 30) \qquad \bar{x} \pm 2.58s/\sqrt{n}. \tag{2.6}$$

For small samples, $n < 30$, the confidence limits are not determined from the normal distribution. The distribution known as Student's t must be used. Table A.2 gives the values of the area under the distribution curve for various values of t. From Table A.2 we see that the t value requires both the specification of area, 95%, 99%, etc., and the number of degrees of freedom v. In this application $v = n - 1$. Also, the standard deviation used is $\hat{s}$ determined from Equation (2.2). Thus, the confidence interval is computed from

$$\bar{x} \pm t \cdot \hat{s}/\sqrt{n} \tag{2.7}$$

where t has $n - 1$ degrees of freedom.

The expression $(s/\sqrt{n})$ or $(\hat{s}/\sqrt{n})$ is called the *standard error of the mean*.

Example

Measurements of systolic blood pressure were made in a small sample of medical students ($n = 8$) and yielded the following (in mm Hg): 130, 141, 120, 110, 118, 124, 146, 128.

From these data find the mean and sample standard deviation, the standard error of the mean, and the 95% confidence interval of the population mean.

Solution.   Application of Equations (2.1) and (2.2) give

$$\bar{x} = 127.$$

$$\hat{s} = 11.9.$$

Hence, standard error = $\hat{s}/\sqrt{n} = 11.9/\sqrt{8} = 4.2$.

The 95% confidence limits are $127 + 4.2t$, where t is determined from Student's t distribution with 7 degrees of freedom. From Table A.2, $t = 2.365$. Thus, the confidence limits are 127 ± 9.97.

Computer Screen

```
              < 2> Mean, Standard Deviation & Confidence Limits
           Pharmacologic Calculation System  -  Version 4.0 - 03/10/86

Input: <K>eyboard, <D>isk, or <E>xit this procedure? K

You may enter 5 'Y' data files. Type 'END' after last file. Enter file name or
<ENTER> for default name:
'FILE1/Y' (or 'END') ? EXAMPLE<ENTER>

You may enter up to 15 observations. Press <ENTER> after the last entry.
       File name:        EXAMPLE
    ------------    --------------
        #  1:  130<ENTER>
        #  2:  141<ENTER>
        #  3:  120<ENTER>
        #  4:  110<ENTER>
        #  5:  118<ENTER>
        #  6:  124<ENTER>
        #  7:  146<ENTER>
        #  8:  128<ENTER>
        #  9:  <ENTER>


'FILE2/Y' (or 'END') ? END<ENTER>
```

```
Data: <E>dit, <L>ist, <S>ave, or <ENTER> to continue? L

       File name:        EXAMPLE
    ------------    --------------
        #  1:            130
        #  2:            141
        #  3:            120
        #  4:            110
        #  5:            118
        #  6:            124
        #  7:            146
        #  8:            128

Data: <E>dit, <L>ist, <S>ave, or <ENTER> to continue? <ENTER>

       File name:        EXAMPLE
    ------------    --------------
            N:             8
      Minimum:            110
         Mean:        127.125
      Maximum:            146
          Sum:           1017
    Std. Dev.:        11.9216
    Std. Err.:        4.21493
      t Value:          2.365
     95% C.L.:         9.9683
```

Computer Report

```
            < 2> Mean, Standard Deviation & Confidence Limits
         Pharmacologic Calculation System - Version 4.0 - 03/10/86


      File name:        EXAMPLE
   --------------   ---------------
          #  1:           130
          #  2:           141
          #  3:           120
          #  4:           110
          #  5:           118
          #  6:           124
          #  7:           146
          #  8:           128


      File name:        EXAMPLE
   --------------   ---------------
              N:            8
      Minimum:            110
         Mean:          127.125
      Maximum:            146
          Sum:           1017
   Std. Dev.:          11.9216
   Std. Err.:           4.21493
     t Value:            2.365
    95% C.L.:           9.9683
```

Procedure 3

Linear Regression I

Linear regression is a method of curve fitting that is widely used in pharmacology and in other disciplines. The objective is to find a straight line that "best fits" a set of data points (x_i, y_i), $i = 1, \ldots, N$. The usual criterion for defining the best fitting straight line is that the sum of the squares of the vertical deviations from the observed point to the corresponding point on the line is a minimum—a least squares method.

One form of the linear equation is

$$y = mx + b. \tag{3.1}$$

In this equation m is the slope of the line (also called the regression coefficient) and b is the y-intercept. It may be shown that the slope of the regression equation is computed from the equation

$$m = \frac{(\sum x_i)(\sum y_i)/N - \sum (x_i y_i)}{(\sum x_i)^2/N - \sum (x_i)^2}, \tag{3.2}$$

and the y-intercept from

$$b = \bar{y} - m\bar{x}, \tag{3.3}$$

where $\bar{x}$ is the mean x value $= \sum x_i/N$, and $\bar{y}$ is the mean y value $= \sum y_i/N$.

Example

Find the regression line for the points: $(-5, -4), (-1, -2), (3, 4), (5, 6), (8, 7), (10, 10)$, and $(15, 12)$. In this example $N = 7$. The data are most conveniently entered in columns as shown below (Table 3.1).

Table 3.1
Format for Data Entry and Computation

Enter x's	Enter y's	Products	Squares
$x_1 = -5$	$y_1 = -4$	$x_1 y_1 = 20$	$x_1^2 = 25$
$x_2 = -1$	$y_2 = -2$	$x_2 y_2 = 2$	$x_2^2 = 1$
3	4	12	9
5	6	30	25
8	7	56	64
10	10	100	100
$x_N = 15$	$y_N = 12$	$x_N y_N = 180$	$x_N^2 = 225$
$\sum x_i = 35$	$\sum y_i = 33$	$\sum x_i y_i = 400$	$\sum x_i^2 = 449$
$N = 7$			
$(\sum x_i)^2 = 1225$			
$\bar{x} = 5$	$\bar{y} = 4.71$		

The slope is

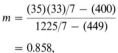

$$m = \frac{(35)(33)/7 - (400)}{1225/7 - (449)}$$

$$= 0.858,$$

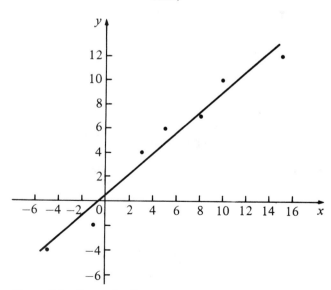

Figure 3.1 Regression line.

and the *y*-intercept is

$$b = 4.71 - (0.858)(5)$$
$$= 0.426.$$

The line is shown in Figure 3.1.

Computer Screen

```
                           < 3> Linear Regression I
              Pharmacologic Calculation System - Version 4.0 - 03/10/86

Input: <K>eyboard, <D>isk, or <E>xit this procedure? K

Enter new variable name(s), or <ENTER> for default(s):
Variable X: 'X' ? <ENTER>
Variable Y: 'Y' ? <ENTER>
Type 'END' after last file. Enter file name or <ENTER> for default name:
'FILE1/XY' (or 'END') ? EXAMPLE<ENTER>

You may enter up to 15 x,y data pairs. Press <ENTER> after the last entry.
    File name:        EXAMPLE
      Variable:          X                Y
-------------- -------------- --------------
        # 1: -5<ENTER>        -4<ENTER>
        # 2: -1<ENTER>        -2<ENTER>
        # 3: 3<ENTER>         33<ENTER>
        # 4: 5<ENTER>         6<ENTER>
        # 5: 8<ENTER>         7<ENTER>
        # 6: 10<ENTER>        10<ENTER>
        # 7: 15<ENTER>        12<ENTER>
        # 8: <ENTER>

'FILE2/XY' (or 'END') ? END<ENTER>
```

```
Data: <E>dit, <L>ist, <S>ave, or <ENTER> to continue? E

Edit: <C>hange, <D>elete, <I>nsert, <L>ist, or <R>ename? C

Change: which entry (1 - 7) in 'EXAMPLE' ? 3<ENTER>

      File name:        EXAMPLE
        Variable:          X                Y
-------------- -------------- --------------
        # 3:              3                33
        # 3: <ENTER>       4<ENTER>
Change: which entry (1 - 7) in 'EXAMPLE' ? <ENTER>

Edit: <C>hange, <D>elete, <I>nsert, <L>ist, or <R>ename? <ENTER>

Data: <E>dit, <L>ist, <S>ave, or <ENTER> to continue? L

      File name:        EXAMPLE
        Variable:          X                Y
-------------- -------------- --------------
        # 1:             -5               -4
        # 2:             -1               -2
        # 3:              3                4
        # 4:              5                6
        # 5:              8                7
        # 6:             10               10
        # 7:             15               12
```

```
Data: <E>dit, <L>ist, <S>ave, or <ENTER> to continue? <ENTER>

        Y =  .857664 * X + .425965

<ENTER> to continue or <L>ist values calculated from regression line? L

     File name:       EXAMPLE
     Variable:           X                    Y   Y Calculated
   ------------    ---------------    ---------------  ---------------
        # 1:            -5              -4          -3.86236
        # 2:            -1              -2          -.431699
        # 3:             3               4           2.99896
        # 4:             5               6           4.71429
        # 5:             8               7           7.28728
        # 6:            10              10           9.00261
        # 7:            15              12          13.2909

  Enter new X to calculate Y or <ENTER> to continue.
  ? 20<ENTER>
                       20                          17.5792
  ? <ENTER>

  Report: <P>rint, <S>ave, or <V>iew?
```

Computer Report

```
                        < 3> Linear Regression I
            Pharmacologic Calculation System - Version 4.0 - 03/10/86

     File name:        EXAMPLE
     Variable:            X                   Y
   -------------   ---------------    ---------------
        # 1:            -5              -4
        # 2:            -1              -2
        # 3:             3               4
        # 4:             5               6
        # 5:             8               7
        # 6:            10              10
        # 7:            15              12


        Y =  .857664 * X + .425965

     File name:        EXAMPLE
     Variable:            X                   Y   Y Calculated
   -------------   ---------------    ---------------  ---------------
        # 1:            -5              -4          -3.86236
        # 2:            -1              -2          -.431699
        # 3:             3               4           2.99896
        # 4:             5               6           4.71429
        # 5:             8               7           7.28728
        # 6:            10              10           9.00261
        # 7:            15              12          13.2909
                       20                          17.5792
```

Procedure 4

Linear Regression II: Lines through Origin

The general regression line is given by $y = mx + b$ (Procedure 3). If the conditions of a problem require that the regression line go through the origin, then the regression line has the form $y = mx$. There is only one parameter to be determined, namely, the slope m. For this case, the least squares criterion leads to

$$m = \frac{\sum_{i=1}^{n} x_i y_i}{\sum_{i=1}^{n} x_i^2}. \tag{4.1}$$

Example

Find the regression line through the origin for the data given below

x	1	2	3	4	5
y	0.20	0.43	0.55	0.70	0.90

Thus

$$m = \frac{(1)(0.20) + (2)(0.43) + (3)(0.55) + (4)(0.70) + (5)(0.90)}{1^2 + 2^2 + 3^2 + 4^2 + 5^2}$$

$$m = \frac{0.20 + 0.86 + 1.65 + 2.8 + 4.5}{55} = 0.18.$$

The regression line is, therefore, $y = 0.18x$.

Computer Screen

```
              < 4> Linear Regression II: Lines Through Origin
              Pharmacologic Calculation System - Version 4.0 - 03/10/86

Input: <K>eyboard, <D>isk, or <E>xit this procedure? K

Enter new variable name(s), or <ENTER> for default(s):
Variable X: 'X' ? <ENTER>
Variable Y: 'Y' ? <ENTER>
Type 'END' after last file. Enter file name or <ENTER> for default name:
'FILE1/XY' (or 'END') ? EXAMPLE<ENTER>

You may enter up to 15 x,y data pairs. Press <ENTER> after the last entry.
     File name:        EXAMPLE
      Variable:          X               Y
     ---------------  --------------  --------------
          # 1: 1<ENTER>      .2<ENTER>
          # 2: 2<ENTER>      .43<ENTER>
          # 3: 3<ENTER>      .55<ENTER>
          # 4: 4<ENTER>      .7<ENTER>
          # 5: 5<ENTER>      .9<ENTER>
          # 6: <ENTER>

'FILE2/XY' (or 'END') ? END<ENTER>
```

```
Data: <E>dit, <L>ist, <S>ave, or <ENTER> to continue? L

    File name:       EXAMPLE
     Variable:          X               Y
   ------------- ------------- -------------
        # 1:            1             .2
        # 2:            2             .43
        # 3:            3             .55
        # 4:            4             .7
        # 5:            5             .9

Data: <E>dit, <L>ist, <S>ave, or <ENTER> to continue? <ENTER>

          Y =  .182 * X

<ENTER> to continue or <L>ist values calculated from regression line? L

    File name:       EXAMPLE
     Variable:          X               Y  Y Calculated
   ------------- ------------- ------------- -------------
        # 1:            1             .2            .182
        # 2:            2             .43           .364
        # 3:            3             .55           .546
        # 4:            4             .7            .728
        # 5:            5             .9            .91
```

```
Enter new X to calculate Y or <ENTER> to continue.
?  6<ENTER>
                             6                      1.092
?  <ENTER>

Report: <P>rint, <S>ave, or <V>iew?
```

Computer Report

```
               < 4> Linear Regression II: Lines Through Origin
            Pharmacologic Calculation System - Version 4.0 - 03/10/86

    File name:       EXAMPLE
     Variable:          X               Y
   ------------- ------------- -------------
        # 1:            1             .2
        # 2:            2             .43
        # 3:            3             .55
        # 4:            4             .7
        # 5:            5             .9

          Y =  .182 * X

    File name:       EXAMPLE
     Variable:          X               Y  Y Calculated
   ------------- ------------- ------------- -------------
        # 1:            1             .2            .182
        # 2:            2             .43           .364
        # 3:            3             .55           .546
        # 4:            4             .7            .728
        # 5:            5             .9            .91
                             6                     1.092
```

Procedure 5

Analysis of the Regression Line

For the regression line $\hat{y} = mx + b$ determined by the points (x_i, y_i), $i = 1, \ldots, N$, the sum of squares about regression SS is given by

$$SS = \sum_{i=1}^{N} (y_i - \hat{y}_i)^2. \tag{5.1}$$

The regression line is found by minimizing SS.

Denoting the mean $\{x_i\}$ by $\bar{x}$, the mean $\{y_i\}$ by $\bar{y}$ and the expression $[SS/(N-2)]^{1/2}$ by s, the estimated standard errors (S.E.) of slope m, y-intercept b, and x-intercept x' are given by the equations below in which each summation is from $i = 1$ to N:

$$\text{S.E.}(m) = s\left[\frac{1}{\sum (x_i - \bar{x})^2}\right]^{1/2} \tag{5.2}$$

$$\text{S.E.}(b) = s\left[\frac{1}{N} + \frac{\bar{x}^2}{\sum (x_i - \bar{x})^2}\right]^{1/2} \tag{5.3}$$

$$\text{S.E.}(x')\dagger = \left|\frac{s}{m}\right|\left[\frac{1}{N} + \frac{(\bar{y}/m)^2}{\sum (x_i - \bar{x})^2}\right]^{1/2}. \tag{5.4}$$

The confidence intervals for each intercept and for the slope of the regression line are obtained by multiplying the respective estimated standard errors by the appropriate value of Student's t for $N - 2$ degrees of freedom.*

The correlation coefficient r is computed from

$$r = \frac{\sum x_i y_i - N\bar{x}\bar{y}}{\sqrt{(\sum x_i^2 - N\bar{x}^2)(\sum y_i^2 - N\bar{y}^2)}}. \tag{5.5}$$

Example

For the data in the example of Procedure 3 it was found that $y = 0.858x + 0.426$ is the regression equation. The estimated standard errors of intercepts and slope and the correlation coefficient are to be determined. The work is arranged as in the table below (Table 5.1).

---

† S.E. (x') is symmetric and approximate. See Bliss, C. I. *Statistics in Biology*, P 439. McGraw-Hill, New York, 1967.

* Table A.2.

Table 5.1
$N = 7$; $\bar{x} = 5.00$; $\bar{y} = 4.71$; $m = 0.858$; $b = 0.426$.

x	y	y^2	$(x - \bar{x})$	$(x - \bar{x})^2$	$(y - \hat{y})$	$(y - \hat{y})^2$
-5	-4	16	-10	100	-0.130	0.0169
-1	-2	4	-6	36	-1.56	2.44
3	4	16	-2	4	1.01	1.01
5	6	36	0	0	1.29	1.66
8	7	49	3	9	-0.284	0.0807
10	10	100	5	25	1.00	1.00
15	12	144	10	100	-1.29	1.66
		365		274		7.87

Thus,

$$SS = 7.87$$

$$s = \left(\frac{7.87}{5}\right)^{1/2} = 1.26$$

$$S.E.(m) = (1.26)\left(\frac{1}{274}\right)^{1/2} = 0.076$$

$$S.E.(b) = (1.26)\left[\frac{1}{7} + \frac{5^2}{274}\right]^{1/2} = 0.607$$

$$S.E.(x') = \left(\frac{1.26}{0.858}\right)\left[\frac{1}{7} + \frac{(4.71/0.858)^2}{274}\right]^{1/2} = 0.736.$$

For calculation of the correlation coefficient, reference to the example of Procedure 5 gives $\sum x_i y_i = 400$, $\sum (x_i^2) = 449$. The other values are obtained from the table above. The correlation coefficient is

$$r = \frac{(400) - 7(5)(4.71)}{\{[449 - (7)(5)^2][365 - (7)(4.71)^2]\}^{1/2}} = 0.981.$$

To get confidence intervals, we obtain t for $7 - 2 = 5$ degrees of freedom. For 95% ($p < 0.05$), the t value is 2.57. Multiplication of t by the estimated standard error yields the half-width of the 95% confidence interval. For the present example,

$$\text{slope} = 0.858 \pm (0.076)(2.57) = 0.858 \pm 0.195$$

$$y\text{-intercept} = 0.426 \pm (0.607)(2.57) = 0.426 \pm 1.57$$

$$x\text{-intercept} = -0.497 \pm (0.736)(2.57) = -0.497 \pm 1.89.$$

Computer Screen

```
                    < 5> Analysis of the Regression Line
              Pharmacologic Calculation System - Version 4.0 - 03/10/86

Input: <K>eyboard, <D>isk, or <E>xit this procedure? D

You may enter 5 'XY' data files. Press <ENTER> after last file name.
File name 1 ? LINE1<ENTER>
File name 2 ? <ENTER>

Data: <E>dit, <L>ist, <S>ave, or <ENTER> to continue? L

    File name:         LINE1
    Variable:            X                    Y
  -------------   ---------------   ---------------
       # 1:             -5                   -4
       # 2:             -1                   -2
       # 3:              3                    4
       # 4:              5                    6
       # 5:              8                    7
       # 6:             10                   10
       # 7:             15                   12

Data: <E>dit, <L>ist, <S>ave, or <ENTER> to continue? <ENTER>
```

```
       Y =  .857664 * X + .425965

       R = .981

   t (95%) = 2.571        5 d.f.

        Variable        Value      Std. Err.    Lower C.L.     Upper C.L.
     -------------   -----------  -----------  ------------  ------------
         Slope:        .857664      .0758287      .662709       1.05262
     Y-Intercept:      .425965      .607306      -1.13542       1.98735
     X-Intercept:     -.496657      .736306      -2.3897        1.39639

   <ENTER> to continue or <L>ist values calculated from regression line? <ENTER>

   Report: <P>rint, <S>ave, or <V>iew?
```

Computer Report

                    < 5> Analysis of the Regression Line
              Pharmacologic Calculation System - Version 4.0 - 03/10/86

    File name: LINE1
    Variable: X   Y
  -------------   ---------------   ---------------
       # 1:   -5   -4
       # 2:   -1   -2
       # 3:   3   4
       # 4:   5   6
       # 5:   8   7
       # 6:   10   10
       # 7:   15   12

       Y = .857664 * X + .425965

       R = .981

   t (95%) = 2.571   5 d.f.

        Variable   Value   Std. Err.   Lower C.L.   Upper C.L.
     -------------   ----------- ----------- ------------ ------------
         Slope: .857664   .0758287   .662709   1.05262
     Y-Intercept: .425965   .607306   -1.13542   1.98735
     X-Intercept: -.496657   .736306   -2.3897   1.39639

Procedure 6

Parallel Lines I: Test for Parallelism

It is often necessary to know whether two lines obtained by linear regression are parallel. This situation arises when comparing drug potencies, when studying the action of antagonists, and in numerous other applications in pharmacology and other branches of science.

This procedure compares the slopes of two regression lines, $L(1)$ and $L(2)$, and uses, therefore, parameters computed from each regression line. The parameters needed in the comparison are tabulated below along with references to the appropriate procedures.

Parameter	Procedure
$m =$ slope	No. 3
$s = \left[\dfrac{\sum (\hat{y}_i - y_i)^2}{N - 2} \right]^{1/2}$	No. 5
$SS_x = \sum (x_i - \bar{x})^2$	No. 5
$N =$ No. of data points	

The test uses Student's t computed from the above parameters for lines (1) and (2).

$$t = \frac{m(1) - m(2)}{s_p [1/SS_x(1) + 1/SS_x(2)]^{1/2}} \tag{6.1}$$

where

$$s_p = \left\{ \frac{[N(1) - 2][S(1)]^2 + [N(2) - 2][S(2)]^2}{N(1) + N(2) - 4} \right\}^{1/2} \tag{6.2}$$

and degrees of freedom $= N(1) + N(2) - 4$. If the computed t value exceeds the tabular value, the slopes differ significantly and the hypothesis of parallelism is rejected.

Example

Lines (1), (2), and (3), shown in Figure 6.1, give the values listed in Table 6.1. Lines (2) and (3) are each to be compared with line (1).

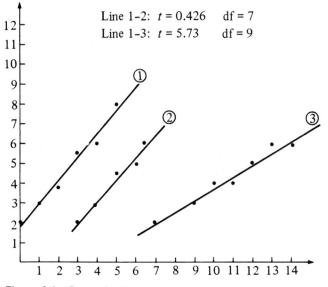

Figure 6.1   Regression lines.

Table 6.1

	N	s	SS_x	m	b
Line (1)	6	0.368	17.5	1.16	1.81
Line (2)	5	0.268	8.2	1.10	−1.31
Line (3)	7	0.293	34.9	0.61	−2.34

Lines (1) *and* (2):

$$s_p = \left\{ \frac{(4)(0.368)^2 + (3)(0.268)^2}{7} \right\}^{1/2} = 0.329$$

$$t = \frac{1.16 - 1.10}{0.329\sqrt{1/17.5 + 1/8.2}} = 0.426.$$

Since $t <$ the tabular value 2.365, the slopes do not differ significantly.

Lines (1) *and* (3):

$$s_p = \left\{ \frac{(4)(0.368)^2 + (5)(0.293)^2}{9} \right\}^{1/2} = 0.328$$

$$t = \frac{1.16 - 0.61}{0.328\sqrt{1/17.5 + 1/34.9}} = 5.73.$$

Since $t >$ the tabular value 2.26, the slopes differ significantly.

Computer Screen

```
                    < 6> Parallel Lines I: Test for Parallelism
                 Pharmacologic Calculation System - Version 4.0 - 03/10/86

Input: <K>eyboard, <D>isk, or <E>xit this procedure? D

You may enter 5 'XY' data files. Press <ENTER> after last file name.
File name 1 ? LINE1<ENTER>
File name 2 ? LINE2<ENTER>
File name 3 ? LINE3<ENTER>
File name 4 ? <ENTER>

Data: <E>dit, <L>ist, <S>ave, or <ENTER> to continue? L

      File name:           LINE1
       Variable:             X                  Y
    ------------    --------------    --------------
          # 1:               0                  2
          # 2:               1                  3
          # 3:               2                  3.8
          # 4:               3                  5.5
          # 5:               4                  6
          # 6:               5                  8
```

```
      File name:           LINE2
       Variable:             X                  Y
    ------------    --------------    --------------
          # 1:               3                  2
          # 2:               4                  3
          # 3:               5                  4.5
          # 4:               6                  5
          # 5:             6.5                  6

      File name:           LINE3
       Variable:             X                  Y
    ------------    --------------    --------------
          # 1:               7                  2
          # 2:               9                  3
          # 3:              10                  4
          # 4:              11                  4
          # 5:              12                  5
          # 6:              13                  6
          # 7:              14                  6

Data: <E>dit, <L>ist, <S>ave, or <ENTER> to continue? <ENTER>

Do you want to show intermediate results (Y/N) ? N
```

```
File name:          LINE1

     Y =  1.16286 * X + 1.80952

File name:          LINE2

     Y =  1.10366 * X -1.30793

File name:          LINE3

     Y =  .610656 * X -2.34426

'LINE1' vs. 'LINE2' :
     t (95%) = 2.365        7 d.f.
     t (99%) = 3.499
    t (calc) = .426    NOT Significant

'LINE1' vs. 'LINE3' :
     t (95%) = 2.262        9 d.f.
     t (99%) = 3.25
    t (calc) = 5.728    Significant at p < 0.01

Report: <P>rint, <S>ave, or <V>iew?
```

Computer Report

```
                        < 6> Parallel Lines I: Test for Parallelism
                 Pharmacologic Calculation System - Version 4.0 - 03/10/86

         File name:              LINE1
          Variable:                X                         Y
     ---------------   ---------------   ---------------
             # 1:                    0                       2
             # 2:                    1                       3
             # 3:                    2                     3.8
             # 4:                    3                     5.5
             # 5:                    4                       6
             # 6:                    5                       8

         File name:              LINE2
          Variable:                X                         Y
     ---------------   ---------------   ---------------
             # 1:                    3                       2
             # 2:                    4                       3
             # 3:                    5                     4.5
             # 4:                    6                       5
             # 5:                  6.5                       6

         File name:              LINE3
          Variable:                X                         Y
     ---------------   ---------------   ---------------
             # 1:                    7                       2
             # 2:                    9                       3
             # 3:                   10                       4
             # 4:                   11                       4
             # 5:                   12                       5
             # 6:                   13                       6
             # 7:                   14                       6


         File name:              LINE1

                 Y =   1.16286 * X + 1.80952

         File name:              LINE2

                 Y =   1.10366 * X -1.30793

         File name:              LINE3

                 Y =   .610656 * X -2.34426


     'LINE1' vs. 'LINE2' :
          t (95%) = 2.365           7 d.f.
          t (99%) = 3.499
          t (calc) = .426    NOT Significant

     'LINE1' vs. 'LINE3' :
          t (95%) = 2.262           9 d.f.
          t (99%) = 3.25
          t (calc) = 5.728   Significant at p < 0.01
```

Procedure 7
Parallel Lines II: Construction of Parallel Lines

Situations are frequently encountered in which two lines, determined by linear regression, are theoretically parallel but, nevertheless, have slightly different slopes m_1 and m_2. If m_1 and m_2 are not significantly different, as determined by the test given in Procedure 6, we can find the common slope m as the weighted mean of the slopes m_1 and m_2:

$$m = \frac{W_1 m_1 + W_2 m_2}{W_1 + W_2}. \tag{7.1}$$

The weighting factors W_1 and W_2 are taken to be the respective reciprocals of the squared standard errors of slope, S.E.(m_1) and S.E.(m_2). Thus

$$W_1 = \frac{1}{[\text{S.E.}(m_1)]^2} \quad \text{and} \quad W_2 = \frac{1}{[\text{S.E.}(m_2)]^2}. \tag{7.2}$$

The standard errors of slopes are found from the analysis of each regression line as given in Procedure 5. From the common slope m, the equations for the parallel lines follow from the mean values of the data points, $(\bar{x}_1, \bar{y}_1)$ for line 1, and $(\bar{x}_2, \bar{y}_2)$ for line 2. Thus, for line 1

$$y = \bar{y}_1 + m(x - \bar{x}_1) \tag{7.3}$$

and for line 2

$$y = \bar{y}_2 + m(x - \bar{x}_2). \tag{7.4}$$

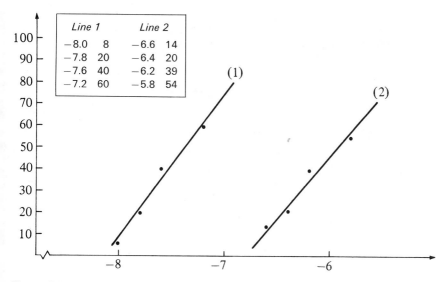

Figure 7.1   Construction of parallel lines.

Example

Isolated strips of rabbit thoracic aorta were dosed with l-norepinephrine and produced the dose–response curve shown as line (1) in Figure 7.1. This same experiment was conducted in the presence of a fixed concentration of the competitive antagonist phentolamine and yielded the line shown as line (2) in Figure 7.1. This curve is shifted to the right of line (1) and is approximately parallel. The regression analysis for each* gave the statistics shown below, from which it is desired to determine the equations of the parallel lines.

Line (1)	Line (2)
$\bar{x}_1 = -7.65$	$\bar{x}_2 = -6.25$
$\bar{y}_1 = 32$	$\bar{y}_2 = 31.75$
$m_1 = 66.3$	$m_2 = 52.4$
$b = 539$	$b = 359$
S.E.$(m_1) = 6.61$	S.E.$(m_2) = 7.44$
$n = 4$	$n = 4$

Thus, for line 1

$$W_1 = \frac{1}{(6.61)^2} = 0.0229$$

and for line 2

$$W_2 = \frac{1}{(7.44)^2} = 0.0181.$$

From Equation (7.1)

$$m = \frac{(0.0229)(66.3) + (0.0181)(52.4)}{0.0229 + 0.0181} = \frac{2.467}{0.0410}$$

$$= 60.2.$$

The parallel lines are given by the equations

$$y = 32.0 + 60.2\,(x + 7.65)$$

and

$$y = 31.75 + 60.2\,(x + 6.25).$$

* See Procedures 3 and 5.

Computer Screen

```
          < 7> Parallel Lines II: Construction of Parallel Lines
             Pharmacologic Calculation System - Version 4.0 - 03/10/86

Input: <K>eyboard, <D>isk, or <E>xit this procedure? D

You may enter 5 'XY' data files. Press <ENTER> after last file name.
File name 1 ? LINE1<ENTER>
File name 2 ? LINE2<ENTER>
File name 3 ? <ENTER>

Data: <E>dit, <L>ist, <S>ave, or <ENTER> to continue? L

    File name:          LINE1
     Variable:            X                    Y
    ------------    --------------    --------------
        # 1:            -8                   8
        # 2:            -7.8                20
        # 3:            -7.6                40
        # 4:            -7.2                60

    File name:          LINE2
     Variable:            X                    Y
    ------------    --------------    --------------
        # 1:            -6.6                14
        # 2:            -6.4                20
        # 3:            -6.2                39
        # 4:            -5.8                54
```

```
Data: <E>dit, <L>ist, <S>ave, or <ENTER> to continue? <ENTER>

Do you want to show intermediate results (Y/N) ? N

    File name:          LINE1

        Y =  66.2875 * X + 539.099

    File name:          LINE2

        Y =  52.4323 * X + 359.452

Common Slope = 60.2165

    File name:          LINE1

        Y =  60.2165 * ( X+ 7.65) + 32

    File name:          LINE2

        Y =  60.2165 * ( X+ 6.25) + 31.75

Report: <P>rint, <S>ave, or <V>iew?
```

Computer Report

```
          < 7> Parallel Lines II: Construction of Parallel Lines
             Pharmacologic Calculation System - Version 4.0 - 03/10/86

    File name:          LINE1
     Variable:            X                    Y
    ------------    --------------    --------------
        # 1:            -8                   8
        # 2:            -7.8                20
        # 3:            -7.6                40
        # 4:            -7.2                60
```

(continued)

```
        File name:              LINE2
         Variable:                X                        Y
    ---------------  ---------------  ---------------
            #  1:              -6.6                      14
            #  2:              -6.4                      20
            #  3:              -6.2                      39
            #  4:              -5.8                      54


        File name:              LINE1

              Y  =   66.2875  *  X  +  539.099

        File name:              LINE2

              Y  =   52.4323  *  X  +  359.452

    Common Slope  =   60.2165

        File name:              LINE1

              Y  =    60.2165  *  (  X+  7.65)  +  32

        File name:              LINE2

              Y  =    60.2165  *  (  X+  6.25)  +  31.75
```

Procedure 8

Graded Dose–Response

The dose–response relation of many agonists yield sigmoidal (**S**-shaped) curves when the response is plotted against the logarithm of the dose (see Figure 8.1). There is no generally accepted theory that explains the shape of such curves*; yet, we find that such curves are often approximately linear between 20% and 80% of the maximum response. In particular, many isolated tissue preparations display this linear segment. The data in the 20%–80% region may therefore be subjected to linear regression as given in Procedure 3, in which y = effect, or percent effect, and x = log dose. The regression line so determined might be used in the comparison of potency (Procedure 10) or in the analysis of the action of a competitive antagonist (Procedure 15). In each of these applications the regression lines are made parallel, and equieffective doses are determined.

The value of the regression technique is that the raw data may not yield a smooth curve. The regression line determined from effect (y) versus log dose (x) is, therefore, an objective method for determining the dose–response relation.

Since this regression line is based on points between (and including) 20% and 80% of E_{max}, it is necessary to know E_{max}. *If this value is not known it must be estimated.* A common procedure for estimating E_{max} is to plot the reciprocal effect ($1/E$) against the reciprocal dose ($1/D$). The rationale for this plot is that

---

* Tallarida, R. J., and Jacob L. S. *The Dose–Response Relation in Pharmacology.* Springer-Verlag, New York, 1979.

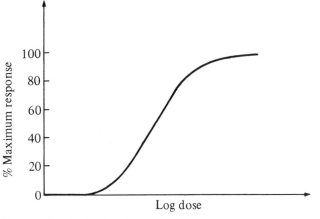

Figure 8.1   Graded log dose–response curve.

many dose–response curves are approximately hyperbolic of the form $E = E_{max} \cdot D/(D + C)$, so that a double reciprocal plot is linear

$$\frac{1}{E} = \frac{C}{E_{max}} \cdot \frac{1}{D} + \frac{1}{E_{max}}. \qquad (8.1)$$

In this equation, C is an empirical constant.*

From Equation (8.1), $1/E_{max}$ is the vertical intercept so that E_{max} is easily estimated. Not infrequently the double reciprocal plot yields an intercept that is negative and, therefore, without meaning since E_{max} must be positive. This occurs usually because small values of dose and effect, when reciprocated, are large. Accordingly, errors in small doses and effects are magnified when reciprocated. One remedy is to weight the data. A more practical remedy is to avoid using the small dose–effect points. We illustrate with the data of Table 8.1 on oxytocin-induced contraction of rat uterus.

Table 8.1
Effect of oxytocin on isolated rat uterus

D	E	$\log D$	$1/D$	$1/E$
0.05	1	−1.30	2.0	1
0.14	5	−0.85	7.14	0.20
0.23	12	−0.64	4.35	0.083
0.40	32	−0.40	2.50	0.031
0.50	38	−0.30	2.00	0.026
1.0	52	0.00	1.00	0.019
1.8	58	0.26	0.56	0.017

[a] Doses are nmol/liter and effects are isotonic contractions (mm).

* The constant C is not necessarily the drug-receptor dissociation constant. See note at end of procedure.

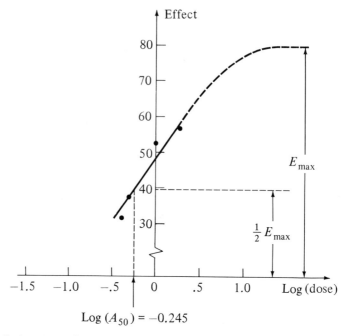

Log $(A_{50}) = -0.245$

Figure 8.2   Log dose–effect curve. Solid curve is the regression line of effect vs. log dose and is given by $E = 40.01$ log dose $+ 49.44$ from which $\log(A_{50}) = -0.245$. (See text.)

Example

With reference to the data in Table 8.1, which, for convenience, also gives values of log D, $1/E$ and $1/D$, the double reciprocal plot yields a regression line with intercept -0.0819. Since this negative intercept is without meaning, we have deleted the data for the three smallest doses. The double reciprocal plot for the four remaining points gave an intercept 0.0126 which translates into an estimated $E_{max} = 79.26$.

With E_{max} now estimated, we use only the points corresponding to effects between 20 and 80% of 79.26 in the regression of E vs. log D. These points are shown in Table 8.2 and plotted in Figure 8.2, which also gives the regression equation in the legend.

Potency of the drug is determined from the left-to-right position of its dose (or log dose) response curve. Thus the value of dose that produces a half maximal effect (A_{50}) is an index of the drug's *potency*. From the regression line of E vs. log dose, shown in Figure 8.2, the value of $\log(A_{50}) = -0.245$, so that $A_{50} = 0.568$ nmol/liter.

Confidence limits of $\log(A_{50})$ are determined as described in Procedure 5. Denoting $\log(A_{50})$ by a, we have the confidence limits of a given approximately by*

$$a \pm t\,[\text{S.E.}(a)] \tag{8.2}$$

* Bliss, C. I. *Statistics in Biology*, p. 439. McGraw-Hill, New York, 1967.

where t is the value of Student's t for $N - 2$ degrees of freedom and S.E.(a) is the standard error of a and is given by

$$S.E.(a) = \left| \frac{s}{m} \right| \sqrt{\frac{1}{N} + \frac{(a - \bar{x})^2}{\sum (x_i - \bar{x})^2}}, \tag{8.3}$$

where all symbols have the same meaning as in Procedure 5.

For the regression line based on the data of Table 8.2, $a = -0.245$, $\bar{x} = -0.110$, $\sum (x_i - \bar{x})^2 = 0.2692$, $N = 4$, $s = 2.48$, and $m = 40.01$. Thus, S.E.$(a) = 0.0345$. The tabular value of t (for 4–2 degrees of freedom and 95%) is 4.303. Accordingly, confidence limits of $\log(A_{50})$ are $-0.245 +/-0.148$ or -0.097 to -0.393. The corresponding confidence limits of A_{50} are 0.404 to 0.799 nmol/liter.

Table 8.2
Log(dose)-effect data
for effects between
20% and 80% of E_{max}

log D	E
−0.40	32
−0.30	38
0.00	52
0.26	58

Computer Screen

```
                    < 8> Graded Dose-Response
           Pharmacologic Calculation System - Version 4.0 - 04/06/86

  Input: <K>eyboard, <D>isk, or <E>xit this procedure? D

  File name: ? EXAMPLE<ENTER>

  Data: <E>dit, <L>ist, <S>ave, or <ENTER> to continue? L

       File name:      EXAMPLE
       Variable:       Dose        Response
     ------------    ----------   ----------
        #  1:           .05           1
        #  2:           .14           5
        #  3:           .23          12
        #  4:           .4           32
        #  5:           .5           38
        #  6:          1            52
        #  7:          1.8          58

  Data: <E>dit, <L>ist, <S>ave, or <ENTER> to continue? <ENTER>

  Do you want to show intermediate results (Y/N) ? Y

  Calculation of A50 requires the knowledge of Emax.  Press <ENTER> to do a
  double reciprocal plot to estimate Emax OR enter Emax ? <ENTER>
```

```
Calculating double reciprocal plot...

     File name:      EXAMPLE
     Variable:        1/Dose    1/Response
   --------------- --------------- ---------------
       #  1:            20             1
       #  2:        7.14286            .2
       #  3:        4.34783         .0833333
       #  4:          2.5           .03125
       #  5:           2           .0263158
       #  6:           1           .0192308
       #  7:        .555556         .0172414


  1/Response =  .0519918 * 1/Dose -.0821034

Emax estimated from double repiprocal plot = -12.1798

Negative Emax! You should delete one or more of the low doses or enter an
estimated Emax.

Emax options: <E>dit data, enter <N>ew estimate, or <K>eep double reciprocal
estimate? E
```

```
Edit: <C>hange, <D>elete, <I>nsert, <L>ist, or <R>ename? D

Delete: which entry (1 - 7) in 'EXAMPLE' ? 1<ENTER>

Delete: which entry (1 - 6) in 'EXAMPLE' ? 1<ENTER>

Delete: which entry (1 - 5) in 'EXAMPLE' ? 1<ENTER>

Delete: which entry (1 - 4) in 'EXAMPLE' ? <ENTER>

Edit: <C>hange, <D>elete, <I>nsert, <L>ist, or <R>ename? <ENTER>

     File name:      EXAMPLE
     Variable:        1/Dose    1/Response
   --------------- --------------- ---------------
       #  1:          2.5           .03125
       #  2:           2           .0263158
       #  3:           1           .0192308
       #  4:        .555556         .0172414


  1/Response =  7.19425E-03 * 1/Dose + .0126182

Emax estimated from double repiprocal plot =  79.2506
```

```
Emax options: <E>dit data, enter <N>ew estimate, or <K>eep double reciprocal
estimate? K

Emax = 79.2506 (estimated from double reciprocal plot)

Log(Dose)-Response regression between 20%-80% of Emax...

     Variable:      Log(Dose)     Response      % Emax
   --------------- --------------- --------------- ---------------
       #  1:        -1.30103          1         1.26182  deleted
       #  2:        -.853872          5         6.3091   deleted
       #  3:        -.638272         12        15.1418   deleted
       #  4:        -.39794          32        40.3782
       #  5:        -.30103          38        47.9492
       #  6:           0            52        65.6146
       #  7:        .255272          58        73.1856

Data points deleted: 3

  Response =  40.0078 * Log(Dose) + 49.4378

        R = .986

  t (95%) = 4.303       2 d.f.
```

```
      Variable         Value      Std. Err.    Lower C.L.    Upper C.L.
  ----------------  ------------  ------------  ------------  ------------
          Slope:      40.0078       4.7507       19.5656       60.4501
  Y-Intercept:        49.4378       1.33134      43.7091       55.1666
  X-Intercept:        -1.2357        .137013      -1.82527      -.646139

  <ENTER> to continue or <L>ist values calculated from regression line?  <ENTER>


          A50          .568505                     .404018       .799961
      Log(A50)        -.245265      .0344723       -.3936        -.0969311

  Report: <P>rint, <S>ave, or <V>iew?  <ENTER>
```

Computer Report

```
                            < 8> Graded Dose-Response
             Pharmacologic Calculation System - Version 4.0 - 04/06/86

      File name:     EXAMPLE
      Variable:        Dose       Response
  ------------    ------------  ------------
        # 1:           .05           1
        # 2:           .14           5
        # 3:           .23          12
        # 4:           .4           32
        # 5:           .5           38
        # 6:          1            52
        # 7:          1.8          58


  Emax = 79.2506 (estimated from double reciprocal plot)

  Log(Dose)-Response regression between 20%-80% of Emax...

      Variable:     Log(Dose)     Response      % Emax
  ------------    ------------  ------------  ------------
        # 1:        -1.30103          1        1.26182  deleted
        # 2:         -.853872         5        6.3091   deleted
        # 3:         -.638272        12       15.1418   deleted
        # 4:         -.39794         32       40.3782
        # 5:         -.30103         38       47.9492
        # 6:          0             52       65.6146
        # 7:          .255272       58       73.1856

  Data points deleted: 3

    Response =   40.0078 * Log(Dose) + 49.4378

      Variable         Value      Std. Err.    Lower C.L.    Upper C.L.
  ------------    ------------  ------------  ------------  ------------
          A50          .568505                     .404018       .799961
      Log(A50)        -.245265      .0344723       -.3936        -.0969311
```

Procedure 9

Quantal Dose–Response: Probits

The quantal, or all-or-none, dose–response relation is obtained by specifying a specific endpoint of drug action and determining the number of subjects that achieve this endpoint as a function of drug dosage.* For example, the endpoint

* Tallarida, R. J., and Jacob, L. S. *The Dose–Response Relation in Pharmacology*, Springer-Verlag, New York, 1979.

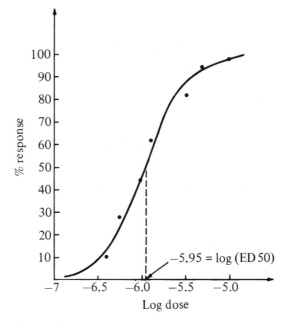

Figure 9.1 Log dose–response curve.

might be the production of sleep as determined by lack of response to a measured noxious stimulus. A fixed amount of a hypnotic drug is given to a group of animals and the number (or percentage) that experience sleep is noted. A larger dose is given and again the number is determined; this number will include all those who experienced sleep with the previous dose, plus the additional number. Thus, the number, or percentage, is cumulative, resulting in the plotted points shown in Figure 9.1 in which the abscissa is log dose.

Another method of plotting the data is to convert the percent who respond to *probits*, or probability units. The probit is related to the percent area under the normalized probability curve. Table A.3 gives the relation between percent and probit.

When the percent (of subjects responding) is converted to probits and plotted against log dose, the resulting plot is linear as in Figure 9.2. Obtaining the linear regression line, and reconverting probits to percent, yields the smooth sigmoid curve of Figure 9.1.

Example

Log dose–response data are given in Table 9.1 and plotted in Figure 9.1. Determine the corresponding graph of probits against log dose.

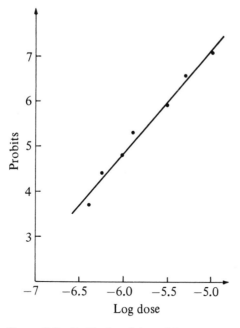

Figure 9.2   Probit plot of data of Figure 9.1.

Table 9.1
Probits for Dose–Response Data

log dose	% response	Probits
−6.4	10	3.7
−6.25	28	4.4
−6.0	44	4.8
−5.9	62	5.3
−5.5	82	5.9
−5.3	94	6.6
−5.0	98	7.1

Column 3 of Table 9.1 contains the corresponding probits as obtained from Table A.3. The regression of probits on log dose is $y = 2.3$ (log dose) $+ 19$, and is plotted in Figure 9.2. The value of y obtained from the regression line is plotted as the smooth curve of Figure 9.1.

The dose that produces a response in 50% of the sample is called *ED*50. The value log(ED50) may be read from the graph. In Figure 9.1 the value is seen to be −5.94. The computer subroutine prints ED50, as well as ED16 and ED84, the effective doses in 16% and 84%, respectively. Logarithms of each are also displayed. (See Procedures 46 or 47 for additional analysis of quantal dose–response curves.)

Computer Screen

```
                    < 9> Quantal Dose-Response: Probits
              Pharmacologic Calculation System - Version 4.0 - 03/10/86

Input: <K>eyboard, <D>isk, or <E>xit this procedure? D

You may enter 5 'XY' data files. Press <ENTER> after last file name.
File name 1 ? LINE1<ENTER>
File name 2 ? <ENTER>

Data: <E>dit, <L>ist, <S>ave, or <ENTER> to continue? L

        File name:           LINE1
        Variable:        Log(Dose)          Response
      --------------   --------------     --------------
            # 1:           -6.4                 10
            # 2:           -6.25                28
            # 3:            -6                  44
            # 4:           -5.9                 62
            # 5:           -5.5                 82
            # 6:           -5.3                 94
            # 7:           -5                   98

Data: <E>dit, <L>ist, <S>ave, or <ENTER> to continue? <ENTER>
```

```
        Probit =   2.28963 * Log(Dose) + 18.6002

                            Dose      Log(Dose)
                        --------------  --------------
        ED16 =       4.22421E-07        -6.37425
        ED50 =       1.1484E-06         -5.93991
        ED84 =       3.12208E-06        -5.50556

<ENTER> to continue or <L>ist values calculated from regression line? L

            Dose        Log(Dose)    % Response        Probit
        --------------  --------------  --------------  --------------
        3.98107E-07       -6.4             10          3.71827
        5.62341E-07       -6.25            28          4.41752
        .000001           -6               44          4.84935
        1.25892E-06       -5.9             62          5.30504
        3.16228E-06       -5.5             82          5.91526
        5.01187E-06       -5.3             94          6.5551
        .00001            -5               98          7.05419

Press <ENTER> to continue, or calculate a new value from: <L>og(dose) or %
<R>esponse? <ENTER>

Report: <P>rint, <S>ave, or <V>iew?
```

Computer Report

```
                    < 9> Quantal Dose-Response: Probits
              Pharmacologic Calculation System - Version 4.0 - 03/10/86

        File name:           LINE1
        Variable:        Log(Dose)          Response
      --------------   --------------     --------------
            # 1:           -6.4                 10
            # 2:           -6.25                28
            # 3:            -6                  44
            # 4:           -5.9                 62
            # 5:           -5.5                 82
            # 6:           -5.3                 94
            # 7:           -5                   98
```

```
Probit =  2.28963 * Log(Dose) + 18.6002
```

	Dose	Log(Dose)
ED16 =	4.22421E-07	-6.37425
ED50 =	1.1484E-06	-5.93991
ED84 =	3.12208E-06	-5.50556

Dose	Log(Dose)	% Response	Probit
3.98107E-07	-6.4	10	3.71827
5.62341E-07	-6.25	28	4.41752
.000001	-6	44	4.84935
1.25892E-06	-5.9	62	5.30504
3.16228E-06	-5.5	82	5.91526
5.01187E-06	-5.3	94	6.5551
.00001	-5	98	7.05419

Procedure 10

Relative Potency I

It is often desired to estimate the relative potencies of a number of drugs in a class that is based on some effect. For example, the agents might be vasodilators, or analgesics, or hormones, etc. Potency refers to the amount (mg, g, moles, etc.) of drug needed to produce a level of effect. Relative potency is the ratio of the amounts of each needed to produce the specified effect. Thus, one drug, the standard (S), is assigned unit potency and the second drug (U) is compared to that of S. The other drugs in the class are similarly compared.

The comparison is best made from the dose–response relations of each, or from the log dose–response relations of each.* The latter will often yield linear graphs as discussed in Procedure 8. If the relative potency is constant at each level of effect, the log dose–response lines will be parallel as in Figure 10.1. In practice, it may be necessary to construct parallel lines from the points of each as described in Procedure 7. The relative potency is determined from the horizontal distance d between the lines:

$$d = \log(\text{dose})_u - \log(\text{dose})_s$$

$$= \log \frac{(\text{dose})_u}{(\text{dose})_s}$$

and

$$\text{relative potency} = \frac{(\text{dose})_u}{(\text{dose})_s} = \text{antilog } d. \tag{10.1}$$

A statistical analysis is given in Procedure 11. With reference to the lines of Figure 10.1, the determination of the relative potency of U to S is illustrated.

---

* In this and the following procedure, graded dose–response data are used. Relative potency is also determined from quantal data as described in Procedure 9. (See also Procedures 46 and 47.)

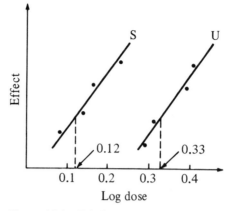

Figure 10.1   Relative potency determination.

The distance d is determined by dropping perpendiculars to the horizontal axis from equieffective points on each line. Thus $d = 0.33 - 0.12 = 0.21$. Hence,

$$\text{relative potency} = \text{antilog}\ (0.21)$$

$$= 1.62.$$

Simpler methods may be used to determine relative potency*. One such method is called a "2 and 2" dose assay. Doses D_1 and D_2 of drug S are administered and the effects $E_s(1)$ and $E_s(2)$ are measured. Identical doses of drug U are given and its effects $E_u(1)$ and $E_u(2)$ are determined. From these values parallel lines are constructed as shown in Figure 10.2. We denote by x the quantity, $\log D_2 - \log D_1 = \log(D_2/D_1)$. The slope m is the average of the slopes. Thus, for U the slope is $[E_u(2) - E_u(1)]/x$ and for S the slope is $[E_s(2) - E_s(1)]/x$. The average slope m is given by $[E_s(2) - E_s(1) + E_u(2) - E_u(1)]/(2x)$. The

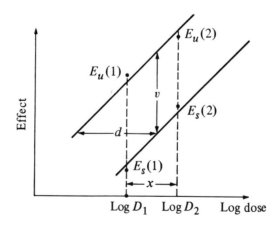

Figure 10.2   The calculation of relative potency for a "2 and 2" dose assay.

* This method is useful because of the simplicity of the computation (Eq. 10.2); procedure 11 is preferred when error estimates of the potency ratio are desired.

average vertical distance v, is $[E_u(2) - E_s(2) + E_u(1) - E_s(1)]/2$. The horizontal distance is d and is given by

$$d = \frac{v}{m} = \left(\frac{E_u(2) - E_s(2) + E_u(1) - E_s(1)}{E_s(2) - E_s(1) + E_u(2) - E_u(1)}\right)(x) \qquad (10.2)$$

and relative potency is antilog d.

Example

Two hypnotics were given to two groups of animals and the effects, denoted by the percentage of each group experiencing sleep, were noted. The doses used (of both drugs) were 5 mg and 25 mg. For drug S the effects were 32% and 61%, whereas these same doses of drug U gave 48% and 84%. From Equation (10.2)

$$d = \frac{84 - 61 + 48 - 32}{61 - 32 + 84 - 48} \cdot \log\left(\frac{25}{5}\right)$$

$$= \left(\frac{39}{65}\right)(\log 5) = 0.419.$$

Thus,

$$\text{relative potency (U/S)} = \text{antilog } 0.419 = 2.6.$$

The corresponding computer subroutine computes the relative potency for the "2 and 2" dose assay or complete dose–response data depending on the number of data points entered. If there are only two data points for each line (2 and 2 dose assay), the program will accept only identical X values (dose) for each line. The two Y values for each line may be either a percentage response (from quantal data) or a mean response (from graded data). In the other case, when more complete dose–response data are entered (more than two X, Y coordinates per line), the data should first be smoothed as described in procedure 8. The program will calculate the dose-ratio (or log dose-ratio) from such data.

Computer Screen

```
                       <10> Relative Potency I
          Pharmacologic Calculation System - Version 4.0 - 03/10/86

This procedure calculates the relative potency of the first dose-response
curve versus one or more additional curves.

Input: <K>eyboard, <D>isk, or <E>xit this procedure? D

You may enter 5 'XY' data files. Press <ENTER> after last file name.
File name 1 ? DrugU<ENTER>
File name 2 ? DrugS<ENTER>
File name 3 ? <ENTER>

Data: <E>dit, <L>ist, <S>ave, or <ENTER> to continue? L

     File name:          DrugU
     Variable:           Dose        Response
  ---------------    -----------   ------------
        # 1:               5            48
        # 2:              25            84

     File name:          DrugS
     Variable:           Dose        Response
  ---------------    -----------   ------------
        # 1:               5            32
        # 2:              25            61
```

```
Data: <E>dit, <L>ist, <S>ave, or <ENTER> to continue? <ENTER>

2 and 2 Dose Assay:

Relative Potency of 'DrugU' versus:

          Curve      Pot. Ratio
      --------------  --------------
          DrugS         2.62653

Report: <P>rint, <S>ave, or <V>iew?
```

Computer Report

```
                         <10> Relative Potency I
            Pharmacologic Calculation System - Version 4.0 - 03/10/86

        File name:          DrugU
        Variable:           Dose            Response
     --------------    --------------    --------------
            # 1:              5               48
            # 2:             25               84

        File name:          DrugS
        Variable:           Dose            Response
     --------------    --------------    --------------
            # 1:              5               32
            # 2:             25               61

   2 and 2 Dose Assay:

   Relative Potency of 'DrugU' versus:

          Curve      Pot. Ratio
      --------------  --------------
          DrugS         2.62653
```

Procedure 11

Relative Potency II: Statistical Analysis (Graded Data)

The relative potency of two drugs is determined as the ratio of equieffective doses (or concentrations) of each from their respective graded dose-response relations.* Frequently, linear regression lines of effect vs. log dose are plotted and made parallel as discussed in Procedure 10. The horizontal distance, L, between the parallel lines is $\log d_1 - \log d_2 = \log(d_1/d_2)$, and $d_1/d_2 = 10^L$ is the relative potency. We now discuss a method for obtaining both the relative potency and its confidence limits. The analysis and computations are considerably simplified if the *same log dose increments are used for each drug* (Figure 11.1), *and the number of observations is the same for each dose and drug.* For each regression line the total number of points will be denoted by N.

The first step in the analysis is the determination of the common slope, m_c as

---

* (See Procedure 47 for relative potency from quantal data.)

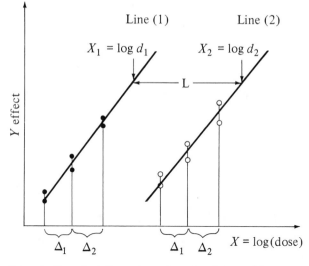

Figure 11.1 Determination of relative potency from the distance L between parallel regression lines. X_1 and X_2 are any two values of log(dose) for the respective drugs that yield the same effect.

described in Procedure 7. Then, from the averages $\bar{X}$ and $\bar{Y}$ for each line, the distance, L, may be computed as

$$L = X_2 - X_1 = (\bar{Y}_1 - \bar{Y}_2)/m_c + (\bar{X}_2 - \bar{X}_1) \tag{11.1}$$

and

$$L - (\bar{X}_2 - \bar{X}_1) = \frac{\bar{Y}_1 - \bar{Y}_2}{m_c} \tag{11.2}$$

Confidence limits are needed for the ratio $Q = (\bar{Y}_1 - \bar{Y}_2)/m_c$. These are computed as the roots of the equation

$$\frac{\bar{Y}_1 - \bar{Y}_2 - Qm_c}{s_p \left[\dfrac{2}{N} + \dfrac{Q^2}{2 \sum (X_i - \bar{X})^2} \right]^{1/2}} = t, \tag{11.3}$$

where t is the value of Student's t for 2N-3 degrees of freedom and s_p^2 is the pooled standard error of estimate from the individual lines which, for equal numbers of points N, is

$$s_p^2 = \tfrac{1}{2}(s_1^2 + s_2^2) \tag{11.4}$$

Thus, the following are needed for each regression line: m, s, $\bar{X}$, $\bar{Y}$, S.E.(m) and $\sum (X_i - \bar{X})^2 = $ SSx.

These are determined as in Procedure 5. The common slope uses the values of m and S.E.(m) for each line as described in Procedure 7.

Values are inserted into Equation (11.3) which is a quadratic, $AQ^2 + BQ + C = 0$, where

$$A = m_c^2 - \frac{t^2 s_p^2}{2 \sum (X_i - \bar{X})^2} \tag{11.5}$$

$$B = 2m_c(\bar{Y}_2 - \bar{Y}_1) \tag{11.6}$$

and

$$C = (\bar{Y}_1 - \bar{Y}_2)^2 - 2t^2 s_p^2/N. \tag{11.7}$$

Thus,

$$Q = -B/2A \pm (B^2 - 4AC)^{1/2}/2A \tag{11.8}$$

and yield upper and lower values, Q_u and Q_l. The upper and lower confidence limits for L are

$$L_u = (\bar{X}_2 - \bar{X}_1) + Q_u \tag{11.9}$$

and

$$L_l = (\bar{X}_2 - \bar{X}_1) + Q_l \tag{11.10}$$

The corresponding values of relative potency are

$$(d_1/d_2) = 10^{L_u} \tag{11.11}$$

and

$$(d_1/d_2) = 10^{L_l} \tag{11.12}$$

Computational Summary

1. From the pair of parallel lines, determine m_c, s_p^2 and $\sum (X_i - \bar{X})^2$; the latter is the same for each line.

2. Using the means $\bar{Y}_1$ and $\bar{Y}_2$, t (tabular) and N, along with the quantities in 1, compute A, B and C from Equations (11.5) to (11.7).

3. The value of A, B and C are used to get the roots Q_u and Q_l according to Equation (11.8).

4. Relative potencies, with upper and lower confidence limits, are determined from Equations (11.9) to (11.12).

Example

Graded log dose–effect data for drugs 1 and 2 gave the data shown below. It is desired to compute the potency ratio and its 95% confidence limits.

	Line 1		Line 2	
	0.9	1.8	1.6	1.5
	0.9	4.1	1.6	2.1
	1.1	3.1	1.8	1.9
	1.1	5.2	1.8	4.4
	1.5	6.7	2.2	5.1
	1.5	9.2	2.2	7.0
	1.8	11	2.5	8.0
	1.8	12.5	2.5	9.9

		Line 1	Line 2
Slope	=	9.815	7.869
y-int	=	-6.305	-10.948
$\bar{X}$	=	1.325	2.025
$\bar{Y}$	=	6.700	4.987
s_s	=	1.318	1.101
SE (slope	=	1.335	1.115
$SSx = \sum (X_1 - \bar{X})^2$	=	0.975	0.975

$1/[SE(slope)]^2 = 0.5611$ 0.8044

$\therefore$ Common slope $= 8.669$

$$L = (6.700 - 4.987)/8.669 + (2.025 - 1.325)$$
$$= 0.1976 + 0.7$$
$$= 0.8976$$

$$s_p^2 = (1.318^2 + 1.101^2)/2$$
$$= (1.737 + 1.212)/2$$
$$= 1.474$$

$t_{95\%}$, $(df = 13) = 2.160$

Quantities

$$A = (8.669)^2 - (2.16)^2(1.474)/0.9750(2)$$
$$= 71.625$$

$$B = (2)(8.669)(4.987 - 6.700)$$
$$= -29.700$$

$$C = (6.7 - 4.981)^2 - (2)(2.160)^2(1.474)/8$$
$$= 2.934 - 13.754/8$$
$$= 1.215$$

Therefore,

$$B^2 - 4AC = 29.700^2 - (4)(71.625)(1.215)$$

$$= 533.99, \text{ and } \sqrt{B^2 - 4AC} = 23.11.$$

$$Q = 29.7/(2)(71.625) \pm 23.11/(2)(71.625)$$

$$= 0.2073 \pm 0.1613$$

$$\therefore \quad Q_u = 0.3686 \quad \text{and} \quad Q_l = 0.0460.$$

$$L_u = (2.025 - 1.325) + 0.3686$$

$$= 1.0686$$

$$L_l = (2.025 - 1.325) + 0.0460$$

$$= 0.7000 + 0.0460$$

$$= 0.7460$$

Therefore, $L = 0.8976$ with range $0.7460 - 1.0686$, so that the potency ratio is 7.90 with range $5.57 - 11.71$.

Computer Screen

```
                    <11> Relative Potency II: Statistical Analysis
              Pharmacologic Calculation System - Version 4.0 - 03/11/86


This procedure calculates the relative potency of the first dose-response curve
    versus one or more additional curves.


Calculation of confidence limits for the potency ratio requires an equal number
    of points (n>2) in each line.

Input: <K>eyboard, <D>isk, or <E>xit this procedure? D


You may enter 5 'XY' data files. Press <ENTER> after last file name.
File name 1 ? LINE1<ENTER>
File name 2 ? LINE2<ENTER>
File name 3 ? <ENTER>


Data: <E>dit, <L>ist, <S>ave, or <ENTER> to continue? L
```

```
   File name:              LINE1
   Variable:          Log(Dose)         Response
-----------------  ---------------  ---------------
      # 1:                 .9                1.8
      # 2:                 .9                4.1
      # 3:                1.1                3.1
      # 4:                1.1                5.2
      # 5:                1.5                6.7
      # 6:                1.5                9.2
      # 7:                1.8                 11
      # 8:                1.8               12.5

   File name:              LINE2
   Variable:          Log(Dose)         Response
-----------------  ---------------  ---------------
      # 1:                1.6                1.5
      # 2:                1.6                2.1
      # 3:                1.8                1.9
      # 4:                1.8                4.4
      # 5:                2.2                5.1
      # 6:                2.2                  7
      # 7:                2.5                  8
      # 8:                2.5                9.9

Data: <E>dit, <L>ist, <S>ave, or <ENTER> to continue? <ENTER>

Do you want to show intermediate results (Y/N) ? N
```

```
   File name:              LINE1

   Response =  9.8154 * Log'Dose) -6.30541

   File name:              LINE2

   Response =  7.86924 * Log(Dose) -10.9477

Common Slope =  8.66887

   File name:              LINE1

     Response =  8.66887 * ( Log(Dose)-1.325) + 6.7

   File name:              LINE2

     Response =  8.66887 * ( Log(Dose)-2.025) + 4.9875


Parallel Line Assay:

Relative Potency of 'LINE1' versus:

          Curve    Pot. Ratio         Lower          Upper
       -----------  ------------  ------------  ------------
          LINE2     7.898517        5.5708       11.71225

Report: <P>rint, <S>ave, or <V>iew? <ENTER>
```

Computer Report

```
            <11> Relative Potency II: Statistical Analysis
       Pharmacologic Calculation System - Version 4.0 - 03/11/86

   File name:              LINE1
   Variable:          Log(Dose)         Response
-----------------  ---------------  ---------------
      # 1:                 .9                1.8
      # 2:                 .9                4.1
      # 3:                1.1                3.1
      # 4:                1.1                5.2
      # 5:                1.5                6.7
      # 6:                1.5                9.2
      # 7:                1.8                 11
      # 8:                1.8               12.5
```

```
File name:           LINE2
Variable:      Log(Dose)        Response
----------     --------------   --------------
      # 1:             1.6             1.5
      # 2:             1.6             2.1
      # 3:             1.8             1.9
      # 4:             1.8             4.4
      # 5:             2.2             5.1
      # 6:             2.2              7
      # 7:             2.5              8
      # 8:             2.5             9.9


File name:           LINE1

Response =   9.8154 * Log(Dose) -6.30541

File name:           LINE2

Response =   7.86924 * Log(Dose) -10.9477

Common Slope =   8.66887

File name:           LINE1

   Response =   8.66887 * ( Log(Dose)-1.325) + 6.7

File name:           LINE2

   Response =   8.66887 * ( Log(Dose)-2.025) + 4.9875


Parallel Line Assay:

Relative Potency of 'LINE1' versus:
```

Curve	Pot. Ratio	Lower	Upper
LINE2	7.898517	5.5708	11.71225

Procedure 12

Dissociation Constant I: Agonists*

An agonist and an antagonist that act on the same receptor are used in this determination. The antagonist must bind irreversibly to the receptor; its presence, therefore, inactivates the receptors to which it combines. If the antagonist concentration is not too great, it will inactivate only a fraction of the total receptor pool and produce a depression of the agonist's dose–response curve. These curves are shown in Figure 12.1, curve (1) for the agonist alone and curve (2) for the agonist in the presence of the antagonist.

Equiactive concentrations $(A_1, A_1'), (A_2, A_2'), \ldots, (A_n, A_n')$ are determined by constructing horizontal lines which intersect both curves, avoiding the extreme points.

The pairs $(1/A_i', 1/A_i)$ are plotted for the n points, producing the (theoretically linear) plot shown in Figure 12.2 from which the slope and y-intercept are

* Furchgott, R. F., and Bursztyn, P. *Ann. N. Y. Acad. Sci.* **144**:882, 1967.

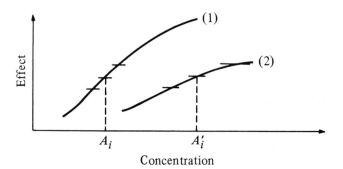

Figure 12.1 Equieffective concentrations for the partially blocked (2) and unblocked (1) preparations.

determined.* The dissociation constant† of the agonist, K_A, is given by the equation

$$K_A = \frac{\text{slope} - 1}{\text{intercept}}. \tag{12.1}$$

Example

The tabulation below gives the values of A and A' obtained from a pair of dose–response curves, and the reciprocals, $1/A$ and $1/A'$. The double-reciprocal plot resulted in the line shown in Figure 12.3 as determined by regression analysis (Procedure 3):

$$1/A = (4.6)(1/A') + 0.16.$$

Thus, the slope = 4.6 and the intercept = 0.16, from which $K_A = 23$ mg/liter.‡ This is the value of K_A determined by a single experiment. A number of similar experiments

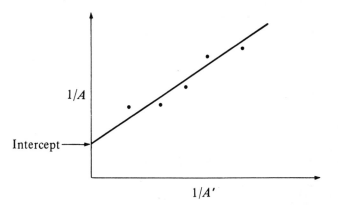

Figure 12.2 Method of partial irreversible blockade.

* The method of least squares (Procedure 3) may be used to find the best straight line.

† The unit of K is that of concentration and will therefore be the same as the concentration units of A and A'.

‡ Values expressed with two significant figures.

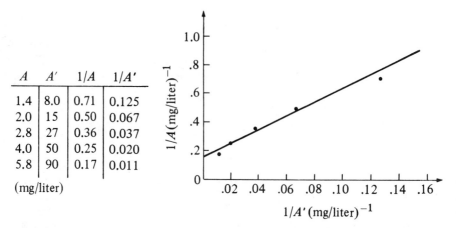

A	A'	$1/A$	$1/A'$
1.4	8.0	0.71	0.125
2.0	15	0.50	0.067
2.8	27	0.36	0.037
4.0	50	0.25	0.020
5.8	90	0.17	0.011

(mg/liter)

Figure 12.3   Determination of K_A from the tabulated data.

should be carried out, determining the K_A value for each. From these individual values one can obtain an estimate of the mean K_A and its confidence interval using Procedure 2.

Note. It is likely that the reciprocated values are not normally distributed; further, the abscissa values ($1/A'$) are subject to error, as are the ordinates ($1/A$). Accordingly, the use of linear regression analysis is not strictly applicable and is, therefore, an approximation. (See also Procedures 8 and 18–20, in which double reciprocal plots are employed.)

Computer Screen

```
                    <12> Dissociation Constant I: Agonists
              Pharmacologic Calculation System - Version 4.0 - 03/11/86

Enter equiactive dose pairs ([A'],[A]).

Input: <K>eyboard, <D>isk, or <E>xit this procedure? D

You may enter 5 'XY' data files. Press <ENTER> after last file name.
File name 1 ? LINE1<ENTER>
File name 2 ? <ENTER>

Data: <E>dit, <L>ist, <S>ave, or <ENTER> to continue? L

        File name:          LINE1
        Variable:           [A']            [A]
    --------------   ---------------   ---------------
        # 1:               8              1.4
        # 2:              15              2
        # 3:              27              2.8
        # 4:              50              4
        # 5:              90              5.8

Data: <E>dit, <L>ist, <S>ave, or <ENTER> to continue? <ENTER>
```

```
Do you want to show intermediate results (Y/N) ? N


        1/[A] =  4.62628 * 1/[A'] + .158373

           Ka = 22.897

Report: <P>rint, <S>ave, or <V>iew? <ENTER>
```

Computer Report

```
                      <12> Dissociation Constant I: Agonists
              Pharmacologic Calculation System - Version 4.0 - 03/11/86

        File name:        LINE1
        Variable:         [A']               [A]
        ----------    --------------    --------------
           # 1:             8              1.4
           # 2:            15               2
           # 3:            27              2.8
           # 4:            50               4
           # 5:            90              5.8


        1/[A] =  4.62628 * 1/[A'] + .158373

           Ka = 22.897
```

Procedure 13

Dissociation Constant II: Partial Agonists

A partial agonist is an agent that requires appreciable receptor occupancy in order to achieve an effect. By way of contrast, full agonists (or strong agonists) have a large spare receptor capacity, that is, these agents produce effects with just a small fraction of their receptors occupied.*

If a strong agonist and a partial agonist act on the same receptor it is possible to determine the apparent dissociation constant K_P of the partial agonist from the concentration–effect curves of each, as shown in Figure 13.1.

Equieffective concentrations of each are determined. These are most conveniently determined by plotting the concentration–effect relations of each on the same set of axes. Thus, P_i and A_i are one pair of equieffective concentrations. If a number (n) of such pairs are determined in this way and plotted as double reciprocals, $1/A_i$ against $1/P_i$, the resulting plot is theoretically linear (see Figure 13.2). The vertical intercept and the slope permit a calculation of K_P, the dissociation constant of the partial agonist, according to the relation†

$$K_P = \frac{\text{slope}}{\text{intercept}}. \tag{13.1}$$

* Stephenson, R. P. *Brit. J. Pharmacol.* **11**:379, 1956.
† Waud, D. R. *J. Pharmacol. Exp. Ther.* **170**:117, 1969.

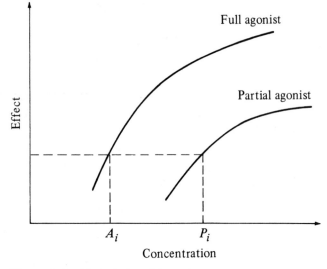

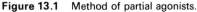

Figure 13.1   Method of partial agonists.

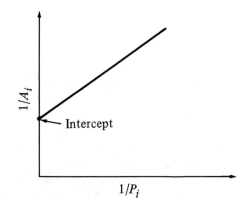

Figure 13.2   Method of partial agonists. The dissociation constant of the partial agonist is the ratio of slope to intercept.

The double reciprocal data are plotted and the regression line determined as described in Procedure 3. The ratio of slope to intercept of the regression line yields K_P.

Example

The table below gives equiactive concentrations of a strong agonist A and a partial agonist P. The respective reciprocals are also given. Units of A and P are molar.

A	P	$1/P$	$1/A$
3×10^{-7}	4.5×10^{-6}	2.2×10^{5}	3.3×10^{6}
4×10^{-7}	6.6×10^{-6}	1.5×10^{5}	2.5×10^{6}
5×10^{-7}	8.0×10^{-6}	1.25×10^{5}	2.0×10^{6}
8×10^{-7}	14×10^{-6}	7.1×10^{4}	1.2×10^{6}
10×10^{-7}	50×10^{-6}	2.0×10^{4}	1.0×10^{6}

The slope and intercept of the regression line are determined as described in Procedure 3. These are 12.1 and 5.80×10^5, respectively, from which K_P may be computed from Equation (13.1):

$$K_P = 12.1/5.8 \times 10^5 = 2.07 \times 10^{-5} \ M.$$

Computer Screen

```
              <13> Dissociation Constant II: Partial Agonists
          Pharmacologic Calculation System - Version 4.0 - 03/11/86

Enter equiactive dose pairs ([Partial Agonist],[Agonist]) in molar units.


Input: <K>eyboard, <D>isk, or <E>xit this procedure? D


You may enter 5 'XY' data files. Press <ENTER> after last file name.
File name 1 ?.LINE1<ENTER>
File name 2 ? <ENTER>


Data: <E>dit, <L>ist, <S>ave, or <ENTER> to continue? L


    File name:          LINE1
    Variable:         [Partial]      [Agonist]
    -------------   -------------   -------------
        # 1:          .0000045        .0000003
        # 2:          .0000066        .0000004
        # 3:          .000008         .0000005
        # 4:          .000014         .0000008
        # 5:          .00005          .000001

Data: <E>dit, <L>ist, <S>ave, or <ENTER> to continue? <ENTER>
```

```
Do you want to show intermediate results (Y/N) ? N


  1/[Agonist] =  12.1242 * 1/[Partial] + 585607


        Kp = 2.07037E-05

Report: <P>rint, <S>ave, or <V>iew? <ENTER>
```

Computer Report

```
              <13> Dissociation Constant II: Partial Agonists
           Pharmacologic Calculation System - Version 4.0 - 03/11/86

      File name:        LINE1
      Variable:       [Partial]        [Agonist]
   --------------   -------------   -------------
        # 1:          .0000045         .0000003
        # 2:          .0000066         .0000004
        # 3:          .000008          .0000005
        # 4:          .000014          .0000008
        # 5:          .00005           .000001


    1/[Agonist] =   12.1242 * 1/[Partial] + 585607

         Kp = 2.07037E-05
```

Procedure 14

Dissociation Constant III: Perturbation Methods (Rate Constants in the Drug–Receptor Reaction)

Consider a drug–receptor reaction

$$D + R \underset{k_2}{\overset{k_1}{\rightleftharpoons}} DR \longrightarrow \cdots \longrightarrow E,$$

where DR is the drug–receptor complex and E the effect at equilibrium. It may be possible to determine the forward and reverse rate constants k_1 and k_2 by the method of chemical relaxation. In this method the system is subjected to a small but sharp variation in some physical parameter upon which the value $K(=k_2/k_1)$ depends. The restoration to equilibrium after this perturbation follows first-order kinetics, that is,

$$\Delta E = \Delta E_{max} e^{-t/\tau}. \tag{14.1}$$

In this Equation (13.1) ΔE is the value of the displacement from equilibrium at any time t, ΔE_{max} is the initial displacement, and τ is the time constant* (see Figure 14.1).

The value of τ may be shown† to depend upon the drug concentration [A] and the constants k_1 and k_2 according to

$$\tau = (k_1[A] + k_2)^{-1}. \tag{14.2}$$

Equation (13.2) shows that $1/\tau$ is linearly related to the drug concentration at equilibrium

$$1/\tau = k_1[A] + k_2. \tag{14.3}$$

* The time constant is that time in which $\Delta E = 1/e \ (\approx 0.37) \ \Delta E_{max}$.

† Tallarida, R. J., Sevy, R. W., and Harakal, C. Bull. Math. Biophysics **32**:65, 1970.

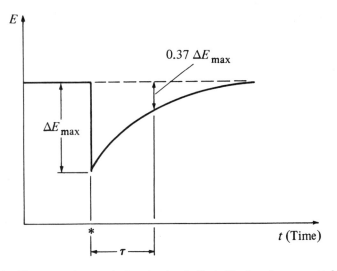

Figure 14.1 The system is perturbed at the time indicated by * and recovers to 0.37 ΔE_{max} at time τ after perturbation.

Thus, if this kind of experiment is carried out at several drug concentrations, and the value of τ determined at each concentration, then the resulting linear plot has slope k_1 and intercept k_2.

Example

In an experiment on isolated vascular smooth muscle* contracted with norepine-phrine in several concentrations, a flash of ultraviolet light was used to perturb the system at each level of concentration. In each case, the restoration to equilibrium was followed, from which the time constant (τ) for recovery was determined. The values of concentration [A] and the time constants τ were as shown below. The values of $1/\tau$ are given also.

$[A](M)$	1.2×10^{-8}	3.5×10^{-8}	1.2×10^{-7}	8.3×10^{-7}
$\tau(sec)$	47	28	17	8
$1/\tau(sec^{-1})$	0.021	0.036	0.059	0.125

The regression line with $1/\tau$ against [A] was determined to be

$$1/\tau = 1.15 \times 10^5 [A] + 0.0316.$$

From Equation (14.3) the slope is k_1 and equals 1.15×10^5 (M^{-1} sec^{-1}) and the intercept $k_2 = 0.0316$ sec^{-1}. From these $K = k_2/k_1 = 2.75 \times 10^{-7}$ M.

*Tallarida, R. J., Sevy, R. W., Harakal, C., and Loughnane, M. H. *IEEE Trans. Biomed. Eng.* **22**:493, 1975.

Computer Screen

```
            <14> Dissociation Constant III: Perturbation Methods
            Pharmacologic Calculation System - Version 4.0 - 03/11/86

Input: <K>eyboard, <D>isk, or <E>xit this procedure? D

You may enter 5 'XY' data files. Press <ENTER> after last file name.
File name 1 ? LINE1<ENTER>
File name 2 ? <ENTER>

Data: <E>dit, <L>ist, <S>ave, or <ENTER> to continue? L

    File name:          LINE1
    Variable:        [Agonist]              tau
    -------------  --------------  --------------
          # 1:        1.2E-08                47
          # 2:        3.5E-08                28
          # 3:        1.2E-07                17
          # 4:        8.3E-07                 8

Data: <E>dit, <L>ist, <S>ave, or <ENTER> to continue? <ENTER>

Do you want to show intermediate results (Y/N) ? N
```

```
      1/tau =  114632 * [Agonist] + .0316317

         R = .974

   t (95%) = 4.303          2 d.f.

      Variable          Value       Std. Err.      Lower C.L.       Upper C.L.
    -------------  --------------  --------------  --------------  --------------
            k1:         114632         18766.1         33880.9          195382
            k2:        .0316317     7.87658E-03    -2.26125E-03        .0655246
    X-Intercept:  -2.75942E-07    1.02219E-07    -7.15788E-07     1.63904E-07

<ENTER> to continue or <L>ist values calculated from regression line? <ENTER>

         K = 2.75942E-07

Report: <P>rint, <S>ave, or <V>iew? <ENTER>
```

Computer Report

```
            <14> Dissociation Constant III: Perturbation Methods
            Pharmacologic Calculation System - Version 4.0 - 03/11/86

         File name:          LINE1
         Variable:        [Agonist]              tau
       -------------  --------------  --------------
             # 1:        1.2E-08                47
             # 2:        3.5E-08                28
             # 3:        1.2E-07                17
             # 4:        8.3E-07                 8

         File name:          LINE1
         Variable:        [Agonist]             1/tau
       -------------  --------------  --------------
             # 1:        1.2E-08             .0212766
             # 2:        3.5E-08             .0357143
             # 3:        1.2E-07             .0588235
             # 4:        8.3E-07                .125
```

```
1/tau =   114632 * [Agonist] + .0316317

    R = .974

t (95%) = 4.303          2 d.f.

    Variable           Value      Std. Err.     Lower C.L.      Upper C.L.
------------------   ------------  ------------  ------------   ------------
          k1:           114632        18766.1        33880.9         195382
          k2:          .0316317   7.87658E-03  -2.26125E-03       .0655246
  X-Intercept:     -2.75942E-07   1.02219E-07  -7.15788E-07    1.63904E-07

    K = 2.75942E-07
```

Procedure 15

*pA*₂ Analysis I: Schild Plot

The pA_2 is a measure of the affinity of a competitive antagonist for its receptor. The determination of the pA_2 is made from experiments in which a fixed concentration of the antagonist is used along with graded concentrations of an agonist acting on the same receptor. The presence of the antagonist shifts the agonist dose–response curve to the right as seen in Figure 15.1.

The agonist dose-ratio A'/A is determined at some level of the effect. This ratio depends upon B according to the relation $A'/A = 1 + B/K_B$, where K_B is the dissociation constant of the antagonist. Thus, for a ratio of 2 we have $B/K_B = 1$ or, taking common logarithms, $\log B - \log K_B = 0$. The pA_2 is defined as the negative common logarithm of B which produces a dose-ratio of 2; hence,

$$pA_2 = -\log B = -\log K_B = \log(1/K_B).$$

Since $1/K_B$ is the affinity constant, the pA_2 may be viewed as a measure of affinity. In these calculations the units are molar.

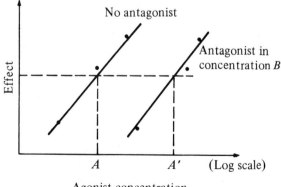

Figure 15.1 Agonist dose–response curve.

It is usually difficult to obtain the pA_2 from an experiment producing a pair of dose–response curves that give a dose-ratio of 2; further, errors in the experiment make such a determination inadvisable. Accordingly, one uses several different antagonist concentrations and determines the agonist dose-ratio for each. Since $A'/A - 1 = B/K_B$

$$\log\left(\frac{A'}{A} - 1\right) = \log B - \log K_B. \qquad (15.1)$$

Thus, if log(ratio − 1) is plotted against log B, a straight line of slope 1 is obtained. The intercept on the abscissa is $\log K_B = -pA_2$. It is convenient to plot the log(ratio − 1) against −log B, in which case the line has slope −1 and the intercept on the abscissa gives a direct reading of pA_2. This plot, often called a "Schild plot," will in most cases yield a set of points which are not colinear; hence, the method of least squares (Procedure 3) is used to get the regression line. The standard error of the intercept on the abscissa gives the standard error of the pA_2 value. The 95% confidence limits may also be determined. Since the Schild plot should have a slope of −1 it is advisable to determine the standard error and confidence limits for the slope of the regression line.

Example

The table below gives the values of agonist dose-ratio A'/A and antagonist molar concentration B determined from an experiment with 4 different concentrations of antagonist. Also tabulated are $\log(A'/A - 1)$ and −log B, the latter having been used in the Schild plot of Figure 15.2. The regression line was determined according to Procedure 3, with $x = -\log B$ from column 3 of the table and $y = \log(A'/A - 1)$ from column 4. The equation of the regression line is $y = -1.19x + 8.25$. Hence, the x-intercept (pA_2) is 6.9. The standard errors of the pA_2 and slope are determined from Equations (5.4) and (5.2), respectively (see Procedure 5.)

$B(M)$	A'/A	$-\log B = x$	$\log(A'/A - 1) = y$
3.16×10^{-7}	4.16	6.5	0.50
1.00×10^{-6}	18.78	6.0	1.25
5.62×10^{-6}	57.23	5.25	1.75
1.00×10^{-5}	317.2	5.0	2.50

These are

$$\text{S.E.}(pA_2) = 0.24$$

and

$$\text{S.E.(slope)} = 0.21.$$

The confidence limits for pA_2 and slope are determined by multiplying the respective standard errors by the value of t for 2 degrees of freedom (N-2). From Table A.2 the value of t for 95% confidence is 4.30. Hence, the confidence limits for the pA_2 are $6.9 \pm (0.24)(4.30) = 6.9 \pm 1.03$.

The confidence limits for the slope are $-1.19 \pm (0.21)(4.30) = 1.19 \pm 0.903$.

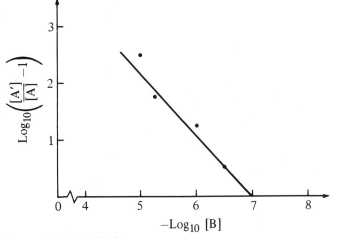

Figure 15.2 Schild plot.

Computer Screen

```
                        <15> pA2 Analysis I: Schild Plot
              Pharmacologic Calculation System - Version 4.0 - 03/31/86

Computation of pA2 uses molar units of antagonist. You may enter antagonist
concentrations in several ways:
 1 = Molar, 2 = ug/ml or mg/kg, 3 = mg/ml, 4 = g/100ml,

Enter option: ? 1

Input: <K>eyboard, <D>isk, or <E>xit this procedure? D

You may enter 5 'XY' data files. Press <ENTER> after last file name.
File name 1 ? LINE1<ENTER>
File name 2 ? <ENTER>

Data: <E>dit, <L>ist, <S>ave, or <ENTER> to continue? L

    File name:        LINE1
    Variable:         [B]        [A']/[A]
   ------------    ------------  ------------
       # 1:         3.16E-07        4.16
       # 2:         .000001        18.78
       # 3:         5.62E-06        57.23
       # 4:         .00001         317.2

Data: <E>dit, <L>ist, <S>ave, or <ENTER> to continue? <ENTER>
```

```
Do you want to show intermediate results (Y/N) ? N

Log(A'/A-1) = -1.18691 * -Log([B]) + 8.25061

         R = .971

   t (95%) = 4.303       2 d.f.

    Variable        Value     Std. Err.   Lower C.L.    Upper C.L.
  ------------    --------    --------    ----------    ----------
      Slope:      -1.18691     .207162     -2.07833      -.29549
 Y-Intercept:      8.25061    1.18472      3.15275       13.3485
        pA2:       6.95134     .243884      5.9019        8.00077

<ENTER> to continue or <L>ist values calculated from regression line? <ENTER>

Report: <P>rint, <S>ave, or <V>iew? <ENTER>
```

Computer Report

```
                         <15> pA2 Analysis I: Schild Plot
              Pharmacologic Calculation System - Version 4.0 - 03/31/86

     File name:        LINE1
     Variable:          [B]      [A']/[A]
   -----------    -----------    ---------
          # 1:     3.16E-07         4.16
          # 2:      .000001        18.78
          # 3:     5.62E-06        57.23
          # 4:       .00001        317.2


   Log(A'/A-1) = -1.18691 * -Log([B]) + 8.25061

           R = .971

      t (95%) = 4.303        2 d.f.

        Variable        Value    Std. Err.    Lower C.L.    Upper C.L.
     -----------   -----------   ---------    ---------     ---------
          Slope:     -1.18691      .207162     -2.07833      -.29549
    Y-Intercept:      8.25061     1.18472      3.15275      13.3485
           pA2:       6.95134      .243884      5.9019       8.00077
```

Procedure 16

pA_2 Analysis II: Time-Dependent Method*

The pA_2, or affinity of an antagonist drug, is generally determined from measurements of equieffective agonist dose-ratios at equilibrium in the absence and presence of a fixed concentration of antagonist. As discussed in Procedure 15, several different doses of the antagonist are used and a Schild plot is constructed for the actual determination. In contrast to that method, the method presented here employs a single dose of the antagonist and examines the agonist dose-ratio as a function of the *time* after peak concentrations.

The dissociation constant K_B for a competitive antagonist in concentration B obeys†

$$\log_{10}(A'/A - 1) = \log_{10} B - \log_{10} K_B. \qquad (16.1)$$

In Equation (15.1) A' and A are equiactive concentrations of agonist in the presence and the absence of the antagonist. The values of A', A, and B are those at equilibrium; hence, in experiments of this kind the dosing schedule must be such that at the time of measurement the concentrations of agonist and antagonist are maximal. If measurements are made at a time t after that of peak concentrations, the values of A', A, and B will change. (Time $t = 0$ is taken to be that at which concentrations are maximal.)

---

* Tallarida, R. J., Harakal, C., Maslow, J., Geller, E. B., and Adler, M. W. *J. Pharmacol. Exp. Ther.* **206**:38–45, 1978.

† See Procedure 15 for a discussion of dose-ratio A'/A.

If both A and B decay exponentially, $A = A_0 e^{-\alpha t}$ and $B = B_0 e^{-\beta t}$, where A_0 and B_0 are the maximum concentrations, Equation (16.1) can be put into time-dependent form:

$$\log(A_0'/A_0 - 1) = \log_{10} B_0 - \beta \log_{10}(e)t - \log_{10} K_B. \qquad (16.2)$$

In practice, the concentrations A_0', A_0, and B_0 are replaced by administered concentrations which are assumed proportional to the maximal concentrations.

Equation (15.2) is linear in $\log_{10}(A_0'/A_0 - 1)$ and t. The slope is $-\beta \log_{10} e$, and the vertical intercept is $(\log_{10} B_0 - \log_{10} K_B)$. Since $pA_2 = -\log_{10} K_B$, we have

$$pA_2 = \text{intercept} - \log_{10} B_0. \qquad (16.3)$$

Thus, in the time-dependent method, a single fixed dose of the antagonist is used and the dose-ratio of agonist is determined. [Although a determination at one time permits a calculation of $-\log_{10} K_B$ from Equation (16.1), inherent errors in the experiment advise that a more extensive experimental procedure be carried out.] Dose-ratios determined at various times after peak levels are plotted and analyzed from Equation (16.2) as previously described. Administration of agonist and antagonist should be timed so that their levels peak at the same time.

Example

A certain analgesic is known to achieve its peak brain concentration 30 min after a subcutaneous injection. A competitive antagonist is known to peak 15 min after the injection. The dosage schedule used is shown in the diagram below, in which we have denoted $t = 0$ to be the time at which both agents achieve their respective maximal concentrations.

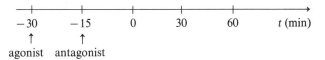

The agonist dose-ratio A'/A is determined at $t = 0$ and at $t = 30, 60$, and 90 min. The values are tabulated below. The antagonist concentration was $B_0 = 6 \times 10^{-7}$ M. The values of $\log_{10}(A'/A - 1)$ are computed for each and plotted.

t	0	30	60	90
(A'/A)	80.4	32.6	16.8	8.9
$\log_{10}(A'/A - 1)$	1.9	1.5	1.2	0.90

The regression gave slope $= -0.011$ and intercept $= 1.87$. From Equation (16.3),

$$pA_2 = 1.87 - \log_{10}(6 \times 10^{-7})$$
$$= 1.87 + 6.22$$
$$= 8.09.$$

Note. This analysis permits a determination of the antagonist elimination rate constant β and, hence, its half-life $= \ln 2/\beta$.

Computer Screen

```
                    <16> pA2 Analysis II: Time-Dependent Method
                  Pharmacologic Calculation System - Version 4.0 - 03/11/86

The Time-Dependent Method requires dose ratio data to be collected over several
   time periods for a single concentration of antagonist.

Enter concentration of antagonist in molar units? 6E-7<ENTER>

Concentration of antagonist = .0000006 M

Input: <K>eyboard, <D>isk, or <E>xit this procedure? D

You may enter 5 'XY' data files. Press <ENTER> after last file name.
File name 1 ? LINE1<ENTER>
File name 2 ? <ENTER>

Data: <E>dit, <L>ist, <S>ave, or <ENTER> to continue? L

      File name:          LINE1
       Variable:          time        [A']/[A]
   -------------     -------------   -------------
          # 1:             0             80.4
          # 2:            30             32.6
          # 3:            60             16.8
          # 4:            90              8.9
```

```
Data: <E>dit, <L>ist, <S>ave, or <ENTER> to continue? <ENTER>

Do you want to show intermediate results (Y/N) ? N


  Log(A'/A-1) = -.0110254 * time + 1.87009

        pA2 = 8.09194

Half-life of antagonist = 27.3034


Report: <P>rint, <S>ave, or <V>iew? <ENTER>
```

Computer Report

```
                    <16> pA2 Analysis II: Time-Dependent Method
                  Pharmacologic Calculation System - Version 4.0 - 03/11/86

Concentration of antagonist = .0000006 M

      File name:          LINE1
       Variable:          time        [A']/[A]
   -------------     -------------   -------------
          # 1:             0             80.4
          # 2:            30             32.6
          # 3:            60             16.8
          # 4:            90              8.9

  Log(A'/A-1) = -.0110254 * time + 1.87009

        pA2 = 8.09194

Half-life of antagonist = 27.3034
```

Procedure 17

pA_2 Analysis III: Constrained Plot

The regression line $y = mx + b$, discussed in Procedure 3, gives the values of m and b that best fit the data points (x_i, y_i). In some situations one of the two parameters, m or b, is known, or the theoretical relation between the x_i and y_i imposes a constraint on the value of m or b. A situation of this kind occurs in the theory underlying the determination of "pA_2" for a competitive antagonist* (see Procedure 15).

In the determination of the pA_2, the Schild plot is often used. This plot is based on the agonist dose-ratio A'/A for several different antagonist concentrations B:

$$\log_{10}(A'/A - 1) = -(-\log_{10} B) + pA_2.$$

Denoting the left side by Y and the value $-\log B$ by X, we have a linear relation

$$Y = -X + pA_2. \tag{17.1}$$

Hence, pA_2 is determined as the intercept in a linear plot of slope -1. Given below are the formulas for determining the intercept (or pA_2) and its confidence limits.

For the set of n points (x_i, y_i) constrained to slope -1, the intercept b is given by

$$b = \bar{x} + \bar{y}, \tag{17.2}$$

where $\bar{x} = (\sum x_i)/n$ and $\bar{y} = (\sum y_i)/n$. The estimated standard error of b is given by

$$\text{S.E.}(b) = s/\sqrt{n} \tag{17.3}$$

where

$$s = \left[\frac{\sum_1^n [(y_i - \bar{y}) + (x_i - \bar{x})]^2}{n - 1} \right]^{1/2}. \tag{17.4}$$

The 95% confidence interval for the intercept (pA_2) is

$$b \pm (t_{n-1})[\text{S.E.}(b)] \tag{17.5}$$

where t_{n-1} is the value of Student's t-distribution for $n - 1$ degrees of freedom.

Example

The following values of B, A'/A, $x \, (= -\log B)$, and $y = \log(A'/A - 1)$ were obtained from an experiment with a narcotic analgesic and a competitive antagonist of that agent.

---

* Tallarida, R. J., Cowan, A., and Adler, M. W. *Life Sci.* **25**:637, 1979.

B (M)	x	A'/A	y
2.5 × 10⁻⁸	7.60	3.8	0.447
1.25 × 10⁻⁷	6.90	8.9	0.898
2.5 × 10⁻⁷	6.60	32.6	1.50
6.25 × 10⁻⁷	6.20	80	1.90

We have $\bar{x} = 6.83$ and $\bar{y} = 1.19$. The computation for determining s is arranged below; b is given by $\bar{x} + \bar{y} = 8.01$.

$(y_i - \bar{y})$	$(x_i - \bar{x})$	$[(y_i - \bar{y}) + (x_i - \bar{x})]^2$
−0.739	0.775	0.001296
−0.288	0.075	0.045369
0.314	−0.225	0.007921
0.714	−0.625	0.007921
		$\sum = 0.062507$

Thus,

$$s = \left[\frac{0.062507}{(4-1)}\right]^{1/2} = 0.144,$$

and

$$S.E.(b) = 0.144/\sqrt{4} = 0.072.$$

Multiplying 0.072 by 3.182, the value of t (from Table A.2) gives 0.23. Thus, the 95% confidence interval is 8.01 ± 0.23.

Computer Screen

```
                <17> pA2 Analysis III: Constrained Plot
        Pharmacologic Calculation System - Version 4.0 - 03/11/86

Computation of pA2 uses molar units of antagonist. You may enter antagonist
concentrations in several ways:
 1 = Molar, 2 = ug/ml or mg/kg, 3 = mg/ml, 4 = g/100ml,

Enter option: ? 1

Input: <K>eyboard, <D>isk, or <E>xit this procedure? D

You may enter 5 'XY' data files. Press <ENTER> after last file name.
File name 1 ? LINE1<ENTER>
File name 2 ? <ENTER>

Data: <E>dit, <L>ist, <S>ave, or <ENTER> to continue? L

    File name:        LINE1
    Variable:          [B]        [A']/[A]
    ------------    ------------  ------------
        # 1:          2.5E-08        3.8
        # 2:         1.25E-07        8.9
        # 3:          2.5E-07       32.6
        # 4:         6.25E-07        80

Data: <E>dit, <L>ist, <S>ave, or <ENTER> to continue? <ENTER>
```

```
Do you want to show intermediate results (Y/N) ? N

  Log(A'/A-1) = -1 x -Log([B]) + 8.01336

     t (95%) = 3.182          3 d.f.

        Variable          Value      Std. Err.    Lower C.L.    Upper C.L.
   ------------------   -----------   ---------   -----------   -----------
            pA2:          8.01336      .0719532      7.7844       8.24231


  Report: <P>rint, <S>ave, or <V>iew? <ENTER>
```

Computer Report

```
                    <17> pA2 Analysis III: Constrained Plot
            Pharmacologic Calculation System - Version 4.0 - 03/11/86

        File name:       LINE1
        Variable:         [B]         [A']/[A]
      --------------   -----------   ----------
          # 1:          2.5E-08         3.8
          # 2:          1.25E-07        8.9
          # 3:          2.5E-07        32.6
          # 4:          6.25E-07        80


  Log(A'/A-1) = -1 x -Log([B]) + 8.01336

     t (95%) = 3.182          3 d.f.

        Variable          Value      Std. Err.    Lower C.L.    Upper C.L.
   ------------------   -----------   ---------   -----------   -----------
            pA2:          8.01336      .0719532      7.7844       8.24231
```

Procedure 18

Enzyme Kinetics I: Michaelis–Menten Equation

Enzyme activity is measured after mixing the enzyme with its substrate S under controlled conditions. The reaction is followed as a function of time. The rate of disappearance of the substrate, denoted by v, is proportional to the concentration of substrate up to a certain substrate concentration. With increasing substrate concentrations, a plateau is reached as the enzyme becomes saturated; at this point the maximum velocity V_{max} is reached.

The Michaelis–Menten equation describes the relation between the velocity v, the substrate concentration [S], and the maximum velocity V_{max}:

$$v = \frac{V_{max}[S]}{[S] + K_M}. \tag{18.1}$$

The constant K_M is known as the Michaelis constant.

Commonly, Equation (18.1) is transformed into linear form by reciprocating both sides:

$$\frac{1}{v} = \frac{K_M}{V_{max}} \frac{1}{[S]} + \frac{1}{V_{max}}. \tag{18.2}$$

Equation (18.2) is known as the Lineweaver–Burk form.

The intercept on the ordinate gives $1/V_{max}$, whereas the slope is K_M/V_{max}. Hence, the data are plotted as $1/v$ against $1/[S]$ and may be fitted by the methods of linear regression (Procedure 3) in order to determine K_M and V_{max} from the regression line.

Example

Values of substrate concentration [S] (mM) and the corresponding product velocities v (mg/min) for an enzyme-catalyzed reaction are given in the table below. Find the maximum velocity V_{max} and the Michaelis constant K_M.

[S]	1.25	1.67	2.50	5.00	10.0	20.0
v	0.101	0.130	0.156	0.250	0.303	0.345

The reciprocal values are given below.

1/[S]	0.800	0.599	0.400	0.200	0.100	0.050
$1/v$	9.90	7.69	6.41	4.00	3.30	2.90

Linear regression (Procedure 3) gives slope = 9.32, and intercept = 2.36. Thus, $1/V_{max} = 2.36$, or $V_{max} = 0.424$ mg/min, and $K_M = $ (slope) $\times$ (V_{max}) = 3.95 mM.

Computer Screen

```
                    <18> Enzyme Kinetics I: Michaelis-Menten Equation
                  Pharmacologic Calculation System - Version 4.0 - 03/11/86


    Input: <K>eyboard, <D>isk, or <E>xit this procedure? D


    You may enter 5 'XY' data files. Press <ENTER> after last file name.
    File name 1 ? LINE1<ENTER>
    File name 2 ? <ENTER>


    Data: <E>dit, <L>ist, <S>ave, or <ENTER> to continue? L


        File name:             LINE1
        Variable:    [Substrate]        Velocity
    ------------  --------------  --------------
          # 1:           1.25            .101
          # 2:           1.67            .13
          # 3:           2.5             .156
          # 4:           5               .25
          # 5:           10              .303
          # 6:           20              .345


    Data: <E>dit, <L>ist, <S>ave, or <ENTER> to continue? <ENTER>
```

```
Do you want to show intermediate results (Y/N) ? N


   1/Velocity =   9.32487 * 1/[Substrate] + 2.36086

         Vmax = .423575
          Km = 3.94978


Report: <P>rint, <S>ave, or <V>iew? <ENTER>
```

Computer Report

```
              <18> Enzyme Kinetics I: Michaelis-Menten Equation
           Pharmacologic Calculation System - Version 4.0 - 03/11/86

      File name:        LINE1
      Variable:      [Substrate]        Velocity
     -------------  -------------    -------------
         # 1:          1.25             .101
         # 2:          1.67             .13
         # 3:          2.5              .156
         # 4:          5                .25
         # 5:          10               .303
         # 6:          20               .345


   1/Velocity =   9.32487 * 1/[Substrate] + 2.36086

         Vmax = .423575
          Km = 3.94978
```

Procedure 19

Enzyme Kinetics II: Competitive Inhibition

A competitive inhibitor combines with the enzyme and inhibits its catalytic activity. The inhibitory activity is reversed if the substrate concentration is increased. If the inhibition is due to the inhibitor combining with the active site of the enzyme in such a way as to prevent substrate combination then, for a fixed concentration I of inhibitor, the double-reciprocal relation, $1/v$ against $1/[S]$, is given by

$$\frac{1}{v} = \frac{K_M}{V_{max}}\left(1 + \frac{I}{K_I}\right)\frac{1}{[S]} + \frac{1}{V_{max}}. \tag{19.1}$$

In Equation (19.1) K_I is the dissociation constant of the enzyme–inhibitor complex. Comparison of Equations (18.2) and (19.1) reveals that both double-reciprocal plots are linear and have the same intercept, namely, $1/V_{max}$. However, Equation (19.1) produces a greater slope $(K_M/V_{max})[1 + (I/K_I)]$ (see Figure 19.1). Determination of the slope in the presence of a fixed concentration I of inhibitor permits a determination of K_I.

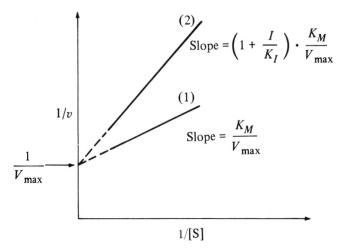

Figure 19.1 Competitive enzyme inhibition. The greater slope, line (2), is due to the inhibitor.

Example

For the same enzyme-catalyzed reaction given in the Example in Procedure 18, and for the same concentrations of substrate (shown again below), the addition of 40 mM of an inhibitor produced the velocities shown below for each value of [S]. Find K_I.

The values of $1/v$ are computed in the last row of the table and, for convenience, the values of $1/[S]$ are reproduced here.

[S]	1.25	1.67	2.50	5.00	10.0	20.0
v	0.061	0.074	0.106	0.169	0.227	0.313
1/[S]	0.800	0.599	0.400	0.200	0.100	0.050
$1/v$	16.4	13.5	9.43	5.92	4.40	3.19

The best fitting line has slope = 17.7 and intercept = 2.46. From the expression for the slope, we have

$$17.7 = \frac{K_M}{V_{max}}\left(1 + \frac{I}{K_I}\right).$$

Using the value of K_M from the Example in Procedure 18, namely, 3.95 mM, $V_{max} = 0.424$, and $I = 40$ mM, we find $K_I = 44.4$ mM. It should be noted that the intercepts of the two Lineweaver–Burk plots, shown in Figure 19.1, are slightly different, whereas theoretically they should be the same. This slight difference is not significant as may be seen by determining the standard errors of the intercept for each line (Procedure 5).

Computer Screen

```
                <19> Enzyme Kinetics II: Competitive Inhibition
               Pharmacologic Calculation System - Version 4.0 - 03/11/86

You must input data for two curves. The first must be without an inhibitor, and
  the second must be in the presence of a competitive inhibitor.

Enter concentration of inhibitor ? 40<ENTER>

Concentration of competitive inhibitor = 40

Input: <K>eyboard, <D>isk, or <E>xit this procedure? D

You may enter 2 'XY' data files. Press <ENTER> after last file name.
File name 1 ? LINE1<ENTER>
File name 2 ? LINE2<ENTER>

Data: <E>dit, <L>ist, <S>ave, or <ENTER> to continue? L

      File name:            LINE1
      Variable:    [Substrate]      Velocity
     ------------- -------------  -------------
          # 1:          1.25           .101
          # 2:          1.67           .13
          # 3:          2.5            .156
          # 4:          5              .25
          # 5:          10             .303
          # 6:          20             .345
```

```
      File name:            LINE2
      Variable:    [Substrate]      Velocity
     ------------- -------------  -------------
          # 1:          1.25           .061
          # 2:          1.67           .074
          # 3:          2.5            .106
          # 4:          5              .169
          # 5:          10             .227
          # 6:          20             .313

Data: <E>dit, <L>ist, <S>ave, or <ENTER> to continue? <ENTER>

Do you want to show intermediate results (Y/N) ? N

      File name:            LINE1

  1/Velocity =  9.32487 * 1/[Substrate] + 2.36086

      File name:            LINE2

  1/Velocity =  17.743 * 1/[Substrate] + 2.45534
```

```
      File name:            LINE1
     ------------- -------------
         Vmax = .423575
           Km = 3.94978

      File name:            LINE2
     ------------- -------------
         Vmax = .407276
           Km = 7.22631

           Ki = 44.3084

Report: <P>rint, <S>ave, or <V>iew? <ENTER>
```

Computer Report

```
                    <19> Enzyme Kinetics II: Competitive Inhibition
                  Pharmacologic Calculation System - Version 4.0 - 03/11/86

    Concentration of competitive inhibitor = 40

            File name:          LINE1
            Variable:      [Substrate]         Velocity
          ------------- --------------- ---------------
               # 1:             1.25            .101
               # 2:             1.67            .13
               # 3:             2.5             .156
               # 4:             5               .25
               # 5:             10              .303
               # 6:             20              .345

            File name:          LINE2
            Variable:      [Substrate]         Velocity
          ------------- --------------- ---------------
               # 1:             1.25            .061
               # 2:             1.67            .074
               # 3:             2.5             .106
               # 4:             5               .169
               # 5:             10              .227
               # 6:             20              .313


            File name:          LINE1

       1/Velocity =  9.32487 * 1/[Substrate] + 2.36086

            File name:          LINE2

       1/Velocity =  17.743 * 1/[Substrate] + 2.45534

            File name:          LINE1
          ------------- ---------------
               Vmax = .423575
                 Km = 3.94978

            File name:          LINE2
          ------------- ---------------
               Vmax = .407276
                 Km = 7.22631

                 Ki = 44.3084
```

Procedure 20

Enzyme Kinetics III: Noncompetitive Inhibition

In competitive inhibition (according to the kinetic model of Procedure 19), the inhibitor molecule reacts reversibly with the enzyme at the site normally occupied by the substrate. There are several mechanisms of noncompetitive inhibition. In one such mechanism the inhibitor can alter the activity of the enzyme without blocking the active site. In other words, I (the inhibitor) can combine with E (the enzyme) or ES (the enzyme–substrate complex), the dissociation constant in either case being denoted by K_I. As in the previous discussions, we denote by K_M the Michaelis constant for the reaction $E + S \rightleftharpoons ES$.

In this case of noncompetitive inhibition the velocity v is given by

$$v = \frac{V_{max}[S]}{([S] + K_M)(1 + I/K_I)}. \qquad (20.1)$$

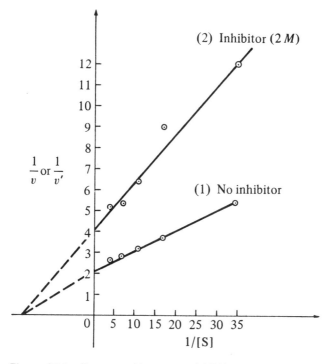

Figure 20.1 Noncompetitive enzyme inhibition.

In the double-reciprocal form,

$$\frac{1}{v} = \left(1 + \frac{I}{K_I}\right)\left(\frac{K_M}{V_{max}} \cdot \frac{1}{[S]} + \frac{1}{V_{max}}\right). \tag{20.2}$$

It is seen that both the slope and the intercept are multiplied by the same factor, namely $1 + I/K_I$, as shown in Figure 20.1. Note that in this case the linear plots in the presence and absence of inhibitor have the same intercept on the abscissa, namely, $-1/K_M$. The data are plotted as $1/v$ against $1/[S]$. The vertical intercept of the resulting plot (for a fixed concentration I) is determined by linear regression (Procedure 3), from which K_I is computed.

Example

The enzymatic hydrolysis of a sugar was followed by determining the initial rate v at various initial concentrations of the sugar S. In the presence of a fixed concentration (2 M) of an inhibitor, the rate v' was reduced at every concentration of the sugar as shown in the table below. It is desired to determine K_I for the inhibitor.

[S]	0.0292	0.0584	0.0876	0.146	0.234
v	0.182	0.265	0.311	0.349	0.371
v'	0.083	0.111	0.154	0.186	0.188

The double-reciprocal plots are shown in Figure 19.1. The regression lines yielded slope m and intercept b as given below.

Line 1	Line 2
$m = 0.0945$	$m = 0.236$
$b = 2.22$	$b = 4.150$

The difference in the intercepts indicates that the antagonism is noncompetitive. In such cases both the slope and the intercept are increased by the same factor. However, in this case, the ratio of slopes is 2.50, whereas the ratio of intercepts is 1.87. The mean of these ratios is 2.18 and may be taken as an approximation to the factor $1 + I/K_I$. Since I is $2\ M$, K_I is approximately 1.69 M.

Computer Screen

```
          <20> Enzyme Kinetics III: Noncompetitive Inhibition
          Pharmacologic Calculation System - Version 4.0 - 03/11/86

You must input data for two curves. The first must be without an inhibitor, and
   the second must be in the presence of a Non-competitive inhibitor.

Enter concentration of inhibitor ? 2<ENTER>

Concentration of Non-competitive inhibitor = 2

Input: <K>eyboard, <D>isk, or <E>xit this procedure? D

You may enter 2 'XY' data files. Press <ENTER> after last file name.
File name 1 ? LINE1<ENTER>
File name 2 ? LINE2<ENTER>

Data: <E>dit, <L>ist, <S>ave, or <ENTER> to continue? L

      File name:         LINE1
      Variable:     [Substrate]      Velocity
    --------------  --------------  --------------
        # 1:            .0292           .182
        # 2:            .0584           .265
        # 3:            .0876           .311
        # 4:            .146            .349
        # 5:            .234            .371
```

```
      File name:         LINE2
      Variable:     [Substrate]      Velocity
    --------------  --------------  --------------
        # 1:            .0292           .083
        # 2:            .0584           .111
        # 3:            .0876           .154
        # 4:            .146            .186
        # 5:            .234            .188

Data: <E>dit, <L>ist, <S>ave, or <ENTER> to continue? <ENTER>

Do you want to show intermediate results (Y/N) ? N


  File name:          LINE1

1/Velocity =   .0947393 * 1/[Substrate] + 2.20845


  File name:          LINE2

1/Velocity =   .237618 * 1/[Substrate] + 4.13686
```

```
 File name:            LINE1
------------- -------------
     Vmax = .452806
       Km = .0428985

 File name:            LINE2
------------- -------------
     Vmax = .241729
       Km = .0574391

       Ki = 1.67974

Report: <P>rint, <S>ave, or <V>iew? <ENTER>
```

Computer Report

```
              <20> Enzyme Kinetics III: Noncompetitive Inhibition
            Pharmacologic Calculation System - Version 4.0 - 03/11/86

Concentration of Non-competitive inhibitor = 2

        File name:            LINE1
        Variable:    [Substrate]        Velocity
      --------------- --------------- --------------
           # 1:          .0292            .182
           # 2:          .0584            .265
           # 3:          .0876            .311
           # 4:          .146             .349
           # 5:          .234             .371

        File name:            LINE2
        Variable:    [Substrate]        Velocity
      --------------- --------------- --------------
           # 1:          .0292            .083
           # 2:          .0584            .111
           # 3:          .0876            .154
           # 4:          .146             .186
           # 5:          .234             .188

        File name:            LINE1

   1/Velocity =  .0947393 * 1/[Substrate] + 2.20845

        File name:            LINE2

   1/Velocity =  .237618 * 1/[Substrate] + 4.13686

        File name:            LINE1
      --------------- ---------------
          Vmax = .452806
            Km = .0428985

        File name:            LINE2
      --------------- ---------------
          Vmax = .241729
            Km = .0574391

            Ki = 1.67974
```

Procedure 21

First-Order Drug Decay

Consider a drug A which decomposes according to the reaction $A \to B + C$. The original concentration of A is denoted by a. After time t the number of moles decomposed is x; hence, the amount of A is $a - x$, and x moles of B or C have been formed. The differential equation for the reaction is

$$\frac{dx}{dt} = k(a - x).$$

The solution of the above differential equation is

$$\ln\left(\frac{a}{a - x}\right) = kt. \tag{21.1}$$

The ratio in Equation (21.1) is amount at time 0 divided by amount at time t. (Concentrations may be used instead of amounts.) If the natural logarithm of this ratio is plotted against time t, a straight line through the origin of slope k is obtained. Thus, such a plot gives the rate constant for the decomposition of A. The straight line through the origin is determined from the regression technique of Procedure 4.

The associated computer program uses as input the original amount (or concentration) of A and the amounts (or concentrations) at times $t_1, t_2, \ldots, t_n$. Output is the slope of the regression line which is numerically equal to the decomposition rate constant k.

Example

A certain drug is administered in an isolated tissue bath preparation and rapidly achieves a tissue concentration of 3.5 $\mu g/g$ tissue. The table below gives the concentrations measured in the tissue at various times after administration. Determine k.

Time (min) = t	Concentration (μg/g tissue)	$\ln\left(\dfrac{a}{a - x}\right) = y$
0	3.5	
6	2.5	0.34
12	1.7	0.72
18	1.4	0.92
24	1.0	1.3

Column 3 of the table gives ln(initial conc./conc. at time t). From Procedure 4 (Equation 4.1),

$$\text{slope} = k = \frac{(6)(0.34) + (12)(0.72) + (18)(0.92) + (24)(1.3)}{6^2 + 12^2 + 18^2 + 24^2}$$

$$= 0.054 \ (\text{min}^{-1}).$$

Computer Screen

```
                        <21> First Order Drug Decay
                Pharmacologic Calculation System - Version 4.0 - 03/11/86

The first entry must be the tissue concentration or amount at time = 0.


Input: <K>eyboard, <D>isk, or <E>xit this procedure? D


You may enter 5 'XY' data files. Press <ENTER> after last file name.
File name 1 ? LINE1<ENTER>
File name 2 ? <ENTER>


Data: <E>dit, <L>ist, <S>ave, or <ENTER> to continue? L

      File name:         LINE1
      Variable:          Time    Tissue Conc
    ------------    --------------  --------------
          # 1:            0             3.5
          # 2:            6             2.5
          # 3:           12             1.7
          # 4:           18             1.4
          # 5:           24             1


Data: <E>dit, <L>ist, <S>ave, or <ENTER> to continue? <ENTER>
```

```
    ln (A/A-X) =  .0530037 * Time


<ENTER> to continue or <L>ist values calculated from regression line? <ENTER>


        K = .0530037

Report: <P>rint, <S>ave, or <V>iew? <ENTER>
```

Computer Report

```
                        <21> First Order Drug Decay
                Pharmacologic Calculation System - Version 4.0 - 03/11/86

      File name:         LINE1
      Variable:          Time    Tissue Conc
    ------------    --------------  --------------
          # 1:            0             3.5
          # 2:            6             2.5
          # 3:           12             1.7
          # 4:           18             1.4
          # 5:           24             1


    ln (A/A-X) =  .0530037 * Time


        K = .0530037
```

Procedure 22

Scatchard Plot*

The combination of a small molecule A with a protein P is viewed as an equilibrium reaction $A + P \rightleftharpoons C$.

In this reaction C denotes the complex that represents the bound molecule. The dissociation constant $K = (A)(P)/(C)$, where (A), (P), and (C) represent equilibrium concentrations of the reacting molecule, protein, and complex, respectively. The ratio of bound to free substance is (C)/(A) and is related to the total protein concentration $(P)_t$ by the equation

$$\frac{(C)}{(A)} = -\frac{1}{K}(C) + \frac{(P)_t}{K}. \tag{22.1}$$

Thus, a plot of the bound-to-free ratio against the bound concentration (C) is linear with slope $= -1/K$ and intercept $(P)_t/K$. Linear regression (Procedure 3) permits a determination of K and $(P)_t$. In many cases this analysis is used to determine the binding of a drug to some tissue, in which case $(P)_t$ represents the total concentration of binding sites. Confidence limits for $(P)_t$ (x-intercept) are computed as in Procedure 5.

Note. Since $K = |1/\text{slope}|$, and the slope and its variance V ($=$ square of std. error) are calculated from regression, we can get 95% confidence limits for K. The basis of the calculation is given in Procedure 41. The confidence limits are *asymmetric* about K and are determined as follows:

A quantity C is first calculated

$$C = \frac{(\text{slope})^2}{(\text{slope})^2 - Vt^2}, \tag{22.2}$$

where t is the value of Student's t for $N - 2$ degrees of freedom using the N points in the regression analysis. Then the confidence limits are computed from

$$C|K| \pm |K|\sqrt{(C-1)(C)} \tag{22.3}$$

Example

In an experiment on the binding of naloxone to a washed membrane preparation of rat brain, the data in the following table† (rounded for illustrative purposes) were obtained.

The regression line gave slope $= -0.57$, intercept $= 0.30$, and correlation coefficient $r = -0.99$. Thus, $K = 1/0.57 = 1.75$ nM. From these data an estimate of $(P)_t$, total concentration of binding sites, is $(K) \times (\text{intercept}) = 1.75$ nM $\times 0.30 = 0.53$ nM.

---

* Scatchard, G. *Ann. N. Y. Acad. Sci.* **51**:660, 1949.

† Hewlett, W. A., Akil, H., and Barchas, J. In *Endogenous and Exogenous Opiate Agonists and Antagonists* (E. L. Way, Ed.), page 95. Pergamon, New York, 1980.

Concentration of [^{3}H]naloxone, bound (nM)	[^{3}H]naloxone, bound/free
0.5	0.015
0.4	0.065
0.3	0.14
0.2	0.18

In this example, slope^2 = $(0.57)^2$, V = $(0.0453)^2$ and t^2 = $(4.30)^2$. Hence C = 1.13 and confidence limits for K are

$$1.13\left(\frac{1}{0.57}\right) \pm \left(\frac{1}{0.57}\right)\sqrt{(0.13)(1.13)}$$

or

$$1.98 \pm 0.67$$

which means 1.31–2.65. Note, these are *not* symmetric about K = 1.75.

Note. It may be shown that the upper and lower confidence limits for K are equivalent to $1/(\text{slope} - L)$ and $1/(\text{slope} + L)$, respectively, where L is the halfwidth of the confidence interval of the slope.

Computer Screen

```
                        <22> Scatchard Plot
              Pharmacologic Calculation System - Version 4.0 - 03/11/86

Input: <K>eyboard, <D>isk, or <E>xit this procedure? D

You may enter 5 'XY' data files. Press <ENTER> after last file name.
File name 1 ? LINE1<ENTER>
File name 2 ? <ENTER>

Data: <E>dit, <L>ist, <S>ave, or <ENTER> to continue? L

        File name:          LINE1
        Variable:          [Bound]    [Bnd]/[Free]
     --------------    --------------  --------------
           # 1:             .5             .015
           # 2:             .4             .065
           # 3:             .3             .14
           # 4:             .2             .18

Data: <E>dit, <L>ist, <S>ave, or <ENTER> to continue? <ENTER>

Do you want to show intermediate results (Y/N) ? N
```

```
[Bnd]/[Free] = -.57 * [Bound] + .2995

        Variable          Value     Std. Err.     Lower C.L.     Upper C.L.
     --------------    -----------  ------------  ------------   ------------
          K :          1.75439                     1.30749        2.66543
        (P)t* :        .525439    1.652486E-02     .4543319       .5965448

* Estimated concentration of binding sites.

Report: <P>rint, <S>ave, or <V>iew? <ENTER>
```

Computer Report

```
                          <22> Scatchard Plot
              Pharmacologic Calculation System - Version 4.0 - 06/24/86

         File name:          LINE1
         Variable:       [Bound]   [Bnd]/[Free]
        ------------    ---------  -------------
            # 1:            .5          .015
            # 2:            .4          .065
            # 3:            .3          .14
            # 4:            .2          .18


    [Bnd]/[Free] = -.57 * [Bound] + .2995

         Variable          Value     Std. Err.    Lower C.L.    Upper C.L.
        -----------    ---------   -----------   -----------   -----------
            K :          1.75439                   1.30749       2.66543
          (P)t* :         .525439  1.652486E-02    .4543319      .5965448

      * Estimated concentration of binding sites.
```

Procedure 23

Henderson–Hasselbalch Equation

Many drugs are weak acids or bases and are, therefore, ionized to some extent in the medium in which they become concentrated in the body. In general, these compounds are more fat soluble in the nonionized form. Consequently, the nonionized form is more permeable to the cell membrane. It is important, therefore, to know the extent of ionization of the drug in the medium from which it is being absorbed. This will depend upon the pH of the medium and the pK of the drug. The pK of the drug is the negative logarithm of the equilibrium constant and is a constant for each drug under physiological conditions. Knowledge of the pK of the drug and the pH of the medium permits a determination of the ratio of ionized (c_i) to unionized (c_u) concentrations of the drug. The ratio is given by the Henderson–Hasselbalch equations:

For weak acids:

$$\log_{10}\left(\frac{c_i}{c_u}\right) = \text{pH} - \text{p}K. \tag{23.1}$$

For weak bases:

$$\log_{10}\left(\frac{c_u}{c_i}\right) = \text{pH} - \text{p}K. \tag{23.2}$$

Example 1

Aspirin (acetylsalicylic acid) has a pK of 3.5. What is the ratio of ionized to unionized concentrations in gastric juice of pH 2.0?

From Equation (23.1), $\log(c_i/c_u) = 2.0 - 3.5 = -1.5$. Thus,

$$c_i/c_u = \text{antilog}(-1.5) = 0.032.$$

Therefore, only a small percentage of the drug is ionized.

Example 2

A weakly basic drug, with $pK = 8$ is placed in an acidic solution of pH $= 3$.
From Equation (23.2) $c_i/c_u = 10^5$; that is, there is extensive ionization.

Computer Screen

```
                    <23> Henderson-Hasselbalch Equation
            Pharmacologic Calculation System - Version 4.0 - 03/11/86

Enter A for weak Acid or B for weak Base ? A
Enter pK of drug ? 3.5<ENTER>
Enter pH of medium? 2<ENTER>

The drug is a weak acid with a pK of 3.5.
The pH of the medium is 2.
The ratio of ionized to unionized drug =  .0316228

Run again (Y/N) ? Y
Enter A for weak Acid or B for weak Base ? B
Enter pK of drug ? 8<ENTER>
Enter pH of medium? 3<ENTER>

The drug is a weak base with a pK of 8.
The pH of the medium is 3.
The ratio of ionized to unionized drug =  100000

Run again (Y/N) ? N

Report: <P>rint, <S>ave, or <V>iew? <ENTER>
```

Computer Report

```
                    <23> Henderson-Hasselbalch Equation
            Pharmacologic Calculation System - Version 4.0 - 03/11/86


The drug is a weak acid with a pK of 3.5.
The pH of the medium is 2.
The ratio of ionized to unionized drug =  .0316228


The drug is a weak base with a pK of 8.
The pH of the medium is 3.
The ratio of ionized to unionized drug =  100000
```

Procedure 24
Exponential Growth and Decay

The values of A and k for the exponential

$$x = Ae^{-kt} \tag{24.1}$$

are determined from the n data points (t_i, x_i) by plotting the natural logarithm of x_i against t_i. The resulting plot is linear with slope $-k$ and intercept $\ln A$. Linear regression (Procedure 3) is used on the pairs $(t_i, \ln x_i)$. The value of k is related to the half-life $t_{1/2}$ as $k = \ln 2/t_{1/2} \approx 0.693/t_{1/2}$.

Example

The tabulation below gives the values of t and x; for each x the value of $\ln x$ is first computed.

t	1	2	5	8	10	15
x	65	60	35	25	15	8
$\ln x$	4.17	4.09	3.56	3.22	2.71	2.08

Application of the method of least squares (Procedure 3) to the pairs $(t, \ln x)$ gives slope $= -0.154$ and intercept of 4.36. Hence $k = -0.154$ and $\ln A = 4.36$, from which A is 78. Thus, the equation

$$x = 78e^{-0.154t}$$

best fits the data. Confidence limits of the half-life (4.50) are computed from the standard error of slope (shown to be 0.0068) and 4 degrees of freedom ($t = 2.78$). Hence

$$t_{1/2}(upper) = \frac{0.693}{0.154 - (0.0068)(2.78)} = 5.13$$

and

$$t_{1/2}(lower) = \frac{0.693}{0.154 + (0.0068)(2.78)} = 4.01$$

(See note at the end of Procedure 22.)

Computer Screen

```
                        <24> Exponential Growth & Decay
              Pharmacologic Calculation System - Version 4.0 - 03/11/86

Input: <K>eyboard, <D>isk, or <E>xit this procedure? D

You may enter 5 'XY' data files. Press <ENTER> after last file name.
File name 1 ? LINE1<ENTER>
File name 2 ? <ENTER>

Data: <E>dit, <L>ist, <S>ave, or <ENTER> to continue? L

      File name:          LINE1
      Variable:           time                  X
    ------------     ------------     ------------
       # 1:               1                65
       # 2:               2                60
       # 3:               5                35
       # 4:               8                25
       # 5:              10                15
       # 6:              15                 8

Data: <E>dit, <L>ist, <S>ave, or <ENTER> to continue? <ENTER>

Do you want to show intermediate results (Y/N) ? N
```

```
    ln(X) = -.153746 * time + 4.35568

       R = .996

   t (95%) = 2.776         4 d.f.

      Variable        Value      Std. Err.    Lower C.L.    Upper C.L.
    ------------   ------------  -----------  ------------  ------------
           K:        -.153746   6.78983E-03    -.172595      -.134898
    Y-Intercept:      4.35568     .0567401      4.19816       4.51319
    X-Intercept:     28.3303      .972837      25.6297       31.0309

    half-life:        4.50838                   4.01604       5.13832

       X = 77.9194 * E^ -.153746 t

Report: <P>rint, <S>ave, or <V>iew? <ENTER>
```

Computer Report

```
                        <24> Exponential Growth & Decay
              Pharmacologic Calculation System - Version 4.0 - 03/11/86

    File name:        LINE1
    Variable:          time               X
    ------------   ------------   ------------
      #  1:             1               65
      #  2:             2               60
      #  3:             5               35
      #  4:             8               25
      #  5:            10               15
      #  6:            15                8


    ln(X) = -.153746 * time + 4.35568

       R = .996

   t (95%) = 2.776         4 d.f.

      Variable        Value      Std. Err.    Lower C.L.    Upper C.L.
    ------------   ------------  -----------  ------------  ------------
           K:        -.153746   6.78983E-03    -.172595      -.134898
    Y-Intercept:      4.35568     .0567401      4.19816       4.51319
    X-Intercept:     28.3303      .972837      25.6297       31.0309

    half-life:        4.50838                   4.01604       5.13832

       X = 77.9194 * E^ -.153746 t
```

Procedure 25

Area under a Curve: Trapezoidal and Simpson's Rules

Simpson's rule is a method for evaluating the area under a curve from values of the ordinate and the abscissa. Thus, this method accomplishes the same objective as that of the trapezoidal rule (discussed subsequently). It may be shown,

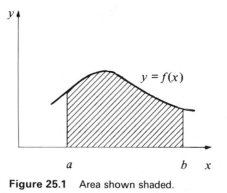

Figure 25.1   Area shown shaded.

however, that Simpson's rule gives a closer approximation to the area, than does the trapezoidal rule.

The shaded region of Figure (25.1) represents the area to be measured. The area, or integral, is $\int_a^b f(x)dx$.

The interval $[a, b]$ of the x-axis is divided into an even number ($2n$) of sub-intervals, each of width $\Delta x = (b - a)/2n$. The corresponding points of the x-axis are $x_0 = a, x_1 = a + \Delta x, x_2 = a + 2\Delta x$, etc., and the corresponding ordinates are y_0, y_1, etc.

The area $A = \int_a^b f(x)dx$ is (approximately)

$$A \approx \Delta x/3(y_0 + 4y_1 + 2y_2 + 4y_3 + 2y_4 + \cdots + 2y_{2n-2} + 4y_{2n-1} + y_{2n}).$$

$$(25.1)$$

Equation (25.1) is Simpson's rule.

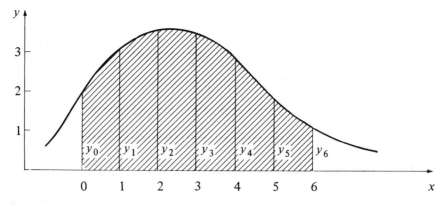

Figure 25.2   Numerical approximation of area using six subintervals.

Example 1

Evaluate the area shown shaded in Figure 25.2, taking $2n = 6$.

The measured values of $y_0, y_1, \ldots, y_6$ are 1.87, 3.12, 3.56, 3.44, 2.87, 1.87, and 1.12, respectively. Thus, Simpson's rule gives

$$A = \tfrac{1}{3}[1.87 + 4(3.12) + 2(3.56) + 4(3.44)$$

$$+ 2(2.87) + 4(1.87) + 1.12]$$

$$= \tfrac{1}{3}[1.87 + 12.48 + 7.12 + 13.76 + 5.74 + 7.48 + 1.12]$$

$$= \tfrac{1}{3}[49.57] = 16.5 \text{ (three significant figures)}.$$

The trapezoidal rule may also be used. This rule is given by

$$A \approx \frac{\Delta x}{2}(y_0 + 2y_1 + 2y_2 + \cdots + 2y_{n-1} + y_n). \tag{25.2}$$

When applied to the previous example, the trapezoidal rule gives

$$A \approx \tfrac{1}{2}[1.87 + 2(3.12) + 2(3.56) + 2(3.44) + 2(2.87) + 2(1.87) + 1.12]$$

$$= 16.4 \text{ (three significant figures)}.$$

Computer Screen

```
            <25> Area Under a Curve: Trapezoidal & Simpson's Rules
            Pharmacologic Calculation System - Version 4.0 - 03/11/86

For the greatest accuracy, the area under the curve should be divided into an
even number (n) of EQUALLY spaced subintervals. Enter n+1 pairs of X and Y
values from the curve.

If the X interval width is divided into UNEQUAL subintervals, the area will be
based on an approximation using the Trapezoidal rule.  Enter X values first.

Input: <K>eyboard, <D>isk, or <E>xit this procedure? D

You may enter 5 'XY' data files. Press <ENTER> after last file name.
File name 1 ? EXAMPLE1<ENTER>
File name 2 ? <ENTER>

Data: <E>dit, <L>ist, <S>ave, or <ENTER> to continue? L
```

```
    File name:       EXAMPLE1
    Variable:            X                Y
  ------------   ---------------   ---------------
      # 1:             0              1.87
      # 2:             1              3.12
      # 3:             2              3.56
      # 4:             3              3.44
      # 5:             4              2.87
      # 6:             5              1.87
      # 7:             6              1.12

Data: <E>dit, <L>ist, <S>ave, or <ENTER> to continue? <ENTER>

Area under Y( X ) between Y( 0 ) and Y( 6 ) :

Using equal subintervals:
    Trapezoidal Rule -   Area = 16.355
    Simpson's Rule -     Area = 16.5233


Report: <P>rint, <S>ave, or <V>iew? <ENTER>
```

Computer Report

```
              <25> Area Under a Curve: Trapezoidal & Simpson's Rules
              Pharmacologic Calculation System - Version 4.0 - 03/11/86

    File name:       EXAMPLE1
    Variable:            X                Y
  ------------   ---------------   ---------------
      # 1:             0              1.87
      # 2:             1              3.12
      # 3:             2              3.56
      # 4:             3              3.44
      # 5:             4              2.87
      # 6:             5              1.87
      # 7:             6              1.12

Area under Y( X ) between Y( 0 ) and Y( 6 ) :

Using equal subintervals:
    Trapezoidal Rule -   Area = 16.355
    Simpson's Rule -     Area = 16.5233
```

When the interval width $[a, b]$ is divided into *unequal* intervals $[x_0, x_1]$, $[x_1, x_2], \ldots, [x_{n-1}, x_n]$, the trapezoidal rule becomes

$$A \approx \tfrac{1}{2}(y_0 + y_1)(x_1 - x_0) + \tfrac{1}{2}(y_1 + y_2)(x_2 - x_1)$$
$$+ \cdots + \tfrac{1}{2}(y_{n-1} + y_n)(x_n - x_{n-1}) \tag{25.3}$$

Example 2

Use the trapezoidal rule to estimate $\int_1^2 x^2 \, dx$ using the five subintervals given below:

x_i	1	1.2	1.3	1.5	1.8	2
y_i	1	1.44	1.69	2.25	3.24	4.0

$$A \approx 2.342.$$

Note. The exact area is $7/3 \approx 2.333$.

Computer Screen

```
                <25> Area Under a Curve: Trapezoidal & Simpson's Rules
                Pharmacologic Calculation System - Version 4.0 - 03/11/86

For the greatest accuracy, the area under the curve should be divided into an
even number (n) of EQUALLY spaced subintervals. Enter n+1 pairs of X and Y
values from the curve.

If the X interval width is divided into UNEQUAL subintervals, the area will be
based on an approximation using the Trapezoidal rule.  Enter X values first.

Input: <K>eyboard, <D>isk, or <E>xit this procedure? D

You may enter 5 'XY' data files. Press <ENTER> after last file name.
File name 1 ? EXAMPLE2<ENTER>
File name 2 ? <ENTER>

Data: <E>dit, <L>ist, <S>ave, or <ENTER> to continue? L

    File name:      EXAMPLE2
    Variable:          X              Y
    -------------  -------------  -------------
        # 1:             1              1
        # 2:            1.2           1.44
        # 3:            1.3           1.69
        # 4:            1.5           2.25
        # 5:            1.8           3.24
        # 6:             2              4
```

```
Data: <E>dit, <L>ist, <S>ave, or <ENTER> to continue? <ENTER>

Area under Y( X ) between Y( 1 ) and Y( 2 ) :

Approximation using unequal intervals:
    Trapezoidal Rule -  Area = 2.342


Report: <P>rint, <S>ave, or <V>iew? <ENTER>
```

Computer Report

```
                <25> Area Under a Curve: Trapezoidal & Simpson's Rules
                Pharmacologic Calculation System - Version 4.0 - 03/11/86

    File name:      EXAMPLE2
    Variable:          X              Y
    -------------  -------------  -------------
        # 1:             1              1
        # 2:            1.2           1.44
        # 3:            1.3           1.69
        # 4:            1.5           2.25
        # 5:            1.8           3.24
        # 6:             2              4

Area under Y( X ) between Y( 1 ) and Y( 2 ) :

Approximation using unequal intervals:
    Trapezoidal Rule -  Area = 2.342
```

Procedure 26

Pharmacokinetics I: Constant Infusion with First-Order Elimination

Many drugs are eliminated from the blood plasma exponentially, that is, the concentration C at any time t is expressed by the equation

$$C = C_0 e^{-k_e t}. \tag{26.1}$$

In this equation C_0 is the plasma concentration at time $t = 0$ and k_e is the rate constant for elimination, or fraction eliminated per unit time. The constant k_e is related to the half-life $t_{1/2}$ according to the relation

$$k_e = \frac{\ln 2}{t_{1/2}} \approx \frac{0.693}{t_{1/2}}. \tag{26.2}$$

Thus, knowledge of the half life permits the determination of k_e from Equation (26.2).

We now consider the case in which this same drug is infused at a constant rate R (amount/time) into the blood and is distributed ideally in the plasma. In this situation the plasma concentration will increase in time according to the relation

$$C = \frac{R}{V k_e} (1 - e^{-k_e t}) \tag{26.3}$$

where e is the base of the natural logarithm and V is the plasma volume. The drug concentration thus approaches a plateau $= R/k_e V$. Thus, if the plasma volume is known* one may determine k_e from the measured plasma concentration at times after the beginning of the infusion.

From Equation (26.3) it may be seen that at a time equal to $t_{1/2}$, the elimination half-time, the concentration is $R/(2V k_e)$, or one half the maximum. At $t = 4t_{1/2}$ the concentration is $\frac{15}{16}$ ($\approx 94\%$) of the maximum concentration.

For a fixed rate of infusion R, the concentration–time data permit a determination of both k_e and V. The value of V so determined is generally called the *apparent volume of distribution*. Binding of the drug to tissue or blood cells will lower the plasma concentration, resulting in apparently large volumes of distribution.

If at some later time t' (see Figure 26.1) the infusion is stopped, the concentration will fall exponentially with the same rate constant k_e, or half-time $t_{1/2} = 0.693/k_e$.

---

* The plasma volume may be determined with the use of a high molecular weight dye such as Evans Blue which is almost entirely confined to the plasma.

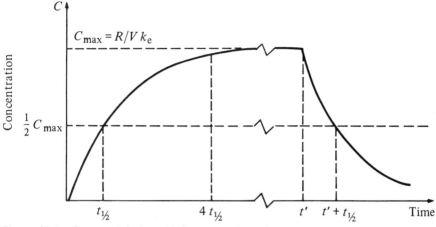

Figure 26.1   Constant infusion with first order elimination.

Example 1

A substance is infused at a constant rate of 10 mg/hr to an adult male. The saturation level of the substance in blood plasma is determined to be 8 μg/ml, and the apparent volume of distribution is known to be 3.5 liters. What is k_e?

From Equation (26.3), the saturation level is R/Vk_e; hence, 8×10^{-3} mg/ml = 10 mg/hr/3.5×10^3 ml (k_e), and $k_e = 0.36$ hr^{-1}.

The computer subroutine permits a variety of computations. For example, it will compute k_e from measured concentrations $C(t)$ at various times and $C(t)_{max}$, the concentration at the steady state, utilizing a least squares curve fitting procedure that fits a regression line through the origin as explained below.

Equation (26.3) may be written

$$C/C_{max} = 1 - e^{-k_e t}$$

which may be put in the form

$$\ln(1 - C/C_{max}) = -k_e t. \tag{26.4}$$

Thus, if the values $(1 - C/C_{max})$ are determined, and their natural logarithms are plotted against time, the resulting plot is linear with slope $-k_e$ and intercept 0.

The best fitting line *through the origin* (in the sense of least squares) gives the slope as previously shown (Procedure 4). Denoting $\ln(1 - C/C_{max})$ by Y, we then have the linear form $Y = -k_e t$ and the slope $-k_e$ is given by

$$-k_e = \frac{\sum tY}{\sum t^2}. \tag{26.5}$$

Computer Screen

```
      <26> Pharmacokinetics I: Constant Infusion, 1st Order Elimination
            Pharmacologic Calculation System - Version 4.0 - 03/11/86


Enter values or press <ENTER> if unknown.
Saturation concentration (Default=1) ... ? 8<ENTER>
Elimination rate constant (1/hr), Ke ... ? <ENTER>
Elimination half-time, t1/2 ........... ? <ENTER>
Infusion rate (mg/hr) ................. ? 10<ENTER>
Apparent volume of distribution (liters) ? 3.5<ENTER>


Results:
Saturation concentration (Default=1) ... = 8
Elimination rate constant (1/hr), Ke ... = .357143
Elimination half-time, t1/2 ........... = 1.94081
Infusion rate (mg/hr) ................. = 10
Apparent volume of distribution (liters) = 3.5


<ENTER> to continue or <L>ist values calculated from regression line? <ENTER>


Report: <P>rint, <S>ave, or <V>iew? <ENTER>
```

Computer Report

```
      <26> Pharmacokinetics I: Constant Infusion, 1st Order Elimination
            Pharmacologic Calculation System - Version 4.0 - 03/11/86


Results:
Saturation concentration (Default=1) ... = 8
Elimination rate constant (1/hr), Ke ... = .357143
Elimination half-time, t1/2 ........... = 1.94081
Infusion rate (mg/hr) ................. = 10
Apparent volume of distribution (liters) = 3.5
```

Example 2

Measurement of plasma concentration at three times (after start of infusion), $t = 5$, 15, and 30 min, yielded 0.1, 0.3, and 0.6, respectively, as fractions of the maximum. Thus, we have the table below.

t(min)	$Y = \ln(1 - C/C_{\max})$	tY	t^2
5	−0.11	−0.55	25
15	−0.36	−5.4	225
30	−0.92	−27.6	900
		−33.6	1150

From Equation (26.5) k_e is given by

$$-k_e = -33.6/1150$$

$$\therefore \quad k_e = 0.029 \text{ min}^{-1}.$$

Other options are given as prompting statements in the computer program.

Computer Screen

```
        <26> Pharmacokinetics I: Constant Infusion, 1st Order Elimination
             Pharmacologic Calculation System - Version 4.0 - 03/11/86

Enter values or press <ENTER> if unknown.
Saturation concentration (Default=1) ... ? <ENTER>
Elimination rate constant (1/hr), Ke ... ? <ENTER>
Elimination half-time, t1/2 ............ ? <ENTER>
Infusion rate (mg/hr) .................. ? <ENTER>
Apparent volume of distribution (liters) ? <ENTER>

More information is required.  Do you want to enter plasma concentrations at
various time intervals (Y/N) ? Y
Enter each concentration as a fraction of the saturation concentration, 1

Input: <K>eyboard, <D>isk, or <E>xit this procedure? K

Type 'END' after last file. Enter file name or <ENTER> for default name:
'FILE1/XY' (or 'END') ? LINE1<ENTER>
```

```
You may enter up to 15 x,y data pairs. Press <ENTER> after the last entry.
     File name:          LINE1
     Variable:          Time            Conc.
-------------     -------------     -------------
       # 1: 5<ENTER>        .1<ENTER>
       # 2: 15<ENTER>       .3<ENTER>
       # 3: 30<ENTER>       .6<ENTER>
       # 4: <ENTER>


Data: <E>dit, <L>ist, <S>ave, or <ENTER> to continue? L

     File name:          LINE1
     Variable:          Time            Conc.
-------------     -------------     -------------
       # 1:               5               .1
       # 2:              15               .3
       # 3:              30               .6

Data: <E>dit, <L>ist, <S>ave, or <ENTER> to continue? <ENTER>

ln(1-C/Cmax) = -.0290136 * Time

<ENTER> to continue or <L>ist values calculated from regression line? <ENTER>
```

```
Results:
Saturation concentration (Default=1) ... = 1
Elimination rate constant (1/hr), Ke ... = .0290136
Elimination half-time, t1/2 ............ = 23.8904

<ENTER> to continue or <L>ist values calculated from regression line? <ENTER>


Report: <P>rint, <S>ave, or <V>iew? <ENTER>
```

Computer Report

```
            <26> Pharmacokinetics I: Constant Infusion, 1st Order Elimination
               Pharmacologic Calculation System - Version 4.0 - 03/11/86


        File name:              LINE1
        Variable:               Time              Conc.
    ----------------  ----------------    ----------------
           # 1:                   5                .1
           # 2:                  15                .3
           # 3:                  30                .6


    ln(1-C/Cmax) = -.0290136 * Time



    Results:
    Saturation concentration (Default=1) ... = 1
    Elimination rate constant (1/hr), Ke ... = .0290136
    Elimination half-time, t1/2 ............ = 23.8904
```

Procedure 27

Pharmacokinetics II: Multiple Intravenous Injections

If a drug that is eliminated exponentially from the plasma is administered intravenously in repeated doses of amount I, at time intervals equal to t', the plasma
concentration–time relation will be as shown in Figure 27.1. We have denoted by

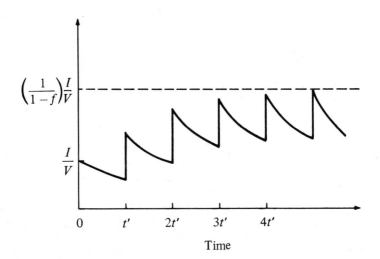

Figure 27.1   Multiple intravenous injections of amount I which distributes in volume V.
The peaks approach the limit $(1/1 - f)(I/V)$ where f is the fraction remaining after each time
interval.

V the apparent volume of distribution and by C the plasma concentration of the drug. After time t', but before the second dose I is given, the concentration falls to some fraction f of the original concentration. (It is assumed that the drug distributes rapidly.) The fraction f is related to the elimination rate constant k_e according to

$$f = e^{-k_e t'}. \tag{27.1}$$

Successive peaks immediately after dosing are given by $(I/V)(1 + f + f^2 + \cdots + f^{n-1})$, where n is the number of doses. The sum of the progression is given by

$$(1 + f + f^2 + \cdots + f^{n-1}) = \frac{1 - f^n}{1 - f}. \tag{27.2}$$

Hence, the peak concentration $C(n)_{max}$ after the nth dose, given at time $(n - 1)t'$, is

$$C(n)_{max} = \frac{I}{V}\frac{1 - f^n}{1 - f}. \tag{27.3}$$

Since $f < 1$, the term f^n approaches 0 as n becomes large, and the *peaks* approach a steady state upper bound C_u given by

$$C_u = \frac{I}{V(1 - f)}, \tag{27.4}$$

whereas the troughs approach a steady state lower bound C_1 given by

$$C_1 = fC_u = \frac{If}{V(1 - f)}. \tag{27.5}$$

Thus, the concentration alternates between C_u and C_1 after a sufficiently long time, with a mean concentration given by $\bar{C}$:

$$\bar{C} = \frac{-I}{V \ln(f)}. \tag{27.6}$$

Example

A drug with plasma elimination rate constant $= 0.25/\text{hr}$ is given in a dose of 10 mg (i.v.) every 4 hr. The drug distributes in a plasma volume of 3.5 liters. Determine the peak level C_u, the trough level C_1, and the mean level $\bar{C}$ during the steady state.

We have $I = 10$ mg and $V = 3.5$ liters. We determine f from Equation (25.1):

$$f = e^{-(0.25)(4)} \approx 0.368.$$

From Equations (27.4), (27.5), and (27.6)

$$C_u = \frac{10 \text{ mg}}{(3.5)(10)^3 \text{ ml}} \frac{1}{(1 - 0.368)} = 4.5 \times 10^{-3} \text{ mg/ml},$$

$$C_1 = (0.368)(4.5 \times 10^{-3}) = 1.7 \times 10^{-3} \text{ mg/ml},$$

and

$$\bar{C} = -\frac{10 \text{ mg}}{(3.5)(10)^3 \ln(0.368)} = 2.9 \times 10^{-3} \text{ mg/ml}.$$

For the same drug in the above example, it is desired to determine the number of doses n that are necessary in order for the peak $C(n)_{max}$ to achieve 95% of the upper plateau level C_u (see Figure 27.2).

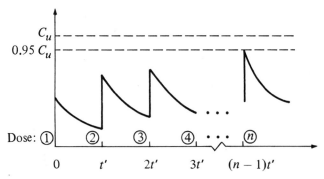

Figure 27.2   Illustrating the number (n) of doses that are required to achieve 95% C_u.

We require $C(n)_{max}/C_u = 0.95$. From Equations (27.3) and (27.4) we have

$$\frac{(I/V)(1 - f^n/1 - f)}{(I/V)(1/1 - f)} = 1 - f^n = 0.95,$$

or since $f = 0.368$,

$$1 - (0.368)^n = 0.95$$

or

$$(0.368)^n = 0.05.$$

Thus, $n = 2.99 \approx 3$ doses.

The accompanying program permits a variety of computations. Prompting statements are included in order to guide the user.

Computer Screen

```
            <27> Pharmacokinetics II: Multiple Intravenous Injections
            Pharmacologic Calculation System - Version 4.0 - 03/11/86

Enter values or press <ENTER> if unknown.
Elimination rate constant (1/hr), Ke ... ? .25<ENTER>
Number of doses ........................ ? <ENTER>
Dosing interval (hrs) .................. ? 4<ENTER>
Desired level as % of upper limit ......   95
Single dose plasma concentration (mg/ml) ? <ENTER>
Dose of drug (mg) ...................... ? 10<ENTER>
Apparent volume of distribution (liters) ? 3.5<ENTER>

Results:
Elimination rate constant (1/hr), Ke ... = .25
Number of doses ........................ = 3
Dosing interval (hrs) .................. = 4
Desired level as % of upper limit ...... = 95
Single dose plasma concentration (mg/ml) = 2.85714E-03
Dose of drug (mg) ...................... = 10
Apparent volume of distribution (liters) = 3.5
Fraction remaining ..................... = .367879
Plasma concentration (mg/ml) ........... :
        Peak = 4.51993E-03
        Mean = 2.85714E-03
        Lower = 1.66279E-03

Report: <P>rint, <S>ave, or <V>iew? <ENTER>
```

Computer Report

```
            <27> Pharmacokinetics II: Multiple Intravenous Injections
            Pharmacologic Calculation System - Version 4.0 - 03/11/86

Results:
Elimination rate constant (1/hr), Ke ... = .25
Number of doses ........................ = 3
Dosing interval (hrs) .................. = 4
Desired level as % of upper limit ...... = 95
Single dose plasma concentration (mg/ml) = 2.85714E-03
Dose of drug (mg) ...................... = 10
Apparent volume of distribution (liters) = 3.5
Fraction remaining ..................... = .367879
Plasma concentration (mg/ml) ........... :
        Peak = 4.51993E-03
        Mean = 2.85714E-03
        Lower = 1.66279E-03
```

Procedure 28

Pharmacokinetics III: Volume of Distribution

When an amount A of drug is administered *intravenously* (i.v.) the simple first order elimination model predicts an exponential decay with a single half life ($t_{1/2}$) equal to $\ln(2)/K_e$, where K_e is the rate constant for elimination. The value of $\ln(2)$ is approximately 0.693; thus, $t_{1/2} \doteq 0.693/K_e$. This kinetic pattern has been discussed in Procedure 21.

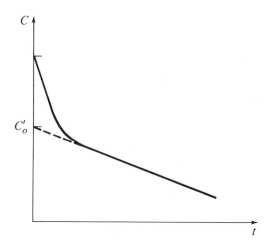

Figure 28.1   Concentration following intravenous administration.

If the drug is transported to tissue binding sites there will be an initial rapid drop in plasma concentration followed by a more prolonged decay due to elimination (excretion and metabolism). (See Figure 28.1.) These two phases are most obvious when the concentration is plotted on a logarithmic scale. The second phase is extrapolated to $t = 0$ (shown as the broken line). The extrapolated intercept C'_o and the amount A are used to calculate the volume of distribution V_d:

$$V_d = \frac{A}{C'_o} \tag{28.1}$$

Data at times after administration ($t = 0$) are collected. These concentrations (C) may be plotted on semilogarithmic paper against time (linear scale) or ln C may be plotted against time (linear scales). If the latter is used, linear regression can be used. The intercept is then ln C'_o, so that $C_o = e^{(\text{intercept})}$. Equation (28.1) is used to calculate V_d.

Example

Two grams of a drug were administered as an i.v. bolus. The plasma concentration (C_p) at various times is given below (Table 28.1) and is also shown graphically (Fig. 28.2). The graph suggests that equilibrium is attained after approximately one hour. Regression of ln(C_p) against time for values at one hour and later gave the equation ln(C_p) = $-0.51t + 2.04$. Hence, ln(C_p) at zero time = 2.04 and $C_p(0) = 7.69$. Accordingly V_d is computed: $V_d = 2g/7.69$ mg/liter $\doteq 260$ liters.

Table 28.1

Time (hr)	C_p(mg/l)	$\ln(C_p)$
0.1	22	
0.25	15	
0.50	9	
0.75	6	
1.0	4.5	1.50
1.5	4.0	1.39
2.0	2.6	0.956
2.5	2.3	0.833
3.0	1.5	0.405
4.0	0.92	−0.083
5.0	0.65	−0.431

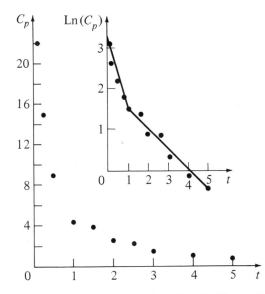

Figure 28.2 Graph of plasma concentration against time. Equilibrium is attained at $t = 1$ (estimated). The values of C_p vs. t at times $t = 1$ and later are used in the regression of $\ln(C_p)$ vs. t. (Inset: $\ln(C_p)$ vs. t.)

The additional point to be made here is that it is often desirable to obtain the area under the curve (0 to ∞) when, actually, the data exist only up to some time T (Fig. 28.3). It is necessary, therefore, to estimate the area from $t = T$ to $t = \infty$ (shaded in the figure). It may be shown that the shaded area is equal to the last ordinate $A(T)$ divided by K_e. (See also Procedure 29.)

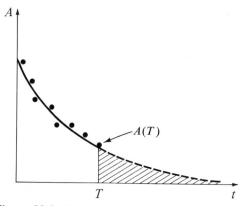

Figure 28.3   The shaded area (to infinity) = $A(T)/K_e$.

Computer Screen

```
             <28> Pharmacokinetics III: Volume of Distribution
         Pharmacologic Calculation System - Version 4.0 - 03/11/86

This procedure calculates the volume of distribution, Vd, from a single i.v.
bolus of a drug and values of its plasma concentration, Cp, over several time
periods.

Enter the drug dose (i.v. bolus, mg) ? 2000<ENTER>

Intravenous bolus dose (mg) = 2000

Input: <K>eyboard, <D>isk, or <E>xit this procedure? D

File name: ? LINE1<ENTER>

Data: <E>dit, <L>ist, <S>ave, or <ENTER> to continue? L

    File name:           LINE1
    Variable:            time                Cp
   ------------    ---------------    ---------------
      # 1:              .1                 22
      # 2:              .25                15
      # 3:              .5                  9
      # 4:              .75                 6
```

```
      # 5:               1                 4.5
      # 6:              1.5                 4
      # 7:               2                 2.6
      # 8:              2.5                 2.3
      # 9:               3                 1.5
     # 10:               4                 .92
     # 11:               5                 .65

Data: <E>dit, <L>ist, <S>ave, or <ENTER> to continue? <ENTER>

Do you want to show intermediate results (Y/N) ? N

Enter time at which phase 2 begins ? 1<ENTER>

Regression from time = 1 to 5:

    ln(Cp) = -.511274 * time + 2.04062

    ln(Co) = 2.04062          Co = 7.69534          R = .992719

       Vd = 259.898

Report: <P>rint, <S>ave, or <V>iew? <ENTER>
```

Computer Report

```
                    <28> Pharmacokinetics III: Volume of Distribution
                 Pharmacologic Calculation System - Version 4.0 - 03/11/86

Intravenous bolus dose (mg) = 2000

        File name:           LINE1
         Variable:            time                   Cp
  --------------    --------------    --------------
          # 1:              .1                  22
          # 2:             .25                  15
          # 3:              .5                   9
          # 4:             .75                   6
          # 5:               1                 4.5
          # 6:             1.5                   4
          # 7:               2                 2.6
          # 8:             2.5                 2.3
          # 9:               3                 1.5
         # 10:               4                 .92
         # 11:               5                 .65

  Regression from time = 1 to 5:

      ln(Cp) = -.511274 * time + 2.04062

      ln(Co) = 2.04062          Co = 7.69534          R = .992719

          Vd = 259.898
```

Procedure 29

Pharmacokinetics IV: *Absorptive Route of Administration**
Plasma Concentration-Time Data

Plasma concentration-time data are useful for determining the rate constants for absorption and elimination (and, hence, the corresponding half lives) following administration via an absorptive route. The elimination rate constant (K_e) and the apparent volume of distribution (V_d) are best obtained from concentration-time data following intravenous administration as described in Procedure 26. However, if the only data available are from administration that uses an absorptive route, the plasma-time data are still useful. The two-compartment model (illustrated in Figure 29.1) is frequently used.

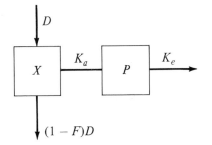

Figure 29.1   Two-compartment model.

*This computational algorithm is based on the standard two-compartment model in which the loss of drug from the plasma is due only to elimination via excretion and metabolism.

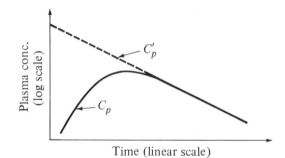

Time (linear scale)

Figure 29.2   Plasma concentration versus time following administration via an absorptive route.

In the most common model both absorption and elimination are first order. A dose (D) is administered of which a fraction (F) is absorbed into plasma, denoted by P in Figure 29.1. X represents the compartment from which absorption takes place such as the gut. The concentration in plasma, C_p, is a function of time and is given by

$$C_p = \frac{FDK_a}{V_d(K_a - K_e)} (e^{-K_e t} - e^{-K_a t}) \tag{29.1}$$

Usually, absorption is more rapid than elimination (i.e., $K_a > K_e$) so that $e^{-K_a t}$ approaches 0 more rapidly than $e^{-K_e t}$. At some time after the time of peak concentration $e^{-K_a t} \doteq 0$ and the plasma concentration is given by C_p':

$$C_p' = \frac{FDK_a}{V_d(K_a - K_e)} e^{-K_e t} \tag{29.2}$$

Note that $C_p' \geq C_p$; accordingly C_p' (shown as the broken curve of Figure 29.2) will be above or coincident with the smooth curve that represents the best fit of the data.

The difference $C_p' - C_p$ is given by

$$C_p' - C_p = \frac{FDK_a}{V_d(K_a - K_e)} e^{-K_a t} \tag{29.3}$$

Taking natural logarithms of both sides of Equation (29.3) yields

$$\ln(C_p' - C_p) = \ln\left(\frac{FDK_a}{V_d(K_a - K_e)}\right) - K_a t \tag{29.4}$$

Hence the slope of a plot of $\ln(C_p' - C_p)$ vs time yields K_a (as the negative slope). With both K_a and K_e determined from the preceding analysis following dose (D) there still remains the problem of determining the ratio (F/V_d). This can be determined by "smoothing" the concentration time data; however it is more common to estimate this ratio from the area under the curve (AUC)$_0^\infty$ as follows. It may be shown that

$$F/V_d = \frac{(AUC)_0^\infty \cdot K_e}{D} \tag{29.5}$$

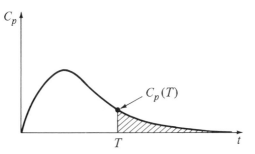

Figure 29.3 The total area (0 to ∞) is the sum of A (determined from the trapezoidal rule) and the shaded area. The latter is equal to the ordinate at T divided by K_e.

The trapezoidal rule may be used to calculate the area (A) under the curve from zero to some time (T). The total area $(AUC)_0^\infty$ is given by

$$(AUC)_0^\infty = A + \frac{C_p(T)}{K_e} \tag{29.6}$$

where $C_p(T)$ is the concentration at time T. (Figure 29.3). The time to peak (t^*) is given by

$$t^* = \frac{\ln(K_e/K_a)}{K_e - K_a} \tag{29.7}$$

Summary of calculations

1. Use values of C_p for several times *after the time of peak concentration* to determine K_e. This may be accomplished by linear regression of $\ln(C_p)$ against t for the last few points and extrapolating as in Figure 29.2. (If C_p is plotted on a logarithmically calibrated scale, the extrapolated values C_p' are read directly). Values of C_p' for all times at which C_p is known are determined.
2. At each time (beginning with time = 0) determine $(C_p' - C_p)$ and $\ln(C_p' - C_p)$. Plot the latter against time and read the slope which is $-K_a$; equivalently, linear regression of $\ln(C_p' - C_p)$ vs. time may be used.
3. With K_a, K_e, and D known, it remains only to determine the ratio F/V_d (unless these have been determined from other studies). For this purpose, we use Equations (29.5) and (29.6).
4. The model equation for plasma concentration is obtained by substitution of the calculated values in Equation (29.1).

Example

An oral dose of lithium carbonate equivalent to 16.2 mMol of lithium was administered orally to volunteers and resulted in the following mean plasma concentrations C_p at times t after administration.

t(hrs.)	0	1	2	3	4	12	24	48	72
C_p(mMol/L)	0	0.08	0.13	0.18	0.26	0.19	0.12	0.05	0.02

Solutions

Values of $\ln(C_p)$ and t for $t = 12, 24, 48$, and 72, were used in regression analysis and yielded slope $= -K_e = -0.0373$ and intercept $= -1.2$ (whose antilog $= 0.301$) so that $C' = 0.301 \exp(-0.0373t)$. From this equation the values for C' corresponding to all measured times were calculated. These are listed in the following table. Also listed are $(C' - C)$ and $\ln(C' - C)$.

time (hrs)	0	1	2	3	4	12	24	48	72
C (mM/L)	0	0.08	0.13	0.18	0.26	0.19	0.12	0.05	0.02
C'	0.301	0.29	0.28	0.27	0.26	0.19	0.12	0.05	0.02
$C' - C$	0.301	0.21	0.15	0.09	0	0	0	0	0
$\ln(C' - C)$	-1.20	-1.56	-1.90	-2.4					

Regression analysis applied to $\ln(C' - C)$ against time yields slope $= -0.40$, so that $K_a = 0.40 \, \text{hr}^{-1}$. Thus the time of peak concentration t^* is computed from (29.7):

$$t^* = \frac{\ln(K_e/K_a)}{K_e - K_a} = \frac{\ln(0.093)}{0.0373 - 0.4}$$

$$= 6.5 \, \text{hr.}$$

The trapezoidal rule, applied to the area (A) between $t = 0$ and $t = 72$ hrs yielded: $A = 7.06$. Also, $C_p(72) = 0.02$. so that $(\text{AUC})_0^\infty = 7.06 + 0.02/0.0373 = 7.60$. From Equation (29.5)

$$F/V_d = \frac{(7.60)(0.0373)}{16.2}$$

$$= 0.0175 \, \text{L}^{-1}.$$

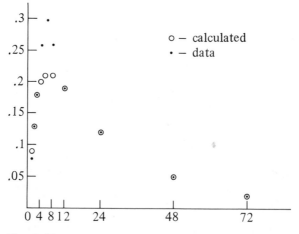

Figure 29.4

With all parameters determined substitution in Equation (29.1) yields

$$C_p = 0.313(e^{-0.0373t} - e^{-0.40t}). \qquad (29.8)$$

The function given by Equation (29.8) is graphed along with the data in Figure 29.4.

Computer Screen

```
        <29> Pharmacokinetics IV: Plasma Concentration-Time Data
        Pharmacologic Calculation System - Version 4.0 - 03/11/86

Input: <K>eyboard, <D>isk, or <E>xit this procedure? D

File name: ? LINE1<ENTER>

Data: <E>dit, <L>ist, <S>ave, or <ENTER> to continue? L

    File name:          LINE1
    Variable:           time              Cp
   -------------   --------------   --------------
       # 1:              0                 0
       # 2:              1                .08
       # 3:              2                .13
       # 4:              3                .18
       # 5:              4                .26
       # 6:             12                .19
       # 7:             24                .12
       # 8:             48                .05
       # 9:             72                .02

Data: <E>dit, <L>ist, <S>ave, or <ENTER> to continue? <ENTER>
```

```
Enter amount of single oral dose given? 16.2<ENTER>

Single oral dose = 16.2

The greatest Cp measured is .26 and occurs at time = 4.

How many periods after peak time do you want to begin analysis of Ke
(default=1) ? <ENTER>

Ke analysis begins at t = 12

      ln(Cp) = -.0373892 * time -1.21401

<ENTER> to continue or <L>ist values calculated from regression line? <ENTER>


      Ke =  .0373892

      Cp' =  .297004 exp(-.0373892 time)

  ln(Cp'-Cp) = -.408351 * time -1.18237

<ENTER> to continue or <L>ist values calculated from regression line? <ENTER>
```

```
      Ka =  .408351            Tp = 6.44472

A.U.C.(Trapezoidal approximation) = 7.06

A.U.C.(t = 72 to infinity) = .534914

   Total A.U.C. =  7.59492          F/Vd =  .0175289

Cp = .312589 x (exp(-.0373892t) - exp(-.408351t) )
```

Computer Report

```
                      <29> Pharmacokinetics IV: Plasma Concentration-Time Data
                    Pharmacologic Calculation System - Version 4.0 - 03/11/86
```

File name: Variable:	LINE1 time	Cp
# 1:	0	0
# 2:	1	.08
# 3:	2	.13
# 4:	3	.18
# 5:	4	.26
# 6:	12	.19
# 7:	24	.12
# 8:	48	.05
# 9:	72	.02

Single oral dose = 16.2

The greatest Cp measured is .26 and occurs at time = 4.

Ke analysis begins at t = 12

$$\ln(Cp) = -.0373892 * time -1.21401$$

$$Ke = .0373892$$

$$Cp' = .297004 \exp(-.0373892 \; time)$$

$$\ln(Cp'-Cp) = -.408351 * time -1.18237$$

$$Ka = .408351 \qquad Tp = 6.44472$$

A.U.C.(Trapezoidal approximation) = 7.06

A.U.C.(t = 72 to infinity) = .534914

Total A.U.C. = 7.59492   F/Vd = .0175289

$$Cp = .312589 \times (\exp(-.0373892t) - \exp(-.408351t))$$

Procedure 30

Pharmacokinetics V: Renal Clearance

Method A

The calculation of renal clearance is made from determinations of the amount of unchanged drug excreted over a time interval (t_1 to t_2) and samples of the plasma concentration of the unchanged drug over the time interval t_1 to t_2. The renal clearance, Cl_r, is given by the equation

$$Cl_r = [\text{amount excreted}]_{t_1}^{t_2} \bigg/ \int_{t_1}^{t_2} C_p \, dt, \qquad (30.1)$$

where C_p is the concentration in plasma of the unchanged drug in the time interval. In the event that plasma concentrations are determined at only the two times, t_1 and t_2, the integral is approximated by $\frac{1}{2}(C_{t_1} + C_{t_2})(t_2 - t_1)$. If plasma concentrations are made at intermediate times the trapezoidal rule (Procedure 25) may be used to evaluate the integral. The above calculation does not depend on the route of administration.

(*Note*: The time interval t_1 to t_2 may be 0 to ∞ in which case the integral is the *total* area under the plasma concentration-time curve. See discussion in Procedure 28).

Method B

The renal excretion rate of unchanged drug, dU/dt, and the plasma concentration C_p are used in the calculation of renal clearance Cl_r:

$$Cl_r = \frac{dU/dt}{C_p} \qquad (30.2)$$

In practice urine concentrations are determined at times (following administration) $t_1, t_2, \ldots, t_n$, and the derivative is approximated by $(U_i - U_{i-1})/(t_i - t_{i-1})$, where $i = 1$ to n, and $t_0 = 0$. The concentration in plasma C_p is that determined at the midpoint of each time interval, that is, $t_1/2, (t_1 + t_2)/2, \ldots, (t_{n-1} + t_n)/2$. A plot of the derivative against concentration at midpoint time is linear through the origin with slope equal to the renal clearance. The least squares criteria constrained through the origin may be used to evaluate the slope.

Example 1

A drug is administered subcutaneously and both urine and plasma samples are taken at time $t = 1, 2, 3,$ and 4 hours after dosing. The amounts of unchanged drug in urine samples at the above times are 14, 7, 3 and 1.5 mg, respectively. The plasma concentration (mg/liter) were as shown in the table below:

time	0	1	2	3	4
concentration	0	0.65	0.24	0.14	0.07

From these, the renal clearance is

$$\frac{(14 + 7 + 3 + 1.5)}{\int_0^4 C_p \, dt}.$$

The integral is estimated from the trapezoidal rule (Procedure 25) and is $1/2(1)[0 + (2)(0.65) + 2(0.24) + 2(0.14) + 0.07] = 1.06$ mg./L hr. Thus,

$$Cl_r = \frac{25.5 \text{ mg}}{1.06 \frac{\text{mg}}{\text{L}} \text{hr}} = 23.9 \text{ L/hr}$$

Computer Screen

```
                    <30> Pharmacokinetics V: Renal Clearance
              Pharmacologic Calculation System - Version 4.0 - 03/11/86

  Two methods are available.

  Method A requires plasma concentration of drug (mg/1), and amount of drug in
  urine (mg) over several time periods (hr).

  Method B requires amount of drug in urine (mg) over several time periods (hr)
  and the plasma concentration of drug (mg/1) obtained at the midpoints of each
  collection interval.

  Enter method <A> or <B> ? A

  Input: <K>eyboard, <D>isk, or <E>xit this procedure? D

  File name: ? EXAMPLE1<ENTER>

  Data: <E>dit, <L>ist, <S>ave, or <ENTER> to continue? L

        File name:      EXAMPLE1
        Variable:      Time (hr)      Cp (mg/1)    Amount (mg)
      --------------  -------------- ------------- --------------
           # 1:            0              0              0
           # 2:            1             .65            14
           # 3:            2             .24             7
           # 4:            3             .14             3
           # 5:            4             .07            1.5
```

```
  Data: <E>dit, <L>ist, <S>ave, or <ENTER> to continue? <ENTER>

  Method A:

  Integral of Cp over time = 1.065 (mg x hr)/liter

  Total amount collected in urine = 25.5 mg

  Renal clearance = 23.9437 liters/hr

  Report: <P>rint, <S>ave, or <V>iew? <ENTER>
```

Computer Report

```
                    <30> Pharmacokinetics V: Renal Clearance
              Pharmacologic Calculation System - Version 4.0 - 03/11/86

        File name:      EXAMPLE1
        Variable:      Time (hr)      Cp (mg/1)    Amount (mg)
      --------------  -------------- ------------- --------------
           # 1:            0              0              0
           # 2:            1             .65            14
           # 3:            2             .24             7
           # 4:            3             .14             3
           # 5:            4             .07            1.5

  Method A:

  Integral of Cp over time = 1.065 (mg x hr)/liter

  Total amount collected in urine = 25.5 mg

  Renal clearance = 23.9437 liters/hr
```

Example 2

An antibiotic is administered and the unchanged amount is determined in urine collected at time 2, 4, 6 and 8 hours after administration. Plasma concentrations, obtained at the midpoint of each collection interval (1, 3, 5, and 7 hours), were also obtained. The values are given in the table below:

	time interval (hr.)	0–2	2–4	4–6	6–8
	amoung (mg)	19.0	12.4	10.0	4.8
(calculated)	excretion rate (mg/hr.)	9.5	6.2	5.0	2.4
	plasma conc. (at mid-pt.)(mg/l)	1.6	1.2	1.0	0.47

A regression line (through the origin) of excretion rate against plasma concentration yields the renal clearance from the slope of the line. Applying Procedure 4 gives 5.52 for the renal clearance as shown below:

$$\text{slope} = \text{clearance} = \frac{(0.47)(2.4) + (1.0)(5.0) + (1.2)(6.2) + (1.6)(9.5)}{(0.47)^2 + (1.0)^2 + (1.2)^2 + (1.6)^2}$$

$$= 5.52 \text{ l/hr.}$$

Computer Screen

```
              <30> Pharmacokinetics V: Renal Clearance
         Pharmacologic Calculation System - Version 4.0 - 03/11/86

Two methods are available.

Method A requires plasma concentration of drug (mg/l), and amount of drug in
urine (mg) over several time periods (hr).

Method B requires amount of drug in urine (mg) over several time periods (hr)
and the plasma concentration of drug (mg/l) obtained at the midpoints of each
collection interval.

Enter method <A> or <B> ? B

Input: <K>eyboard, <D>isk, or <E>xit this procedure? K


Type 'END' after last file. Enter file name or <ENTER> for default name:
'FILE1/XYZ' (or 'END') ? EXAMPLE2<ENTER>

You may enter up to 15 x,y,z data sets. Press <ENTER> after the last entry.
     File name:      EXAMPLE2
     Variable:     Time (hr)      Cp (mg/l)     Amount (mg)
   ------------   -----------   -----------   -------------
     # 1: 2<ENTER>      1.6<ENTER>      19<ENTER>
     # 2: 4<ENTER>      1.2<ENTER>      12.4<ENTER>
     # 3: 6<ENTER>      1<ENTER>        10<ENTER>
     # 4: 8<ENTER>      .47<ENTER>      4.8<ENTER>
     # 5: <ENTER>
```

```
Data: <E>dit, <L>ist, <S>ave, or <ENTER> to continue? L

   File name:      EXAMPLE2
   Variable:       Time (hr)    Cp (mg/l)   Amount (mg)
------------   -------------  -----------  -------------
     # 1:             2           1.6            19
     # 2:             4           1.2          12.4
     # 3:             6            1             10
     # 4:             8           .47           4.8

Data: <E>dit, <L>ist, <S>ave, or <ENTER> to continue? <ENTER>

Method B:

   File name:      EXAMPLE2
   Variable:       Cp (mg/l)   Rate (mg/hr)
------------   -------------  -------------
     # 1:           1.6           9.5
     # 2:           1.2           6.2
     # 3:            1             5
     # 4:           .47           2.4
```

```
Rate (mg/hr) =  5.51016 * Cp (mg/l)

<ENTER> to continue or <L>ist values calculated from regression line? <ENTER>


Renal clearance = 5.51016 liters/hr


Report: <P>rint, <S>ave, or <V>iew? <ENTER>
```

Computer Report

```
                        <30> Pharmacokinetics V: Renal Clearance
                Pharmacologic Calculation System - Version 4.0 - 03/11/86

   File name:      EXAMPLE2
   Variable:       Time (hr)    Cp (mg/l)   Amount (mg)
------------   -------------  -----------  -------------
     # 1:             2           1.6            19
     # 2:             4           1.2          12.4
     # 3:             6            1             10
     # 4:             8           .47           4.8

Method B:

   File name:      EXAMPLE2
   Variable:       Cp (mg/l)   Rate (mg/hr)
------------   -------------  -------------
     # 1:           1.6           9.5
     # 2:           1.2           6.2
     # 3:            1             5
     # 4:           .47           2.4

Rate (mg/hr) =  5.51016 * Cp (mg/l)

Renal clearance = 5.51016 liters/hr
```

Procedure 31

Pharmacokinetics VI: Renal Excretion Data Following Intravenous Administration

Following intravenous administration, the amount of *unchanged* drug excreted in the urine is determined from urine samples obtained at times $t_i(i = 1$ to $N)$ after administration at time 0. The excretion rate dU/dt is given by the equation

$$dU/dt = k_r D e^{-k_e t}, \tag{31.1}$$

where D is the dose, t is the time, and k_r and k_e are rate constants for renal excretion and total elimination, respectively. (A rate constant is a fraction per unit time.) Taking logarithms (base e) of Equation (31.1), we get

$$\ln(dU/dt) = \ln(k_r \cdot D) - k_e t. \tag{31.2}$$

The logarithm of the excretion rate is a linear function of the time, with slope $-k_e$ and (vertical) intercept $= \ln(k_r \cdot D)$. Since the dose D is known, both k_e and k_r may be determined. In practice, urine is collected at times $t_1, t_2, \ldots, t_n$, yielding amounts of unchanged drug $U_1, U_2, \ldots, U_n$, respectively, so that dU/dt may be approximated by values U_1/t_1, $U_2/(t_2 - t_1)$, $U_3/(t_3 - t_2)$, etc. Also, the logarithms of these are plotted against the midpoint of the collection time interval. These midpoints are $t_1/2$, $(t_2 + t_1)/2$, $(t_3 + t_2)/2$, etc. Linear regression (Procedure 3 or 5) is used to obtain the slope and intercept and, hence, the values of k_e and k_r. If the apparent volume of distribution V_d is also known, then the renal clearance (Cl_r) can be calculated from

$$Cl_r = k_r \cdot V_d. \tag{31.3}$$

Note: An alternative method, using accumulated drug in the urine is sometimes used. Following intravenous administration the amount of *unchanged* drug in the urine is collected at various times and summed. That is, at time t_i, *the total accumulated drug* up to that time is determined and denoted $U(t_i)$. After a sufficiently long time $U(t)$ will be a constant (U_∞), meaning that the excretion of unchanged drug is complete. It may be shown that the following model equation applies:

$$U(t_i) = U_\infty(1 - e^{-k_e t_i}).$$

Thus,

$$U_\infty - U(t_i) = U_\infty e^{-k_e t_i},$$

or

$$\ln(U_\infty - U(t_i)) = -k_e t_i + \ln(U_\infty),$$

yielding a straight-line plot when $\ln(U_\infty - U(t_i))$ is plotted against time t_i. This method is more difficult to use and is not recommended for routine use by non-specialists. Accordingly, computer programs are not included for this alternate method.

Example

A drug was given as an intravenous bolus (100 mg) and urine samples were collected at times t_i after administration. These samples yielded urine volumes and *unchanged* drug concentration as given in the table below. The table also contains the midpoint time of the collection interval (calculated from the collection times), the amount excreted during the collection interval (calculated from the data), the approximate values of dU/dt and the logarithms of these.

time (hr)	1	2	4	6	10	14
volume of urine (ml)	80	120	130	200	340	300
concentration (mg/l)	250	125	77	32.5	7.9	3.67
(calculated) midpoint time (hr)	0.5	1.5	3	5	8	12
(calculated) amount excreted (mg)	20	15	10	6.5	2.7	1.1
(calculated) dU/dt (mg/hr)	20	15	5	3.25	0.675	0.275
(calculated) $\ln(dU/dt)$	2.99	2.71	1.61	1.18	−0.39	−1.29

A linear regression (Procedure 5) of $\ln(dU/dt)$ against midpoint time gave slope $= -0.385$ and intercept $= 3.06$. Thus $k_e = 0.385$ and $\ln(k_r D) = 3.06$ so that $k_r = 0.213$. (It is noteworthy that the amount excreted as unchanged drug at the end of 14 hrs is approximately 55 mg, much less than the 100 mg administered. Hence, there is appreciable metabolism of this drug.

Computer Screen

```
<31> Pharmacokinetics VI: Renal Excretion Data Following I.V. Administration
          Pharmacologic Calculation System - Version 4.0 - 03/12/86

Enter the dose of drug administered intravenously (mg) ? 100<ENTER>

Enter the collection time (hr), volume of urine collected, and the
concentration of drug in the urine.

Input: <K>eyboard, <D>isk, or <E>xit this procedure? D

File name: ? EXAMPLE<ENTER>

Data: <E>dit, <L>ist, <S>ave, or <ENTER> to continue? L

      File name:        EXAMPLE
      Variable:       Time (hr)  Volume (ml)  Conc.(mg/l)
    -----------     -----------  -----------  -----------
        # 1:             1            80          250
        # 2:             2           120          125
        # 3:             4           130           77
        # 4:             6           200         32.5
        # 5:            10           340          7.9
        # 6:            14           300         3.67
```

```
Data: <E>dit, <L>ist, <S>ave, or <ENTER> to continue? <ENTER>

   File name:      EXAMPLE
   Variable:           t     ln(dU/dt)          dU/dt
 -------------  -----------  -------------  -------------
     # 1:            .5       2.99573             20
     # 2:           1.5       2.70805             15
     # 3:            3        1.61044          5.005
     # 4:            5        1.17866          3.25
     # 5:            8        -.398241          .6715
     # 6:           12       -1.29008           .27525


   ln(dU/dt) = -.385239 * t + 3.06029

 <ENTER> to continue or <L>ist values calculated from regression line? <ENTER>

 Dose of drug given i.v. (mg) = 100

 Drug excreted at the end of 14 hours (mg) = 55.297

 Ke = .385239          Kr = .213337


 Report: <P>rint, <S>ave, or <V>iew? <ENTER>
```

Computer Report

```
<31> Pharmacokinetics VI: Renal Excretion Data Following I.V. Administration
        Pharmacologic Calculation System - Version 4.0 - 03/12/86

   File name:      EXAMPLE
   Variable:    Time (hr)   Volume (ml)   Conc.(mg/l)
 -------------  -----------  -------------  -------------
     # 1:           1            80            250
     # 2:           2           120            125
     # 3:           4           130             77
     # 4:           6           200           32.5
     # 5:          10           340            7.9
     # 6:          14           300           3.67

   File name:      EXAMPLE
   Variable:           t     ln(dU/dt)          dU/dt
 -------------  -----------  -------------  -------------
     # 1:            .5       2.99573             20
     # 2:           1.5       2.70805             15
     # 3:            3        1.61044          5.005
     # 4:            5        1.17866          3.25
     # 5:            8        -.398241          .6715
     # 6:           12       -1.29008           .27525


 ln(dU/dt) = -.385239 * t + 3.06029

 Dose of drug given i.v. (mg) = 100

 Drug excreted at the end of 14 hours (mg) = 55.297

 Ke = .385239          Kr = .213337
```

Procedure 32

Pharmacokinetics VII: Multiple Dosing from Absorptive Site

When a drug that is eliminated exponentially is administered via an absorptive route in equal doses D at equal time intervals T, the plasma concentration will fluctuate (Figure 32.1). The mean concentration approaches an upper limit.

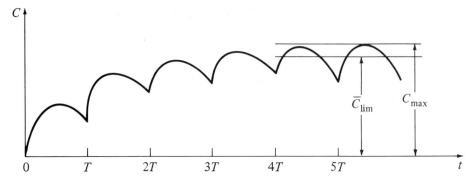

Figure 32.1   Drug concentration (C) with administration of the same dose at equal time intervals (T) using an absorptive route. The mean concentration, after a sufficiently long time, is denoted $\bar{C}_{\text{lim}}$, whereas the peaks approach the limit C_{max}. (See text.)

When the absorptive rate constant is unknown the calculation of this limit is very approximate. This case is considered first. For this we need the fractional absorption F, and either the clearance, Cl, or both the volume of distribution and half-life. We denote the dose by D and the time interval by T; then $\bar{C}_{\text{lim}}$ is given by

$$\bar{C}_{\text{lim}} = \frac{F \cdot D}{T \cdot Cl}. \tag{32.1}$$

Clearance is related to volume of distribution V_d and half-life $t_{1/2}$ according to

$$Cl = \ln 2 \cdot V_d/t_{1/2} \approx 0.693 V_d/t_{1/2} \tag{32.2}$$

Thus $\bar{C}_{\text{lim}}$ may be expressed

$$\bar{C}_{\text{lim}} = \frac{1 \cdot 44 F \cdot D \cdot t_{1/2}}{T \cdot V_d}. \tag{32.3}$$

The time to attain 95% $\bar{C}_{\text{lim}}$ is given by

$$t_{95} = 4.3 t_{1/2}. \tag{32.4}$$

When the elimination rate constant (k) is known, the half-life is computed as $\ln(2)/k$.

When the absorptive rate constant α is known, as in the two-compartment model of Figure 32.2, the concentration as a function of time is computed, and

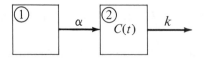

Figure 32.2   Two-compartment model. Drug is absorbed from compartment (1) with rate constant α and is eliminated from plasma (compartment (2)) with rate constant k.

both the mean and peak values are also determinable. For convenience we denote by $C(t)$ the concentrations in the first time interval $0 < t < T$:

$$C(t) = \frac{\alpha DF}{V_d(k - \alpha)} [e^{-\alpha t} - e^{-kt}] \qquad (32.5)$$

In this equation α is the fractional absorption per unit time (absorptive rate constant) and is *different from k*. Further, it is convenient to define constants A and g:

$$A = C(T) \qquad (32.6)$$

$$g = e^{-kT} \qquad (32.7)$$

Then, for subsequent intervals we have:

$$C(T + t) = C(t) + Ae^{-kt}$$

$$C(2T + t) = C(t) + A(1 + g)e^{-kt}$$

$$C(3T + t) = C(t) + A(1 + g + g^2)e^{-kt}$$

$$\vdots$$

etc.

After a sufficiently long time the progression $(1 + g + g^2 + \cdots)$ approaches a limit $1/(1 - g)$. Hence, the concentration limit is

$$C(t)_{\lim} = C(t) + \frac{A}{1 - g} e^{-kt} \qquad (32.8)$$

The mean value is

$$\bar{C}_{\lim} = \frac{\alpha DF}{V_d(k - \alpha)} \cdot \frac{1}{T} \left\{ \frac{1}{\alpha} (1 - e^{-\alpha T}) - \frac{1}{k} (1 - e^{-kT}) \right\} + \frac{A}{Tk} \qquad (32.9)$$

For $\alpha \gg k$ the mean is approximately*

$$\bar{C}_{\lim} \doteq \frac{FD}{V_d Tk} (1 - e^{-\alpha T}) \qquad (32.10)$$

The upper limit for the peaks is calculated from

$$C_{\max} = M(e^{-\alpha t_c} - e^{-kt_c}) + Se^{-kt_c}, \qquad (32.11)$$

where

$$M = \alpha DF/V_d(k - \alpha), \qquad (32.12)$$

$$S = A/(1 - g), \qquad (32.13)$$

and

$$t_c = \frac{1}{k - \alpha} \log_e \left[\frac{k(M - S)}{\alpha M} \right]. \qquad (32.14)$$

* Comparison with Equation (32.3) shows that they agree when $e^{-\alpha T}$ is negligible.

Example 1

A drug that is completely absorbed ($F = 1$) with oral administration is given in amount 200 mg every four hours. The clearance is 3.01 L/hr. and the elimination half-life is 8 hrs. It is desired to find the limiting concentration and the time to achieve 95% of this value. From Equation (32.1)

$$\bar{C}_{\lim} = \frac{(1)(200)}{(4)(3.0)} = 16.7 \text{ mg/l.}$$

The time to attain 95% of the limit is $4.3 \times 8 = 34$ hours.

Computer Screen

```
     <32> Pharmacokinetics VII: Multiple Dosing from Absorptive Site
           Pharmacologic Calculation System - Version 4.0 - 03/12/86

Enter the following required data (enter t1/2 or Ke):

Dose of drug (mg) ...................... ? 200<ENTER>
Dosing interval (hrs) .................. ? 4<ENTER>
Elimination half-time, t1/2 ........... ? 8<ENTER>

Enter the following data, or press <ENTER> if value is unknown:

Fractional absorption .................. 1? <ENTER>
Apparent volume of distribution (1) ..... ? <ENTER>
Clearance rate (1/hr) .................. 0? 3.0<ENTER>
Absorption rate constant (1/hr), Ka ..... ? <ENTER>

Results:

Dose of drug (mg) ...................... = 200
Dosing interval (hrs) .................. = 4
Elimination half-time, t1/2 ........... = 8
Fractional absorption .................. = 1
Elimination rate constant (1/hr), Ke .... = .0866434
Apparent volume of distribution (1) ..... = 34.6247
Clearance rate (1/hr) .................. = 3
Time to reach 95% of Cm (hr) ........... = 34.5754

Mean limiting concentration (Cm, mg/1) .. = 16.6667 approx.

Report: <P>rint, <S>ave, or <V>iew? <ENTER>
```

Computer Report

```
     <32> Pharmacokinetics VII: Multiple Dosing from Absorptive Site
           Pharmacologic Calculation System - Version 4.0 - 03/12/86

Dose of drug (mg) ...................... = 200
Dosing interval (hrs) .................. = 4
Elimination half-time, t1/2 ........... = 8
Fractional absorption .................. = 1
Elimination rate constant (1/hr), Ke .... = .0866434
Apparent volume of distribution (1) ..... = 34.6247
Clearance rate (1/hr) .................. = 3
Time to reach 95% of Cm (hr) ........... = 34.5754

Mean limiting concentration (Cm, mg/1) .. = 16.6667 approx.
```

A more precise calculation of concentrations requires knowledge of α. If, for example, $\alpha = 1$, then we use Equation (32.10) with the value of V_d determined from Equation (32.2) as $V_d = t_{1/2} \cdot Cl/0.693 = 34.6$, from which $\bar{C}_{\lim} = 16.4$ mg/l. Substitution into Equations (31.11)–(31.14) yields

$$M = -6.33, S = 14.89, t_c = 1.35 \text{ and } C_{\max} = 17.24.$$

Example 2

A drug that is completely absorbed from the gastrointestinal tract has an absorptive rate constant $= 0.5$ and an elimination rate constant $= 0.02$. The drug has a volume of distribution of 5 liters and is given in a dose of 10 mg every six hours.

Thus, $D = 10$, $\alpha = 0.5$, $k = 0.02$, $F = 1$, $V_d = 5$ and $T = 6$, from which it follows that $M = -2.1$, $A = 1.7$ and $S = 15.4$. Hence,

$$t_c = \frac{1}{0.02 - 0.5} \log_e \left[\frac{(0.02)(-2.1 - 15.4)}{(0.5)(-2.1)} \right] = 2.27$$

$$\bar{C}_{\lim} = \frac{(1)(10)}{(5)(6)(0.02)} (1 - e^{-(0.5)(6)}) = 15.8 \text{ mg/l.}$$

$$C_{\max} = (-2.1)[e^{-(0.5)(2.27)} - e^{-(0.02)(2.27)}] + 15.4 e^{-(0.02)(2.27)}$$

$$= 16.1 \text{ mg/l.}$$

(It is noteworthy that the use of Equation (32.3) gives $\bar{C}_{\lim} = 16.7$.)

Computer Screen

```
        <32> Pharmacokinetics VII: Multiple Dosing from Absorptive Site
            Pharmacologic Calculation System - Version 4.0 - 03/12/86

Enter the following required data (enter t1/2 or Ke):

Dose of drug (mg) ...................... ? 10<ENTER>
Dosing interval (hrs) .................. ? 6<ENTER>
Elimination half-time, t1/2 ............ ? <ENTER>
Elimination rate constant (1/hr), Ke .... ? .02<ENTER>

Enter the following data, or press <ENTER> if value is unknown:

Fractional absorption .................. 1? <ENTER>
Apparent volume of distribution (l) ..... ? 5<ENTER>
Clearance rate (1/hr) .................. .1? <ENTER>
Absorption rate constant (1/hr), Ka ..... ? 0.5<ENTER>

Results:
```

```
Dose of drug (mg) ...................... = 10
Dosing interval (hrs) .................. = 6
Elimination half-time, t1/2 ............ = 34.6574
Fractional absorption .................. = 1
Absorption rate constant (1/hr), Ka ..... = .5
Elimination rate constant (1/hr), Ke .... = .02
Apparent volume of distribution (l) ..... = 5
Clearance rate (1/hr) .................. = .1
Time to reach 95% of Cm (hr) ........... = 149.787

Mean limiting concentration (Cm, mg/l) .. = 15.8369

Maximum plasma concentration (Cmax, mg/l) = 16.0597

Report: <P>rint, <S>ave, or <V>iew? <ENTER>
```

Computer Report

```
            <32> Pharmacokinetics VII: Multiple Dosing from Absorptive Site
               Pharmacologic Calculation System - Version 4.0 - 03/12/86

      Dose of drug (mg) ........................ = 10
      Dosing interval (hrs) .................... = 6
      Elimination half-time, t1/2 ............. = 34.6574
      Fractional absorption ................... = 1
      Absorption rate constant (1/hr), Ka ..... = .5
      Elimination rate constant (1/hr), Ke .... = .02
      Apparent volume of distribution (l) ..... = 5
      Clearance rate (1/hr) ................... = .1
      Time to reach 95% of Cm (hr) ........... = 149.787

      Mean limiting concentration (Cm, mg/l) .. = 15.8369

      Maximum plasma concentration (Cmax, mg/l) = 16.0597
```

Procedure 33

Analysis of Variance I: One-Way

The method known as analysis of variance considers the problem of determining whether, among a set of three or more samples, there are means that differ significantly. We let k denote the number of samples. Sample 1 contains n_1 variates denoted $A_{11}, A_{21}, \ldots, A_{n_1 1}$. Sample 2 contains n_2 variates denoted A_{12}, $A_{22}, \ldots, A_{n_2 2}$, and so on, as seen in Table 33.1. In a sense, this method is a generalization of the test which is used to determine whether the means of two given samples differ significantly.

Table 33.1
Arrangement of data for k samples with unequal sample sizes, $n_1, n_2, \ldots, n_k$

	1st sample	2nd sample		kth sample
	A_{11}	A_{12}	$\cdots$	A_{1k}
	A_{21}	A_{22}	$\cdots$	A_{2k}
	$\vdots$	$\vdots$		$\vdots$
	$A_{n_1 1}$	$A_{n_2 2}$	$\cdots$	$A_{n_k k}$
Totals	T_1	T_2	$\cdots$	T_k
Mean	$\bar{A}_1$	$\bar{A}_2$	$\cdots$	$\bar{A}_k$

Grand total $= T$
Grand mean $= \bar{A}$

From the sample values A_{ij} we determine the total and the mean for each sample and the mean of all means, called the grand mean $\bar{A}$. The *total* sum of squares, S.S., is the sum of the squared differences of each variate from the grand mean $\bar{A}$. Thus, S.S. is given by

$$\text{S.S.} = (A_{11} - \bar{A})^2 + (A_{21} - \bar{A})^2 + \cdots + (A_{n_k k} - \bar{A})^2, \qquad (33.1)$$

An alternate form, more suitable for calculation, will be given subsequently. Also, we define the *between means* sum of squares, denoted S.S.T., by the relation

$$\text{S.S.T.} = n_1(\bar{A}_1 - \bar{A})^2 + n_2(\bar{A}_2 - \bar{A})^2 + \cdots + n_k(\bar{A}_k - \bar{A})^2 \qquad (33.2)$$

and the *within-samples* sum of squares, S.S.E., by the relation

$$\text{S.S.E.} = \sum_1^{n_1} (A_{i1} - \bar{A}_1)^2 + \sum_1^{n_2} (A_{i2} - \bar{A}_2)^2 + \cdots + \sum_1^{n_k} (A_{ik} - \bar{A}_k)^2. \qquad (33.3)$$

More useful computing forms of these quantities are given below:

$$\text{S.S.} = \sum_1^{n_1} A_{i1}^2 + \sum_1^{n_2} A_{i2}^2 + \cdots + \sum_1^{n_k} A_{ik}^2 - \frac{T^2}{n_1 + n_2 + \cdots + n_k} \qquad (33.4)$$

$$\text{S.S.T.} = \frac{T_1^2}{n_1} + \frac{T_2^2}{n_2} + \cdots + \frac{T_k^2}{n_k} - \frac{T^2}{n_1 + n_2 + \cdots + n_k} \qquad (33.5)$$

$$\text{S.S.E.} = \sum_1^{n_1} A_{i1}^2 + \sum_1^{n_2} A_{i2}^2 + \cdots + \sum_1^{n_k} A_{ik}^2 - \left(\frac{T_1^2}{n_1} + \frac{T_2^2}{n_2} + \cdots + \frac{T_k^2}{n_k} \right). \qquad (33.6)$$

It may be shown that the total sum of squares for the set of variates is the sum of the between-means sum of squares and the within-samples sum of squares:

$$\text{S.S.} = \text{S.S.T.} + \text{S.S.E.} \qquad (33.7)$$

The partitioning of S.S. into S.S.E. and S.S.T. is useful in that these provide two estimates of the population variance σ^2. These estimates are denoted by s_p and s_t, where

$$s_p^2 = \text{S.S.E.}/(n_1 + n_2 + \cdots + n_k - k)$$

and

$$s_t^2 = \text{S.S.T.}/(k - 1).$$

The ratio s_t^2/s_p^2 satisfies the F-distribution, where

$$F = s_t^2/s_p^2, \qquad (33.8)$$

with degrees of freedom $v_1 = k - 1$ and $v_2 = n_1 + n_2 + \cdots + n_k - k$.

The value of F obtained from Equation (33.8) is compared with the tabular value (Table A.11) at the specified level of significance (usually 95%). If the computed F exceeds the tabular value, then there is at least one pair of samples whose means differ significantly.

The calculations are usually summarized in an *analysis of variance table*, as shown in Table 33.2.

Tabular value of the F-distribution are read by noting the degrees of freedom for the numerator $(k - 1)$ across the top and the degrees of freedom for the denominator $(n_1 + n_2 + \cdots + n_2 - k)$ down the side as shown in Table A.11.

Table 33.2
Analysis of Variance

Source of variation	Sum of squares	Degrees of freedom	Mean square	F
Total	S.S.	$n_1 + n_2 + \cdots + n_k - 1$		
Between means	S.S.T.	$(k - 1)$	$s_t^2 = \dfrac{\text{S.S.T.}}{k - 1}$	$\dfrac{s_t^2}{s_p^2}$
Within samples	S.S.E.	$(n_1 + n_2 + \cdots + n_k - k)$ $s_p^2 = \dfrac{\text{S.S.E.}}{n_1 + n_2 + \cdots + n_k - k}$		

Example

The values for four samples are given below. Compute F.

	12	12	9	12
	10	16	7	8
	7	15	6	8
	8	9	11	10
	9		7	
	14			
T	60	52	40	38
Mean	10.0	13.0	8.0	9.5

S.S. $= 148$

S.S.T. $= 57$ d.f. $= k - 1 = 3$ (across)

S.S.E. $= 91$ d.f. $= \sum_{i=1}^{k} n_i - k = 19 - 4 = 15$ (down side)

$s_t^2 = 19$; $s_p^2 = 6.07$; $F = 3.13$; $F_{0.95} = 3.29$ (Table A.11).

Since the computed F is less than the tabular value, we cannot conclude that the means differ significantly.

Computer Screen

```
                      <33> Analysis of Variance I: One-way
              Pharmacologic Calculation System - Version 4.0 - 03/12/86

Do you want to show intermediate results (Y/N) ? Y

Input: <K>eyboard, <D>isk, or <E>xit this procedure? D

You may enter 5 'Y' data files. Press <ENTER> after last file name.
File name 1 ? GROUP1<ENTER>
File name 2 ? GROUP2<ENTER>
File name 3 ? GROUP3<ENTER>
File name 4 ? GROUP4<ENTER>
File name 5 ? <ENTER>

Data: <E>dit, <L>ist, <S>ave, or <ENTER> to continue? L

    File name:        GROUP1         GROUP2         GROUP3         GROUP4
   -----------    -----------    -----------    -----------    -----------
       # 1:           12             12             9             12
       # 2:           10             16             7              8
       # 3:           7              15             6              8
       # 4:           8              9             11             10
       # 5:           9                             7
       # 6:           14
```

```
Data: <E>dit, <L>ist, <S>ave, or <ENTER> to continue? <ENTER>

   File name:        GROUP1         GROUP2         GROUP3         GROUP4
   ----------- -------------- -------------- -------------- --------------
         N:              6              4              5              4
   Minimum:              7              9              6              8
      Mean:             10             13              8            9.5
   Maximum:             14             16             11             12
       Sum:             60             52             40             38
 Std. Dev.:        2.60768        3.16228              2        1.91485
 Std. Err.:        1.06458        1.58114        .894427        .957427
  95% C.L.:         2.73704        5.03118        2.48293        3.04653

   Source of       Sum of        Deg. of         Mean
   Variation       Squares       Freedom        Square        F Value
   ----------- -------------- -------------- -------------- --------------
     Total:            148             18
   Between:             57              3             19           3.13
    Within:             91             15        6.06667

   F (95%):           3.29     F (99%):            5.42

 Differences between means: NOT Significant at p < 0.05


 Report: <P>rint, <S>ave, or <V>iew? <ENTER>
```

Computer Report

```
                          <33> Analysis of Variance I: One-way
                  Pharmacologic Calculation System - Version 4.0 - 03/12/86

   File name:        GROUP1         GROUP2         GROUP3         GROUP4
   ----------- -------------- -------------- -------------- --------------
      # 1:             12             12              9             12
      # 2:             10             16              7              8
      # 3:              7             15              6              8
      # 4:              8              9             11             10
      # 5:              9                             7
      # 6:             14

   File name:        GROUP1         GROUP2         GROUP3         GROUP4
   ----------- -------------- -------------- -------------- --------------
         N:              6              4              5              4
   Minimum:              7              9              6              8
      Mean:             10             13              8            9.5
   Maximum:             14             16             11             12
       Sum:             60             52             40             38
 Std. Dev.:        2.60768        3.16228              2        1.91485
 Std. Err.:        1.06458        1.58114        .894427        .957427
  95% C.L.:         2.73704        5.03118        2.48293        3.04653

   Source of       Sum of        Deg. of         Mean
   Variation       Squares       Freedom        Square        F Value
   ----------- -------------- -------------- -------------- --------------
     Total:            148             18
   Between:             57              3             19           3.13
    Within:             91             15        6.06667

   F (95%):           3.29     F (99%):            5.42

 Differences between means: NOT Significant at p < 0.05
```

Procedure 34

Analysis of Variance II: Two-Way, Single Observation

In analysis of variance it might be necessary or desirable to have a second criterion of classification. For example, in the study of effectiveness of a number of different drug treatments, one can ask different physicians to rate the drugs on

Table 34.1

Blocks	1	2	3	$\cdots$	K	Total
		Treatments				
1	A_{11}	A_{12}	A_{13}	$\cdots$	A_{1K}	T'_1
2	A_{21}					T'_2
$\vdots$	$\vdots$					
N	A_{N1}	A_{N2}		$\cdots$	A_{NK}	T'_N
Total	T_1	T_2		$\cdots$	T_K	T

a numerical scale after examining the patients who receive each. Interest is in examining significant differences between the scores of the drugs as well as on the physicians. In accord with common usage we refer to the drugs as "treatments." The layout of the data is in randomized block styles; thus, the physicians constitute the "blocks." Each combination of block and treatment is called a "cell." The entries within cells are single observations. They might represent mean values based on equal sample size for N blocks and K treatments. (In Procedure 35 we consider replications within each cell).

In the statistical literature it is common to refer to the K values of variable 1 (treatment) as "levels." The second variable (block) would also be said to have N levels.

Column totals are denoted $T_i(i = 1$ to $K)$; row totals are denoted $T'_j(j = 1$ to $N)$. The grand total is denoted T. The notations S.S. and S.S.E. are used as in one-way analysis of variance for total sum of squares and sum of squares for error,* respectively. The *between means sum of squares* is determined for blocks and for treatments, and these are denoted S.S.B. and S.S.T., respectively. Computational formulas are given below. The analysis of variance table is shown in Table 34.2.

Computation

$$C = T^2/(NK)$$

$$\text{S.S.} = (A_{11}^2 + A_{21}^2 + \cdots + A_{NK}^2) - C$$

$$\text{S.S.T.} = \frac{T_1^2 + T_2^2 + \cdots + T_K^2}{N} - C$$

$$\text{S.S.B.} = \frac{T_1'^2 + T_2'^2 + \cdots + T_n'^2}{K} - C$$

$$\text{S.S.E.} = \text{S.S.} - \text{S.S.T.} - \text{S.S.B.}$$

The F-value for treatments is compared with the tabular value for degrees of freedom $v_1 = K - 1$ and $v_2 = (n - 1)(K - 1)$. v_1 is read across and v_2 down in the F-tables.

---

* The term "residual sum of squares" is preferred by many writers.

Table 34.2

Source of variation	Sum of squares	Degrees of freedom	Mean square	F
Total	S.S.	$NK - 1$		
Between means (treatment)	S.S.T.	$K - 1$	$S_t^2 = \dfrac{\text{S.S.T.}}{K - 1}$	S_t^2/S_p^2
Between means (blocks)	S.S.B.	$N - 1$	$S_b^2 = \dfrac{\text{S.S.B.}}{N - 1}$	S_b^2/S_p^2
Within samples	S.S.E.	$(N - 1)(K - 1)$	$S_p^2 = \dfrac{\text{S.S.E.}}{(N - 1)(K - 1)}$	

Example

Four physicians examined groups of patients who received one of five different drug treatments for the same illness and rated the treatments on a scale of 0–10, the former meaning no improvement and the latter the maximum improvement. The mean values are given in the matrix below:

			Treatments			
Blocks	1	2	3	4	5	Total
1	6	7	10	3	5	31
2	7	9	10	4	6	36
3	5	8	9	6	7	35
4	7	8	9	6	6	36
Total	25	32	38	19	24	138

Solution

$$C = \frac{138^2}{20} = 952.2$$

$$\text{S.S.} = 6^2 + 7^2 + \cdots + 7^2 + 6^2 - C = 1022 - 952.2$$

$$= 69.8$$

$$\text{S.S.T.} = \frac{25^2 + 32^2 + 38^2 19^2 + 24^2}{4} - C = 1007.5 - 952.2$$

$$= 55.3$$

$$\text{S.S.B.} = \frac{31^2 + 36^2 + 35^2 + 36^2}{5} - C = 955.6 - 952.2 = 3.4$$

$$\text{S.S.E.} = 69.8 - 55.3 - 3.4 = 11.1$$

Summary

Source of variation	Sum of squares	Degrees of freedom	Mean square	F
Total	69.8	19		
Between (treatments)	55.3	4	13.82	14.94
Between (blocks)	3.4	3	1.13	1.22
Within	11.1	12	0.925	

Since the F-value of 14.94 is greater than the tabular value of $F_{0.95}$ for $v_1 = 4$ and $v_2 = 12$, there are significant differences between the mean scores for drugs (treatments). On contrast, the F-value 1.22 is less than the tabular value of $F_{0.95}$ for $v_1 = 3$ and $v_2 = 12$ so that there is no significant difference between the mean scores of physicians. The Duncan multiple range test (Procedure 37) may be used to find which pairs of drugs have significant differences between their means.

Computer Screen

```
            <34> Analysis of Variance II: Two-way, Single Observation
            Pharmacologic Calculation System - Version 4.0 - 03/12/86


For 2-way ANOVA, each file represents a different 'treatment' and entries (mean
  values) across all treatments represent a 'block'.

Do you want to show intermediate results (Y/N) ? N

Input: <K>eyboard, <D>isk, or <E>xit this procedure? D

You may enter 5 'Y' data files. Press <ENTER> after last file name.
File name 1 ? TREATMENT1<ENTER>
File name 2 ? TREATMENT2<ENTER>
File name 3 ? TREATMENT3<ENTER>
File name 4 ? TREATMENT4<ENTER>
File name 5 ? TREATMENT5<ENTER>

Data: <E>dit, <L>ist, <S>ave, or <ENTER> to continue? L

   File name:   TREATMENT1   TREATMENT2   TREATMENT3   TREATMENT4   TREATMENT5
  ------------ ------------ ------------ ------------ ------------ ------------
      # 1:          6            7           10            3            5
      # 2:          7            9           10            4            6
      # 3:          5            8            9            6            7
      # 4:          7            8            9            6            6
```

```
Data: <E>dit, <L>ist, <S>ave, or <ENTER> to continue? <ENTER>

    Source of        Sum of      Deg. of      Mean
    Variation        Squares     Freedom      Square      F Value
 -------------    ------------ ------------  ---------- -----------
       Total:       69.8            19
  Treatments:       55.3             4         13.825       14.95
      Blocks:        3.39996         3          1.13332      1.23
      Within:       11.1            12          .925003

    F (95%):         3.26      F (99%):         5.41

 Differences between treatments: Significant at p < 0.01


    F (95%):         3.49      F (99%):         5.95

 Differences between blocks: NOT Significant at p < 0.05


 Report: <P>rint, <S>ave, or <V>iew? <ENTER>
```

Computer Report

```
        <34> Analysis of Variance II: Two-way, Single Observation
        Pharmacologic Calculation System — Version 4.0 — 03/12/86
```

File name:	TREATMENT1	TREATMENT2	TREATMENT3	TREATMENT4	TREATMENT5
# 1:	6	7	10	3	5
# 2:	7	9	10	4	6
# 3:	5	8	9	6	7
# 4:	7	8	9	6	6

Source of Variation	Sum of Squares	Deg. of Freedom	Mean Square	F Value
Total:	69.8	19		
Treatments:	55.3	4	13.825	14.95
Blocks:	3.39996	3	1.13332	1.23
Within:	11.1	12	.925003	

```
    F (95%):         3.26      F (99%):         5.41

 Differences between treatments: Significant at p < 0.01


    F (95%):         3.49      F (99%):         5.95

 Differences between blocks: NOT Significant at p < 0.05
```

Procedure 35
Analysis of Variance III: Two-Way, with Replication

The number of replicates per "cell" is equal for all cells. The term "cell" is used for a combination of factors, a treatments and b blocks. Thus, the number of cells is the product ab. The number of replicates per cell is denoted r.

Example

Entries are Ca^{++} levels in males and females with and without hormone treatment.

		Treatment		No treatment	
		$\longleftarrow$ $(a = 2)$ $\longrightarrow$			
	male	$\begin{bmatrix} 32 \\ 23.8 \\ 28.8 \\ 25 \\ 29.3 \end{bmatrix}$ $r = 5$		$\begin{bmatrix} 14.5 \\ 11.0 \\ 10.8 \\ 14.3 \\ 10.0 \end{bmatrix}$ $r = 5$	

$(b = 2)$ $\sum = 138.9$ $\sum = 60.6$

| | female | $\begin{bmatrix} 39.1 \\ 26.2 \\ 21.3 \\ 35.8 \\ 40.2 \end{bmatrix}$ $r = 5$ | | $\begin{bmatrix} 16.5 \\ 18.4 \\ 12.7 \\ 14.0 \\ 12.8 \end{bmatrix}$ $r = 5$ | |

$\sum = 162.6$ $\sum = 74.4$

$$N = abr = 20$$

Total (no treatment) $= 60.6 + 74.4 = 135.0$
Total (treatment) $= 162.6 + 138.9 = 301.5$ $\left. \right\} + = 436.5$

Total, block 1 (female) $= 162.6 + 74.4 = 237.0$
Total, block 2 (male) $= 60.6 + 138.9 = 199.5$ $\left. \right\} + = 436.5$

$$\sum \sum \sum X_{ij1} = 436.5$$

$$\sum \sum \sum (X_{ij1})^2 = 11354.31$$

Correction:

$$C = \frac{(\sum \sum \sum X_{ij1})^2}{N} = \frac{436.5^2}{20} = 9526.6$$

$$\text{SS total} = \sum \sum \sum (x_{ij1})^2 - C = 11354.31 - 9526.6$$
$$= 1827.7 \ (df = N - 1 = 19)$$

$$\text{SS}_{\text{cells}} = \frac{(74.4)^2 + (60.6)^2 + (162.6)^2 + (138.9)^2}{5} - 9526.6$$

$(df = ab - 1 = 3) = 1461.3$

$$\text{(Within)} \quad SS_{error} = SS_{total} - SS_{cells} = 1827.7 - 1461.3$$
$$(df = ab(r - 1) = 16) \qquad = 366.4$$

$$SS_{treatments} = \frac{(135.0)^2 + (301.5)^2}{(2) \quad (5)} - 9526.6 = 1386.1*$$
$$(df = a - 1 = 1)$$

$$SS_{blocks} = \frac{(237.0)^2 + (199.5)^2}{(2) \quad (5)} - 9526.6 = 70.3**$$
$$(\text{sex})$$
$$(df = b - 1 = 1)$$

$$SS_{interaction} = SS_{cells} - SS_{treatment} - SS_{blocks}$$
$$(df = (a - 1)(b - 1) = 1) = 1461.3 - 1386.1 - 70.3$$
$$= 4.9$$

Source of variation	Sum of squares	Degree of freedom	Mean square
Total	1827.7	19	
Cells	1461.3	3	
Treatments	1386.1	1	1386.1
Blocks	70.3	1	70.3
Interaction	4.9	1	4.9
Within (error)	366.4	16	22.9

Thus,

1. $F_{treatments} = \dfrac{1386.1}{22.9} = 60.5$; tabular $F_{1,16} = 4.49$

    significant, i.e., treatment effects Ca^{++} level.

2. $F_{blocks} = \dfrac{70.3}{22.9} = 3.1$; tabular $F_{1,16} = 4.49$

    not significant, i.e., no diff. between male and female on Ca^{++} level

3. $F_{interaction} = 4.9 = 0.2$; tabular $F_{1,16} = 4.49$

    not significant, i.e., no interaction between gender and treatment

---

* The denominator, (2)(5), is the product br.
** The denominator, (2)(5), is the product ar.

Computer Screen

```
              <35> Analysis of Variance III: Two-way, with Replication
                 Pharmacologic Calculation System - Version 4.0 - 03/12/86

Two factor ANOVA with replications requires entry of 2 Blocks (e.g. male &
female), each with 2 or more treatments. Each file represents a different
treatment (e.g. dose 1, dose 2, etc.).

Enter Block A now:

Do you want to show intermediate results (Y/N) ? N

Input: <K>eyboard, <D>isk, or <E>xit this procedure? D

You may enter 5 'Y' data files. Press <ENTER> after last file name.
File name 1 ? MTREAT<ENTER>
File name 2 ? MNOT<ENTER>
File name 3 ? <ENTER>

Data: <E>dit, <L>ist, <S>ave, or <ENTER> to continue? L

    File name:        MTREAT           MNOT
   ------------    ------------    ------------
          # 1:           32           14.5
          # 2:         23.8           11
          # 3:         28.8           10.8
          # 4:           25           14.3
          # 5:         29.3           10

Data: <E>dit, <L>ist, <S>ave, or <ENTER> to continue? <ENTER>
```

```
Enter Block B now:

Input: <K>eyboard, <D>isk, or <E>xit this procedure? D

You may enter 2 'Y' data files. Press <ENTER> after last file name.
File name 1 ? FTREAT<ENTER>
File name 2 ? FNOT<ENTER>

Data: <E>dit, <L>ist, <S>ave, or <ENTER> to continue? L

    File name:        FTREAT           FNOT
   ------------    ------------    ------------
          # 1:         39.1           16.5
          # 2:         26.2           18.4
          # 3:         21.3           12.7
          # 4:         35.8           14
          # 5:         40.2           12.8

Data: <E>dit, <L>ist, <S>ave, or <ENTER> to continue? <ENTER>

     Source of       Sum of        Deg. of        Mean
     Variation       Squares       Freedom       Square        F Value
   ------------   ------------   ------------   ------------   ------------
   Treatments:      1386.11            1          1386.11       60.5335
       Blocks:      70.3115            1          70.3115        3.07061
  Interaction:      4.90234            1          4.90234        .214092
        Error:      366.372           16          22.8983
```

```
    Variation       F (95%)       F (99%)              Significance
   ------------   ------------   ------------        ------------
   Treatments:       4.49           8.53               p < 0.01
       Blocks:       4.49           8.53               n.s.
  Interaction:       4.49           8.53               n.s.

Report: <P>rint, <S>ave, or <V>iew? <ENTER>
```

Computer Report

```
        <35> Analysis of Variance III: Two-way, with Replication
           Pharmacologic Calculation System - Version 4.0 - 03/12/86

    File name:        MTREAT              MNOT
    ------------  ------------      ------------
         # 1:              32              14.5
         # 2:            23.8                11
         # 3:            28.8              10.8
         # 4:              25              14.3
         # 5:            29.3                10

    File name:        FTREAT              FNOT
    ------------  ------------      ------------
         # 1:            39.1              16.5
         # 2:            26.2              18.4
         # 3:            21.3              12.7
         # 4:            35.8                14
         # 5:            40.2              12.8

    Source of        Sum of         Deg. of       Mean
    Variation       Squares         Freedom       Square        F Value
    ------------  ------------   ------------  ------------   ------------
    Treatments:     1386.11             1        1386.11        60.5335
       Blocks:      70.3115             1        70.3115        3.07061
  Interaction:      4.90234             1        4.90234        .214092
       Error:       366.372            16        22.8983

    Variation       F (95%)         F (99%)                    Significance
    ------------  ------------   ------------              ------------
    Treatments:       4.49            8.53                      p < 0.01
       Blocks:        4.49            8.53                        n.s.
  Interaction:        4.49            8.53                        n.s.
```

Procedure 36

Newman–Keuls Test

Analysis of variance (Procedure 33) considers the problem of determining, among a set of k samples (three or more), whether there are means that differ significantly. When it is found that there *is* a significant difference it may be desirable to find *which pairs*, among all possible pairs of means, are different. For this purpose a multiple-range-test such as the Newman–Keuls* test is commonly used. For k samples the number of pairs is $k(k - 1)/2$.

The k sample means are first arranged in order of increasing magnitude

$$\bar{A}_1, \bar{A}_2, \ldots, \bar{A}_k.$$

Consider the pair $\bar{A}_k$ vs. $\bar{A}_1$; for these a standard error term (SE) is computed using the respective sample sizes n_k and n_1 and the value s_p^2 (from the previous analysis of variance):

$$\text{SE} = \left[\frac{s_p^2}{2} (1/n_k + 1/n_1) \right]^{1/2}. \tag{36.1}$$

---

* Newman, D. *Biometrika* **31**:20, 1939. Keuls, M. *Euphytica* **1**:112, 1952.

Also needed is the value of the "Studentized range" denoted by q:

$$q = \frac{\bar{A}_k - \bar{A}_1}{\text{SE}} \tag{36.2}$$

and the value, w, equal to the number of means in the range of the pair being tested. (For the pair $\bar{A}_k$, $\bar{A}_1$, the value $w = k$; for the pair $\bar{A}_k$, $\bar{A}_2$, the value $w = k - 1$, etc.). The calculated value of q from Equation (36.2) is then compared with the *critical value* of $q_{\alpha, v, w}$ from Table A.13, using the desired confidence value α (usually 0.05 or 0.01), the "within sample" degrees of freedom v and the value w previously defined. If the calculated $q \geq q_{\alpha, v, w}$, then the pair of means differ significantly at the α level. A similar test is made on each pair of means.

The order of comparison of means is "largest" against "smallest" (k vs. 1), then "largest" against "second-smallest" (k vs. 2), etc; then "second-largest" against "smallest" ($k - 1$ vs. 1), and "second-largest" against "second-smallest" ($k - 1$ vs. 2), etc.*

Example

Four groups are listed below. Analysis of variance demonstrated a significant difference among the means (ANOVA table given below).

I	II	III	IV
5	7	2	12
2	9	2	10
4	4	1	8
2	6	2	5
5	10	4	12
1		3	10
		3	11
		1	

The means are given below along with the number ( ):

I	II	III	IV
3.17	7.20	2.25	9.71
(6)	(5)	(8)	(7)

---

* Although not common, it is possible that the Newman-Keuls test may fail to identify a difference between any pair of means even though analysis of variance suggests that a difference exists.

The analysis of variance table is given below; $F = 22.72$.

Source	Sum of squares	Degrees of freedom	Mean square	F
Between	255.78	3	85.26	22.72
Within	82.56	22	3.76	
Total	338.34			

The means are arranged in ascending order

	III	I	II	IV
$\bar{A}_k$	2.25	3.17	7.20	9.71
	(8)	(6)	(5)	(7)

The comparisons are largest against smallest—then largest against next smallest, etc., and for each, SE, q and w are determined. Note, $s_p^2 = 3.76$ and $v = 22$. We illustrate IV vs. III:

$$SE = \sqrt{\frac{3.76}{2}\left(\frac{1}{8}+\frac{1}{7}\right)} = 0.710$$

$$q = \frac{9.71 - 2.25}{0.710} = 10.51$$

$$w = 4$$

The tabular value of $q_{0.99}$, obtained by extrapolation is 4.96. Since the calculated $q > 4.96$, the means IV and III differ significantly ($p < 0.01$). The remaining calculations are summarized below with tabular values of $q_{0.95}$ and $q_{0.99}$. (* means $p < 0.05$; ** means $p < 0.01$)

Comparison	Difference	SE	q	w	$q_{0.95}$	$q_{0.99}$
IV–III	7.46**	0.710	10.51	4	3.93	4.96
IV–I	6.54**	0.763	8.57	3	3.55	4.60
IV–II	2.51*	0.803	3.13	2	2.93	3.99
II–III	4.95**	0.782	6.33	3	3.55	4.60
II–I	4.03**	0.830	4.86	2	2.93	3.99
I–III	0.92	0.740	1.24	2	2.93	3.99

Computer Screen

```
                         <36> Newman-Keuls Test
              Pharmacologic Calculation System - Version 4.0 - 03/25/86

Do you want to show intermediate results (Y/N) ? N

Input: <K>eyboard, <D>isk, or <E>xit this procedure? D

You may enter 5 'Y' data files. Press <ENTER> after last file name.
File name 1 ? I<ENTER>
File name 2 ? II<ENTER>
File name 3 ? III<ENTER>
File name 4 ? IV<ENTER>
File name 5 ? <ENTER>

Data: <E>dit, <L>ist, <S>ave, or <ENTER> to continue? L

   File name:         I           II          III          IV
   -----------   ----------- ----------- ----------- -----------
        # 1:          5           7           2           12
        # 2:          2           9           2           10
        # 3:          4           4           1            8
        # 4:          2           6           2            5
        # 5:          5          10           4           12
        # 6:          1                       3           10
        # 7:                                  3           11
        # 8:                                  1

Data: <E>dit, <L>ist, <S>ave, or <ENTER> to continue? <ENTER>
```

```
   Source of      Sum of      Deg. of       Mean
   Variation      Squares     Freedom      Square      F Value
   -----------   ---------   ----------   ---------   ---------
      Total:     338.346        25
    Between:     255.784         3        85.2614      22.72
     Within:     82.5619        22        3.75281

   F (95%):        3.05     F (99%):         4.82

Differences between means: Significant at p < 0.01

     Step (w):       2           3           4
   -----------   ---------   ---------   ---------
   q95% ( 22):     2.935       3.555       3.93
   q99% ( 22):     3.99        4.59        4.965

   Filename   vs Filename   Difference   Std. Err.          q
   ---------   -----------   ----------   ---------   ---------
      III           I         .916667      .739787     1.23909
      III          II         4.95         .780918     6.3387
      III          IV         7.46429      .708949    10.5287
       I           II         4.03333      .829467     4.86256
       I           IV         6.54762      .762098     8.59158
      II           IV         2.51429      .802085     3.13469
```

```
Newman-Keuls Test Summary:

                   III          I           II          IV
                   2.25      3.16667        7.2       9.71429
                ----------- ----------- ----------- -----------
      III                     .916667      4.95**     7.46429**
       I                                  4.03333**   6.54762**
      II                                              2.51429*

 * Significant at p < 0.05
** Significant at p < 0.01

Report: <P>rint, <S>ave, or <V>iew? <ENTER>
```

Computer Report

```
                              <36> Newman-Keuls Test
                  Pharmacologic Calculation System - Version 4.0 - 03/25/86
```

File name:	I	II	III	IV
# 1:	5	7	2	12
# 2:	2	9	2	10
# 3:	4	4	1	8
# 4:	2	6	2	5
# 5:	5	10	4	12
# 6:	1		3	10
# 7:			3	11
# 8:			1	

Source of Variation	Sum of Squares	Deg. of Freedom	Mean Square	F Value
Total:	338.346	25		
Between:	255.784	3	85.2614	22.72
Within:	82.5619	22	3.75281	

F (95%):	3.05	F (99%):	4.82

Differences between means: Significant at p < 0.01

Step (w):	2	3	4
q95% (22):	2.935	3.555	3.93
q99% (22):	3.99	4.59	4.965

Filename	vs Filename	Difference	Std. Err.	q
III	I	.916667	.739787	1.23909
III	II	4.95	.780918	6.3387
III	IV	7.46429	.708949	10.5287
I	II	4.03333	.829467	4.86256
I	IV	6.54762	.762098	8.59158
II	IV	2.51429	.802085	3.13469

Newman-Keuls Test Summary:

	III 2.25	I 3.16667	II 7.2	IV 9.71429
III		.916667	4.95**	7.46429**
I			4.03333**	6.54762**
II				2.51429*

```
* Significant at p < 0.05
** Significant at p < 0.01
```

Procedure 37
Duncan Multiple Range Test

Among a set of k samples *of equal size n*, analysis of variance (Procedure 33) indicates a significant difference between the sample means. It is required to determine which pairs of means differ significantly. (See also Procedures 36 and 38.) Duncan* proposed a test that provides a series of shortest significant

---

* Duncan, D. B. *Biometrics 11*:1–42, 1955.

ranges, given by a quantity R_p, in order to compare differences between means. In this test, the k means are arranged in order of magnitude. Quantities R_p are calculated as follows:

$$R_p = Q_p(s_p^2/n)^{1/2} \tag{37.1}$$

where Q_p is obtained from Table A.14 and s_p^2 has the usual meaning from analysis of variance (within means variance). The tables for Q_p depend on the number of means being compared at one time, denoted p, and degrees of freedom $= k(n - 1)$. From the ordering of the means, consider adjacent pairs. If these differ by an amount greater than R_2 the difference is significant. Further, for any triplet, the difference between the largest and smallest must exceed R_3 for significance. In general, take p consecutive means. The difference between the largest and smallest must exceed R_p in order to be significant.

Example

Table 37.1

	A	B	C	D	E
	6	7	10	3	5
	5	9	10	4	6
	7	8	9	6	7
	7	8	9	6	6
Totals	25	32	38	19	24
Means	6.25	8.00	9.50	4.75	6.00

For the data of Table 37.1, application of Duncan's test requires computation of R_2, R_3, R_4, and R_5. We need, therefore, the tabular values, for $k(n - 1) = 15$ degrees of freedom. From Table A.14, these are (for 5% level):

Q_2	Q_3	Q_4	Q_5
3.01	3.16	3.25	3.31

Each Q_p-value is multiplied by $\sqrt{s_p^2/n}$, which, for these data, is $\sqrt{0.967/4} = 0.492$. Hence, the R_p are obtained:

R_2	R_3	R_4	R_5
1.48	1.55	1.60	1.63

The arrangement of means is below.

D	E	A	B	C
4.75	6.00	6.25	8.00	9.50

Comparison of adjacent pairs shows DE and EA are not significantly different. The range among triplets show DA not significantly different,* whereas EB and AC are significant. Pairs in R_4 are DB and EC, each significant. DC is greater than R_5 and therefore is significant.

Computer Screen

```
                         <37> Duncan Multiple Range Test
             Pharmacologic Calculation System - Version 4.0 - 03/12/86

Do you want to show intermediate results (Y/N) ? N

Input: <K>eyboard, <D>isk, or <E>xit this procedure? D

You may enter 5 'Y' data files. Press <ENTER> after last file name.
File name 1 ? A<ENTER>
File name 2 ? B<ENTER>
File name 3 ? C<ENTER>
File name 4 ? D<ENTER>
File name 5 ? E<ENTER>

Data: <E>dit, <L>ist, <S>ave, or <ENTER> to continue? L

    File name:        A            B            C            D            E
   ------------ ------------ ------------ ------------ ------------ ------------
      # 1:          6            7           10            3            5
      # 2:          5            9           10            4            6
      # 3:          7            8            9            6            7
      # 4:          7            8            9            6            6

Data: <E>dit, <L>ist, <S>ave, or <ENTER> to continue? <ENTER>
```

```
    Source of       Sum of       Deg. of       Mean
    Variation       Squares      Freedom       Square       F Value
   ------------ ------------ ------------ ------------ ------------
      Total:        69.8          19
     Between:       55.3           4          13.825        14.3
     Within:        14.5          15          .966667

    F (95%):        3.06      F (99%):        4.89

Differences between means: Significant at p < 0.01

         R2           R3           R4           R5
   ------------ ------------ ------------ ------------
      1.4797       1.55344      1.59769      1.62718

Duncan's Multiple Range Test Summary: Differences

                       D            E            A            B            C
                     4.75          6          6.25          8           9.5
   ------------ ------------ ------------ ------------ ------------ ------------
              D                    1.25         1.5         3.25*        4.75*
              E                                  .25         2*           3.5*
              A                                             1.75*        3.25*
              B                                                          1.5*

* Significant at p < 0.05

Report: <P>rint, <S>ave, or <V>iew? <ENTER>
```

* The range DA is close enough to R_3 that its significance is doubtful. Application of the L.S.D. test (Procedure 38) showed significance at the 0.05 level.

Computer Report

```
                              <37> Duncan Multiple Range Test
                    Pharmacologic Calculation System - Version 4.0 - 03/12/86

      File name:           A               B               C               D               E
    ------------    ------------    ------------    ------------    ------------    ------------
         # 1:             6               7              10               3               5
         # 2:             5               9              10               4               6
         # 3:             7               8               9               6               7
         # 4:             7               8               9               6               6

      Source of        Sum of          Deg. of          Mean
      Variation        Squares         Freedom          Square         F Value
    ------------    ------------    ------------    ------------    ------------
         Total:         69.8             19
       Between:         55.3              4             13.825           14.3
        Within:         14.5             15            .966667

      F (95%):           3.06         F (99%):                          4.89
```

Differences between means: Significant at $p < 0.01$

```
            R2              R3              R4              R5
    ------------    ------------    ------------    ------------
        1.4797         1.55344         1.59769         1.62718
```

Duncan's Multiple Range Test Summary: Differences

```
                              D               E               A               B               C
                            4.75             6             6.25             8             9.5
                        ------------    ------------    ------------    ------------    ------------
            D                            1.25             1.5            3.25*           4.75*
            E                                             .25             2*             3.5*
            A                                                            1.75*           3.25*
            B                                                                            1.5*
```

* Significant at $p < 0.05$

Procedure 38

Least Significant Difference Test

When the F-ratio determined by analysis of variance indicates a significant difference between sample means, it is desirable to determine which means are significantly different. The Newman–Keuls test (Procedure 36) is applicable for this purpose. When the *sample sizes are equal*, additional tests (besides Newman–Keuls) may be used. We discuss here one such test based on calculation of a quantity representing the smallest difference which could exist between two sample means if these means are significantly different. In Procedure 37 we presented an alternative test (Duncan's). Neither of these tests should be applied if the F-value (Procedure 33) does not indicate a significant difference.

The notation is the same as that of Procedure 33. There are k samples, each of size n. The quantity representing the least significant difference (L.S.D.) is given below (Eq. 38.1) and uses the value of student's t at the desired level (such as 0.05) and degrees of freedom $= k(n-1)$ from Table A.2.

$$\text{L.S.D.} = t \cdot \sqrt{2s_p^2/n} \tag{38.1}$$

where s_p is defined in Procedure 33. All possible pairs of means should be taken and the difference compared to L.S.D. Any difference greater than L.S.D. is significant.

Example

Five groups (A to E), each with five values are given in Table 38.1. The associated ANOVA table is given (Table 38.2) from which L.S.D. is calculated as shown.

Table 38.1

	A	B	C	D	E
	6	7	10	3	5
	5	9	10	4	6
	7	8	9	6	7
	7	8	9	6	6
	—	—	—	—	—
Total	25	32	38	19	24
Mean	6.25	8.00	9.50	4.75	6.00

Table 38.2

Analysis of Variance

Source	Sum of squares	Degrees of freedom	Mean square	F
Total	S.S. = 69.8	$nk - 1 = 19$		
Between	S.S.T. = 55.3	$k - 1 = 4$	$s_t^2 = 13.8$	$F = 14.3$
Within	S.S.E. = 14.5	$nk - 1 = 15$	$s_p^2 = 0.967$	

From Table A.11, $F_{0.95} = 3.06$. Since $14.3 > 3.06$, there are means that differ significantly. The least significant difference is obtained from t for 15 degrees of freedom:

$$\text{L.S.D.} = 2.131 \cdot \sqrt{(2)(0.967)/5} = 1.33$$

Examination of all pairs of means shows that the difference between AE and DE are less than the L.S.D. and, therefore, not significant. In all other pairs the means differ significantly. (See footnote, p. 127.)

Computer Screen

```
                    <38> Least Significant Difference Test
               Pharmacologic Calculation System - Version 4.0 - 03/12/86

Do you want to show intermediate results (Y/N) ? N

Input: <K>eyboard, <D>isk, or <E>xit this procedure? D

You may enter 5 'Y' data files. Press <ENTER> after last file name.
File name 1 ? A<ENTER>
File name 2 ? B<ENTER>
File name 3 ? C<ENTER>
File name 4 ? D<ENTER>
File name 5 ? E<ENTER>

Data: <E>dit, <L>ist, <S>ave, or <ENTER> to continue? L

    File name:          A           B           C           D           E
   ------------ ------------ ------------ ------------ ------------ ------------
       # 1:          6           7          10           3           5
       # 2:          5           9          10           4           6
       # 3:          7           8           9           6           7
       # 4:          7           8           9           6           6

Data: <E>dit, <L>ist, <S>ave, or <ENTER> to continue? <ENTER>
```

```
        Source of      Sum of      Deg. of      Mean
        Variation      Squares     Freedom      Square      F Value
       ------------ ------------ ------------ ------------ ------------
         Total:        69.8         19
         Between:      55.3          4         13.825        14.3
         Within:       14.5         15         .966667

       F (95%):        3.06     F (99%):        4.89

Differences between means: Significant at p < 0.01

L.S.D. Test Summary:

L.S.D., p < 0.05 = 1.32511
L.S.D., p < 0.01 = 1.83252

                         D            E            A            B            C
                        4.75          6          6.25          8           9.5
                    ------------ ------------ ------------ ------------ ------------
                D                    1.25         1.5*        3.25**       4.75**
                E                                  .25          2**         3.5**
                A                                              1.75*       3.25**
                B                                                           1.5*

 * Significant at p < 0.05
** Significant at p < 0.01

Report: <P>rint, <S>ave, or <V>iew? <ENTER>
```

Computer Report

```
                    <38> Least Significant Difference Test
               Pharmacologic Calculation System - Version 4.0 - 03/12/86

    File name:          A           B           ·C           D           E
   ------------ ------------ ------------ ------------ ------------ ------------
       # 1:          6           7          10           3           5
       # 2:          5           9          10           4           6
       # 3:          7           8           9           6           7
       # 4:          7           8           9           6           6
```

Source of Variation	Sum of Squares	Deg. of Freedom	Mean Square	F Value
Total:	69.8	19		
Between:	55.3	4	13.825	14.3
Within:	14.5	15	.966667	

F (95%):	3.06	F (99%):	4.89

Differences between means: Significant at p < 0.01

L.S.D. Test Summary:

L.S.D., p < 0.05 = 1.32511
L.S.D., p < 0.01 = 1.83252

	D 4.75	E 6	A 6.25	B 8	C 9.5
D		1.25	1.5*	3.25**	4.75**
E			.25	2**	3.5**
A				1.75*	3.25**
B					1.5*

 * Significant at p < 0.05
** Significant at p < 0.01

Procedure 39
t-Test I: Grouped Data

The *t*-test is often used when it is desired to determine whether two population means differ significantly. If a sample of size N_1, taken from population 1, has a mean $\bar{x}$ and a standard deviation s_x, and a sample of size N_2, taken from population 2, has a mean $\bar{y}$ and a standard deviation s_y, the pooled variance s_p^2 is first determined as follows:

$$s_p^2 = \frac{(N_1 - 1)s_x^2 + (N_2 - 1)s_y^2}{N_1 + N_2 - 2}. \tag{39.1}$$

A more convenient computational formula for s_p^2 uses the raw data $\{x_i\}$ from sample 1 and $\{y_i\}$ from sample 2:

$$s_p^2 = \frac{\sum x_i^2 + \sum y_i^2 - (\sum x_i)^2/N_1 - (\sum y_i)^2/N_2}{N_1 + N_2 - 2}. \tag{39.2}$$

The quantity *t* is computed from the formula

$$t = \frac{\bar{x} - \bar{y}}{s_p\sqrt{1/N_1 + 1/N_2}}. \tag{39.3}$$

The magnitude of t is then compared with the value of t determined from its distribution for a specified level of confidence (usually 95% or 99%) and a number of degrees of freedom v given by

$$v = N_1 + N_2 - 2. \tag{39.4}$$

Table A.2 gives values of t for several confidence levels and $v = 1$ to 30. If the computed t exceeds the tabular value, then the means differ significantly.

Example

In order to test the effectiveness of a new analgesic drug, two groups of rats were used. The first group received saline, whereas the second group received the drug. The test of analgesia measured the time in seconds that each animal could tolerate a painful stimulus. The data for the two groups are given in the table below.

Saline $\{x_i\}$	Drug $\{y_i\}$
18	22
14	18
16	31
11	38
21	26
24	28
19	29
20	40
24	
15	

From the data we find the following values:

$$\bar{x} = 18.2 \qquad \bar{y} = 29.0$$
$$s_y = 4.26 \qquad s_y = 7.43$$
$$N_1 = 10 \qquad N_2 = 8.$$

Equation (39.1) yields for s_P^2

$$s_P^2 = \frac{(9)(4.26)^2 + (7)(7.42)^2}{16}$$

$$= 34.3.$$

Thus

$$t = \frac{18.2 - 29.0}{\sqrt{34.3}\sqrt{\frac{1}{10} + \frac{1}{8}}} = \frac{-10.8}{(5.86)(0.474)}$$

$$= -3.88.$$

From Table A.2 it is seen that the value of t for 16 degrees of freedom and 99% is 2.92. Since the magnitude of the computed value, 3.88, exceeds the tabular value, the difference is significant with $p < 0.01$.

Computer Screen

```
                        <39> t-Test I: Grouped Data
               Pharmacologic Calculation System - Version 4.0 - 03/12/86

Input: <K>eyboard, <D>isk, or <E>xit this procedure? D

You may enter 5 'Y' data files. Press <ENTER> after last file name.
File name 1 ? SALINE<ENTER>
File name 2 ? DRUG<ENTER>
File name 3 ? <ENTER>

Data: <E>dit, <L>ist, <S>ave, or <ENTER> to continue? L

    File name:        SALINE           DRUG
    -----------    ------------    ------------
         # 1:           18              22
         # 2:           14              18
         # 3:           16              31
         # 4:           11              38
         # 5:           21              26
         # 6:           24              28
         # 7:           19              29
         # 8:           20              40
         # 9:           24
        # 10:           15
```

```
Data: <E>dit, <L>ist, <S>ave, or <ENTER> to continue? <ENTER>

    File name:        SALINE           DRUG
    -----------    ------------    ------------
           N:           10               8
     Minimum:           11              18
        Mean:         18.2              29
     Maximum:           24              40
         Sum:          182             232
   Std. Dev.:      4.26354         7.42582
   Std. Err.:      1.34825         2.62543
   95% C.L.:       3.04974         6.20913

'SALINE' vs. ' DRUG':  Pooled Variance = 34.35
    t (95%) = 2.12        16 d.f.
    t (99%) = 2.921
    t (calc) = 3.885    Significant at p < 0.01

Report: <P>rint, <S>ave, or <V>iew? <ENTER>
```

Computer Report

```
                        <39> t-Test I: Grouped Data
               Pharmacologic Calculation System - Version 4.0 - 03/12/86

    File name:        SALINE           DRUG
    -----------    ------------    ------------
         # 1:           18              22
         # 2:           14              18
         # 3:           16              31
         # 4:           11              38
         # 5:           21              26
         # 6:           24              28
         # 7:           19              29
         # 8:           20              40
         # 9:           24
        # 10:           15
```

(continued)

```
File name:           SALINE              DRUG
------------    --------------    -------------
        N:                10                 8
  Minimum:                11                18
     Mean:              18.2                29
  Maximum:                24                40
      Sum:               182               232
Std. Dev.:           4.26354           7.42582
Std. Err.:           1.34825           2.62543
95% C.L.:            3.04974           6.20913

'SALINE' vs. '  DRUG':  Pooled Variance = 34.35
  t (95%) = 2.12        16 d.f.
  t (99%) = 2.921
  t (calc) = 3.885      Significant at p < 0.01
```

Procedure 40

t-Test II: Paired Data

When data are presented in paired fashion the paired *t*-test is often used. For example, we might be interested in the heart rate of a subject before and after receiving some drug. In such cases it is the difference that we are interested in. For each subject we have two values, x_i and y_i, and the difference, $d_i = x_i - y_i$, as outlined below.

Before treatment	After treatment	Difference
x_1	y_1	d_1
x_2	y_2	d_2
$\vdots$	$\vdots$	$\vdots$
x_n	y_n	d_n

The hypothesis being tested is that the mean difference is zero. The mean of the set $\{d_i\}$ is determined along with the standard deviation of the set $\{d_i\}$. Thus,

$$\text{mean}: \bar{d} = \left(\sum d_i\right)/n \tag{40.1}$$

$$\text{standard deviation}: s_d = \sqrt{\frac{\sum (d_i - \bar{d})^2}{n - 1}}. \tag{40.2}$$

The *t* statistic (for $n - 1$ degrees of freedom) is given by

$$t = \frac{\bar{d}}{s_d/\sqrt{n}}. \tag{40.3}$$

Example

The table below gives the heart rates of 8 subjects (beats/min) before and after drug treatment.

Subject	Before	After	Difference
1	75	73	2
2	81	78	3
3	68	69	-1
4	70	64	6
5	85	75	10
6	76	71	5
7	70	63	7
8	73	72	1

The calculations give

$$\bar{d} = 4.12$$

$$s_d = 3.56.$$

Thus

$$t = \frac{4.12}{3.56/\sqrt{8}} = 3.27.$$

The tabular value of *t* for 7 degrees of freedom and 99 % is 3.50, whereas for 95 % it is 2.36.* Hence, the difference is not significant at the 99 % level but it is significant at the 95 % level.

Computer Screen

```
                        <40> t-Test II: Paired Data
              Pharmacologic Calculation System - Version 4.0 - 03/12/86

Enter 2 'Y' data files, the difference will be computed.

Input: <K>eyboard, <D>isk, or <E>xit this procedure? D

You may enter 2 'Y' data files. Press <ENTER> after last file name.
File name 1 ? BEFORE<ENTER>
File name 2 ? AFTER<ENTER>

Data: <E>dit, <L>ist, <S>ave, or <ENTER> to continue? L

    File name:        BEFORE          AFTER
   ------------   -------------   -------------
        # 1:           75             73
        # 2:           81             78
        # 3:           68             69
        # 4:           70             64
        # 5:           85             75
        # 6:           76             71
        # 7:           70             63
        # 8:           73             72

Data: <E>dit, <L>ist, <S>ave, or <ENTER> to continue? <ENTER>
```

* Table A.2.

```
    File name:        BEFORE        AFTER    DIFFERENCE
-----------    -----------   -----------   -----------
        # 1:             75           73             2
        # 2:             81           78             3
        # 3:             68           69            -1
        # 4:             70           64             6
        # 5:             85           75            10
        # 6:             76           71             5
        # 7:             70           63             7
        # 8:             73           72             1

    File name:        BEFORE        AFTER    DIFFERENCE
-----------    -----------   -----------   -----------
           N:              8            8             8
     Minimum:             68           63            -1
        Mean:          74.75       70.625         4.125
     Maximum:             85           78            10
         Sum:            598          565            33
   Std. Dev.:         5.8493      5.15302       3.56321
   Std. Err.:        2.06804      1.82187       1.25978
    95% C.L.:        4.89091      4.30871       2.97939

    t (95%) = 2.365          7 d.f.
    t (99%) = 3.499
    t (calc) = 3.274    Significant at p < 0.05

Report: <P>rint, <S>ave, or <V>iew?  <ENTER>
```

Computer Report

```
                              <40> t-Test II: Paired Data
              Pharmacologic Calculation System - Version 4.0 - 03/12/86

    File name:        BEFORE        AFTER
-----------    -----------   -----------
        # 1:             75           73
        # 2:             81           78
        # 3:             68           69
        # 4:             70           64
        # 5:             85           75
        # 6:             76           71
        # 7:             70           63
        # 8:             73           72

    File name:        BEFORE        AFTER    DIFFERENCE
-----------    -----------   -----------   -----------
        # 1:             75           73             2
        # 2:             81           78             3
        # 3:             68           69            -1
        # 4:             70           64             6
        # 5:             85           75            10
        # 6:             76           71             5
        # 7:             70           63             7
        # 8:             73           72             1

    File name:        BEFORE        AFTER    DIFFERENCE
-----------    -----------   -----------   -----------
           N:              8            8             8
     Minimum:             68           63            -1
        Mean:          74.75       70.625         4.125
     Maximum:             85           78            10
         Sum:            598          565            33
   Std. Dev.:         5.8493      5.15302       3.56321
   Std. Err.:        2.06804      1.82187       1.25978
    95% C.L.:        4.89091      4.30871       2.97939

    t (95%) = 2.365          7 d.f.
    t (99%) = 3.499
    t (calc) = 3.274    Significant at p < 0.05
```

Procedure 41

Ratio of Means

It is common to compare the difference of two means as discussed in Procedure 39 (t-test). Sometimes it is desirable to compare the *ratio* of the means; for example in computing potency ratios. Discussed here is the computation of confidence limits for the ratio of two independent means $\bar{x}_1$ and $\bar{x}_2$. The observed ratio is $\bar{x}_1/\bar{x}_2$, where the numerator is derived from N_1 values of x and the denominator from N_2 values of x. The samples are assumed to be independent and the values x normally distributed. The means $\bar{x}_1$ and $\bar{x}_2$ are also normal with variances V_1 and V_2 and covariance of zero. A theorem due to Fieller* permits a computation of the confidence limits of the ratio R from the roots of a quadratic equation

$$(\bar{x}_1 - R\bar{x}_2)^2 - t^2 V = 0 \tag{41.1}$$

where V is related to the variances of the respective means and R according to

$$V = s_1^2/N_1 + R^2 s_2^2/N_2.$$

In the above equation, t is the tabular value of Student's t for $(N_1 + N_2 - 2)$ degrees of freedom. When the individual standard deviations s_1 and s_2 are approximately the same, the pooled value s_p is used

$$s_p^2 = \frac{(N_1 - 1)s_1^2 + (N_2 - 1)s_2^2}{N_1 + N_2 - 2} \tag{41.2}$$

so that

$$V = s_p^2 \left(\frac{1}{N_1} + \frac{R^2}{N_2} \right) \tag{41.3}$$

is used in Equation (41.1).

The calculation is simplified if we use a methodology due to Bliss.† In this method we calculate V_1 and V_2, either from the pooled variance

$$V_1 = \frac{s_p^2}{N_1} \quad \text{and} \quad V_2 = \frac{s_p^2}{N_2},$$

or from individual sample variances

$$V_1 = \frac{s_1^2}{N_1} \quad \text{and} \quad V_2 = \frac{s_2^2}{N_2}.$$

Also a term C is calculated:

$$C = \frac{\bar{x}_2^2}{\bar{x}_2^2 - V_2 t^2} \tag{41.4}$$

* Fieller, E. C. *Quart. J. Pharmacol.* **17**:117–123, 1944.
† Bliss, C. I. *Biometrics* **12**:491–526, 1956.

The confidence limits of the ratio are computed from

$$CR \pm \sqrt{(C-1)(CR^2 + V_1/V_2)} \qquad (41.5)$$

where the observed ratio $\bar{x}_1/\bar{x}_2$ is used for R. The confidence limits are *not* symmetric around the observed ratio.

Example

Measurement obtained on two samples are given below. It is desired to estimate 95% confidence limits for the ratio.

	Group 1	Group 2
	15, 13.8, 14.2, 15.5	7, 8.5, 6.3, 7.2
	14.8 and 14.9.	9.1, 7.5 and 6.8.

$$\bar{x}_1 = 14.7 \qquad\qquad \bar{x}_2 = 7.49$$
$$s_1 = 0.606 \qquad\qquad s_2 = 0.986$$
$$N = 6 \qquad\qquad\qquad N = 7$$

Thus, $\bar{x}_1/\bar{x}_2 = 14.7/7.49 = 1.96$,
while

$$s_p^2 = [(6)(0.986)^2 + (5)(0.606)^2]/11$$
$$= 0.697.$$

Using s_p^2, V_2 is computed:

$$V_2 = s_p^2/N_2 = 0.697/7$$

$$= 0.0996; \text{ also } V_1 = 0.696/6 = 0.116 \text{ so that } \frac{V_1}{V_2} = 1.167$$

From Table A.2, the value of t for 95% and 11 degrees of freedom is 2.201. The value of C, from Equation (41.4) is

$$C = \frac{7.49^2}{7.49^2 - (0.0996)(2.201)^2} = 1.009.$$

Confidence limits for the ratio are, from Equation (41.5)

$$(1.009)(1.96) \pm \sqrt{(0.009)(1.009 \times 1.96^2 + 1.167)}$$

or 1.98 ± 0.213. The observed ratio 1.96 is *not* at the center of the confidence interval.

Computer Screen

```
                          <41> Ratio of Means
              Pharmacologic Calculation System - Version 4.0 - 03/12/86

Do you want to show intermediate results (Y/N) ? N

Input: <K>eyboard, <D>isk, or <E>xit this procedure? D

You may enter 5 'Y' data files. Press <ENTER> after last file name.
File name 1 ? GROUP1<ENTER>
File name 2 ? GROUP2<ENTER>
File name 3 ? <ENTER>

Data: <E>dit, <L>ist, <S>ave, or <ENTER> to continue? L

    File name:       GROUP1        GROUP2
    -----------   ------------  ------------
        # 1:             15             7
        # 2:           13.8           8.5
        # 3:           14.2           6.3
        # 4:           15.5           7.2
        # 5:           14.8           9.1
        # 6:           14.9           7.5
        # 7:                          6.8

Data: <E>dit, <L>ist, <S>ave, or <ENTER> to continue? <ENTER>
```

```
'GROUP1' vs. 'GROUP2':  Pooled Variance = .697143
    t (95%) = 2.201      11 d.f.
    t (99%) = 3.106


    Variable        Value    95% Limits   Lower C.L.   Upper C.L.
    -----------  ------------              ------------ ------------
      Ratio       1.96374                    1.77124      2.19035

Report: <P>rint, <S>ave, or <V>iew? <ENTER>
```

Computer Report

```
                          <41> Ratio of Means
              Pharmacologic Calculation System - Version 4.0 - 03/12/86

    File name:       GROUP1        GROUP2
    -----------   ------------  ------------
        # 1:             15             7
        # 2:           13.8           8.5
        # 3:           14.2           6.3
        # 4:           15.5           7.2
        # 5:           14.8           9.1
        # 6:           14.9           7.5
        # 7:                          6.8

'GROUP1' vs. 'GROUP2':  Pooled Variance = .697143
    t (95%) = 2.201      11 d.f.
    t (99%) = 3.106


    Variable        Value    95% Limits   Lower C.L.   Upper C.L.
    -----------  ------------              ------------ ------------
      Ratio       1.96374                    1.77124      2.19035
```

Procedure 42

Chi-Square Test

The chi-square (χ^2) test is applicable to many situations in which experimental frequencies are compared to theoretical frequencies based on a hypothesis. For example, in tossing a die many times one expects that each of the values one to six will occur one-sixth of the time. Thus, in 600 tosses the expected frequencies, denoted $e_1, e_2, \ldots, e_6$, are each 100. We denote the actual frequencies, or observed frequencies, by $o_1, o_2, \ldots, o_6$. The statistic chi-square (χ^2) for these six events is given by

$$\chi^2 = \frac{(o_1 - e_1)^2}{e_1} + \frac{(o_2 - e_2)^2}{e_2} + \cdots + \frac{(o_6 - e_6)^2}{e_6}. \tag{42.1}$$

Clearly, the closer the agreement between the observed and expected frequencies, the smaller is the value of χ^2. An application that is often useful in pharmacology is illustrated in the following example.

Example 1

Two hundred and one children and adults of both sexes, all with a history of motion sickness, took an antihistamine drug prior to sailing on the same ocean cruise. It is desired to know whether the drug is equally effective in the four groups based on the frequencies of motion sickness shown underscored in Table 42.1.

Table 42.1
Frequency of motion sickness

	I Male children	II Female children	III Male adults	IV Female adults	
Reported nausea	15 (9.95)	14 (10.7)	6 (9.55)	5 (9.75)	40
No nausea	35 (40.0)	40 (43.3)	42 (38.4)	44 (39.2)	161
Total	50	54	48	49	201

The hypothesis to be tested is that there is *no difference* (a null hypothesis) among the four groups. If the null hypothesis is disproved, as indicated by a large value of x^2 then a significant difference exists. Corresponding to each entry in the table we can determine the expected number under the null hypothesis. For example, if there were no difference among the four groups, then the same fraction 40/201 of the total for each group would report nausea. Thus, for group 1, $(40/201) \times 50$ or 9.95; for group 2, $(40/201) \times 54$, or 10.7; for group 3, $(40/201) \times 48$, or 9.55; and for group 4, $(40/201) \times 49$, or 9.75. These values of the expected numbers are placed in parentheses in Table 42.1. By subtraction from the group totals we obtain the expected number for the second row (no nausea) entries. The value x^2 is

$$\chi^2 = \frac{(15 - 9.95)^2}{9.95} + \frac{(14 - 10.7)^2}{10.7} + \cdots + \frac{(44 - 39.2)^2}{39.2} = 8.97.$$

Associated with the distribution χ^2 is the number of degrees of freedom, d.f. For the two-row, four-column table of the example, d.f. = 3. In general, d.f. is the product $(r - 1) \times (c - 1)$, where r is the number of rows and c is the number of columns. From Table A.8 for d.f. = 3, the value of χ^2 (95%) is 7.82. Since 8.97 > 7.82 we reject the null hypothesis and conclude that there is a significant difference among the four groups.

Computer Screen

```
                            <42> Chi-Square Test
                Pharmacologic Calculation System - Version 4.0 - 03/13/86

Each data file represents a 'Row' in the contingency table. Since data values
across all rows represent a 'Column' in the contingency table, n's for each
file (Row) must be equal.

Input: <K>eyboard, <D>isk, or <E>xit this procedure? D

You may enter 5 'Y' data files. Press <ENTER> after last file name.
File name 1 ? NAUSEA<ENTER>
File name 2 ? NONAUSEA<ENTER>
File name 3 ? <ENTER>

Data: <E>dit, <L>ist, <S>ave, or <ENTER> to continue? L

    File name:         NAUSEA      NONAUSEA
    ------------    ------------  ------------
        # 1:             15            35
        # 2:             14            40
        # 3:              6            42
        # 4:              5            44

Data: <E>dit, <L>ist, <S>ave, or <ENTER> to continue? <ENTER>
```

```
Expected Frequencies:

    NAUSEA        NONAUSEA        Totals
  ------------  ------------   ------------
    9.95025       40.0498          50
   10.7463        43.2537          54
    9.55224       38.4478          48
    9.75124       39.2488          49

Chi-Square, (95%) = 7.815    3 d.f.
Chi-Square, Calc. = 8.969    Significant

Report: <P>rint, <S>ave, or <V>iew? <ENTER>
```

Computer Report

```
                            <42> Chi-Square Test
                Pharmacologic Calculation System - Version 4.0 - 03/13/86

    File name:         NAUSEA      NONAUSEA
  ------------    ------------  ------------
        # 1:             15            35
        # 2:             14            40
        # 3:              6            42
        # 4:              5            44

Expected Frequencies:

    NAUSEA        NONAUSEA        Totals
  ------------  ------------   ------------
    9.95025       40.0498          50
   10.7463        43.2537          54
    9.55224       38.4478          48
    9.75124       39.2488          49

Chi-Square, (95%) = 7.815    3 d.f.
Chi-Square, Calc. = 8.969    Significant
```

The computation of x^2 should be modified in situations in which $r = 2$ and $c = 2$ to the following:

$$x^2 = \sum_{i=1}^{4} \frac{(|o_i - e_i| - 1/2)^2}{e_i}$$ (42.2)

that is, one-half is subtracted from the absolute value of the difference between each "observed" and "expected" value. It is noteworthy that Equation (42.2) may be used when it is desired to compare two proportions and the sample sizes are small. (See also Procedure 43.)

Example 2

It is desired to compare the proportions 12/22 and 6/26. This yields the 2×2 table below:

Table 42.2

12	6
10	20
22	26

When expected numbers are placed (in parentheses) next to each entry we obtain Table 42.3.

Table 42.3

12	(8.25)	6	(9.75)
12	(13.75)	20	(16.25)

Calculation of x^2 from Equation (42.2) leads to $x^2 = 3.78$. The tabular value (for one degree of freedom) and 95% is 3.84. Hence, the proportions are *not* significantly different. (Note: application of the usual formula (Eq. 42.1) leads to $x^2 = 5.03$ and would suggest a significant difference at the 0.05 level.)

Computer Screen

```
                         <42> Chi-Square Test
               Pharmacologic Calculation System - Version 4.0 - 03/13/86

     Each data file represents a 'Row' in the contingency table. Since data values
     across all rows represent a 'Column' in the contingency table, n's for each
     file (Row) must be equal.

     Input: <K>eyboard, <D>isk, or <E>xit this procedure? K

     You may enter 5 'Y' data files. Type 'END' after last file. Enter file name or
     <ENTER> for default name:
     'FILE1/Y' (or 'END') ? PROP1<ENTER>

     You may enter up to 15 observations. Press <ENTER> after the last entry.
         File name:          PROP1
     ------------        ------------
           # 1:  12<ENTER>
           # 2:  10<ENTER>
           # 3:  <ENTER>

     'FILE2/Y' (or 'END') ? PROP2<ENTER>
```

```
You may enter up to 15 observations. Press <ENTER> after the last entry.
  File name:          PROP2
  ------------  ------------
      # 1:  6<ENTER>
      # 2:  20<ENTER>
      # 3:  <ENTER>


'FILE3/Y' (or 'END') ?  END<ENTER>

Data: <E>dit, <L>ist, <S>ave, or <ENTER> to continue?  L

  File name:          PROP1         PROP2
  ------------  ------------  ------------
      # 1:          12             6
      # 2:          10            20

Data: <E>dit, <L>ist, <S>ave, or <ENTER> to continue?  <ENTER>
```

```
2 x 2 contingency table (using adjusted chi-square).

Expected Frequencies:

        PROP1         PROP2         Totals
   ------------  ------------  ------------
       8.25          9.75            18
      13.75         16.25            30

Chi-Square, (95%) = 3.841     1 d.f.
Chi-Square, Calc. = 3.782   Not Significant

Report: <P>rint, <S>ave, or <V>iew?  <ENTER>
```

Computer Report

```
                        <42> Chi-Square Test
             Pharmacologic Calculation System - Version 4.0 - 03/13/86

  File name:          PROP1         PROP2
  ------------  ------------  ------------
      # 1:          12             6
      # 2:          10            20

2 x 2 contingency table (using adjusted chi-square).

Expected Frequencies:

        PROP1         PROP2         Totals
   ------------  ------------  ------------
       8.25          9.75            18
      13.75         16.25            30

Chi-Square, (95%) = 3.841     1 d.f.
Chi-Square, Calc. = 3.782   Not Significant
```

Procedure 43

Proportions: Confidence Limits

If N animals (or subjects) are treated and m of these respond to the treatment, an estimate of the proportion of the population that respond is $p = m/N$. (The percent response is $p \times 100$). For very large N, the standard error of the proportion p is given by $\sqrt{p \cdot q/N}$, where $q = 1 - p$. Confidence limits of the proportion are

$$p \pm 2 \cdot \sqrt{p \cdot q/N} \qquad (43.1)$$

where z has the value 1.96 for 95% confidence or 2.58 for 99%.

Moderate values of N, say Np and Nq at least 5, require the more precise estimate of confidence limits:

$$N/(N + z^2)\{p - 1/2N + z^2/2N - z \cdot \sqrt{R_1}\} \qquad (43.2)$$

and

$$N/(N + z^2)\{p + 1/2N + z^2/2N + z \cdot \sqrt{R_2}\} \qquad (43.3)$$

where

$$R_1 = (p + 1/2N)(1 - p - 1/2N)/N + z^2/4N^2 \qquad (43.4)$$

and

$$R_2 = (p - 1/2N)(1 - p + 1/2N)/N + z^2/4N^2 \qquad (43.5)$$

When two proportions are to be compared the *adjusted chi-square test* (Procedure 42) may be used.

Example

Among 30 animals tested with a test dose of an experimental analgesic, 12 demonstrated appreciable analgesia. Confidence limits (95%) for the proportion estimated as $12/30 = 0.40$ are computed as follows:

$$R_1 = (0.40 + 1/60)(0.60 - 1/60)/30 + 1.96^2/4(30)^2$$
$$= (0.41667)(0.5833)/30 + 0.00107 = 0.00917$$

$$R_2 = (0.40 - 1/60)(0.60 + 1/60)/30 + 1.96^2/4(30)^2$$
$$= (0.3833)(0.6167)/30 + 0.00107 = 0.00895$$

Confidence limits are

$$30/(30 + 1.96^2)\{0.40 - 1/60 + 1.96^2/60 - 1.96 \cdot \sqrt{0.00917}\}$$
$$= 0.886\{0.40 - 0.0167 + 0.0640 - 1.96(0.0958)\}$$
$$= 0.2299$$

and

$$30/(30 + 1.96^2)\{0.40 + 0.0167 + 0.0640 + 1.96 \cdot \sqrt{0.00895}\}$$
$$= 0.886\{0.666\}$$
$$= 0.590$$

Thus, the proportion is 0.40 with 95% confidence limits 0.23 to 0.59.

Computer Screen

```
                    <43> Proportions: Confidence Limits
             Pharmacologic Calculation System - Version 4.0 - 03/13/86

Number of subjects exhibiting the effect ? 12<ENTER>
Enter the total number of subjects ? 30<ENTER>

Number of subjects showing effect = 12
Total number of subjects         = 30

   Proportion    95% C.L.:        Lower         Upper
   -----------   ---------     ----------    ----------
        .4                       .230203       .590472

Report: <P>rint, <S>ave, or <V>iew? <ENTER>
```

Computer Report

```
                    <43> Proportions: Confidence Limits
             Pharmacologic Calculation System - Version 4.0 - 03/13/86

Number of subjects showing effect = 12
Total number of subjects          = 30

   Proportion    95% C.L.:        Lower         Upper
   -----------   ---------     ----------    ----------
        .4                       .230203       .590472
```

Procedure 44

Dunnett's Test (Comparison with a Control)

An experimenter frequently wishes to compare the mean of some control group with that of another group. Methods for doing this are presented in Procedures 39, 40, and 42. When there are *several* (p) groups, and the comparison is between each of these p means and the *control mean*, we may use the Dunnett test. Analysis of variance* may be used in this case also, but it may result in confidence limits that are wider than necessary.

Table 44.1 illustrates the notation. For example, there are N_0 items in the control group; these are denoted $X_{01}, X_{02}, \ldots, X_{0N_0}$. There are N_1 items in group 1, N_2 items in group 2, $\ldots$, N_p items in group p. The totals are denoted T_0 for the control group, T_1 for group 1, etc. The mean values are written $\overline{X}_0$, $\overline{X}_1, \ldots, \overline{X}_p$.

We must first estimate the variance of the $p + 1$ sets of observations.

---

* Procedure 33.

Table 44.1
Comparison with a Control

| | Control | Treatment number | | | | |
		1	2	3	$\cdots$	p
	X_{01}	X_{11}	X_{21}	X_{31}	$\cdots$	X_{p1}
	X_{02}	X_{12}	X_{22}	X_{32}	$\cdots$	X_{p2}
	$\vdots$	$\vdots$	$\vdots$	$\vdots$		$\vdots$
	X_{0N_0}	X_{1N_1}	X_{2N_2}	X_{3N_3}	$\cdots$	X_{pN_p}
Totals:	T_0	T_1	T_2	T_3	$\cdots$	T_p
N:	N_0	N_1	N_2	N_3	$\cdots$	N_p
Means:	$\overline{X}_0$	$\overline{X}_1$	$\overline{X}_2$	$\overline{X}_3$	$\cdots$	$\overline{X}_p$

The within-group sum of squares, s^2, is taken as an independent estimate of the common variance of the $(p + 1)$ sets of observations. Thus, s^2 is given by

$$s^2 = \frac{\sum_{i=1}^{N_0} (X_{0i} - \overline{X}_0)^2 + \sum_{i=1}^{N_1} (X_{1i} - \overline{X}_1)^2 + \cdots + \sum_{i=1}^{N_p} (X_{pi} - \overline{X}_p)^2}{(N_0 + N_1 + \cdots + N_p) - (p + 1)}.$$

(44.1)

The above is more simply computed by summing the squares of all the observations and subtracting each group sum squared divided by the number in the group:

$$s^2 = \frac{\sum_{i=0}^{p} \sum_{j=1}^{N_i} X_{ij}^2 - (T_0^2/N_0) - (T_1^2/N_1) - \cdots - (T_p^2/N_p)}{(N_0 + N_1 + \cdots + N_p) - (p + 1)}.$$

(44.2)

Confidence limits for the difference between each group mean $\overline{X}_j$ and the control group mean $\overline{X}_0$ are obtained by adding and subtracting a quantity designated A as defined below; thus,

$$(\overline{X}_j - \overline{X}_0) \pm A,$$

where A is given by

$$A = (s)(d)\sqrt{\frac{1}{N_j} + \frac{1}{N_0}}.$$

(44.3)

The constant d is taken from tables in which the desired probability, usually $P = 95\%$ or $P = 99\%$ is specified. The number of degrees of freedom is $(N_0 + N_1 + \cdots + N_p) - (p + 1)$.

Two tables are used (Tables A-9), one for $P = 95\%$ and the other for $P = 99\%$.

Example

In an experiment on isolated vascular smooth muscle strips, an agonist drug in concentration 10^{-9} M was given to four strips and produced tensions (in g) as given in column one of the table below. Two higher concentrations (10^{-8} and 10^{-7} M)

were used in order to determine whether the magnitude of the tension was dose-related. These tensions are given in columns 2 and 3.

	Dose 1	Dose 2	Dose 3
	2.8	3.6	4.0
	3.9	3.9	4.5
	2.7	4.3	5.2
	3.2	4.8	3.9
Totals:	12.6	16.6	17.6
N:	4	4	4
Means:	3.15	4.15	4.40

From Equation (44.2)

$$s^2 = \frac{(2.8)^2 + (3.9)^2 + \cdots + (5.2)^2 + (3.9)^2 - (12.6)^2/4 - (16.6)^2/4 - (17.6)^2/4}{(4 + 4 + 4) - (2 + 1)}$$

$$s^2 = \frac{188.8 - 39.7 - 68.9 - 77.4}{9}$$

$$s^2 = 0.31,$$

and

$$s = 0.55.$$

The degrees of freedom are 9. Two-sided limits for $p = 2$ and 95% give $d = 2.61$. Thus, A is computed by Equation (44.3)

$$(0.55)(2.61) \times \sqrt{\tfrac{1}{4} + \tfrac{1}{4}} = 1.02.$$

It may be concluded that the mean response for dose 2, namely, 4.15, exceeds the mean response for dose 1, namely, 3.15, by an amount between

$$(4.15 - 3.15) \pm 1.02 = -0.022 \quad \text{and} \quad 2.02 \text{ g.}$$

The reader may show that the mean response for dose 3, namely, 4.40, exceeds the mean response for dose 1 by an amount between 0.228 and 2.27.

Computer Screen

```
                          <44> Dunnett's Test
             Pharmacologic Calculation System - Version 4.0 - 03/13/86

Input: <K>eyboard, <D>isk, or <E>xit this procedure? D

You may enter 5 'Y' data files. Press <ENTER> after last file name.
File name 1 ? DOSE1<ENTER>
File name 2 ? DOSE2<ENTER>
File name 3 ? DOSE3<ENTER>
File name 4 ? <ENTER>

Data: <E>dit, <L>ist, <S>ave, or <ENTER> to continue? L

     File name:       DOSE1         DOSE2         DOSE3
    --------------  -----------   -----------   -----------
        # 1:           2.8           3.6            4
        # 2:           3.9           3.9           4.5
        # 3:           2.7           4.3           5.2
        # 4:           3.2           4.8           3.9

Data: <E>dit, <L>ist, <S>ave, or <ENTER> to continue? <ENTER>
```

```
     File name:        DOSE1          DOSE2          DOSE3
  ------------    ------------   ------------   ------------
          N:              4              4              4
    Minimum:            2.7            3.6            3.9
       Mean:           3.15           4.15            4.4
    Maximum:            3.9            4.8            5.2
        Sum:           12.6           16.6           17.6
  Std. Dev.:        .544671        .519615        .594419
  Std. Err.:        .272336        .259808        .297209
   95% C.L.:        .866572        .826708         .94572


  S2 = .306668      S = .553776      P = 2

  Enter A.9 Table value for 2 treatments and 9 d.f. ? 2.61
  A.9 Table value for 2 treatments and 9 d.f. =  2.61

  'DOSE1' vs. 'DOSE2':    A = 1.02202

  Mean of 'DOSE2' differs from the mean of 'DOSE1'
  by an amount between: -.0220205 and 2.02202.
```

```
  'DOSE1' vs. 'DOSE3':    A = 1.02202

  Mean of 'DOSE3' differs from the mean of 'DOSE1'
  by an amount between:  .22798 and 2.27202.
```

```
  Report: <P>rint, <S>ave, or <V>iew? <ENTER>
```

Computer Report

```
                                     <44> Dunnett's Test
                  Pharmacologic Calculation System - Version 4.0 - 03/13/86

     File name:        DOSE1          DOSE2          DOSE3
  ------------    ------------   ------------   ------------
        # 1:             2.8            3.6              4
        # 2:             3.9            3.9            4.5
        # 3:             2.7            4.3            5.2
        # 4:             3.2            4.8            3.9

     File name:        DOSE1          DOSE2          DOSE3
  ------------    ------------   ------------   ------------
          N:              4              4              4
    Minimum:            2.7            3.6            3.9
       Mean:           3.15           4.15            4.4
    Maximum:            3.9            4.8            5.2
        Sum:           12.6           16.6           17.6
  Std. Dev.:        .544671        .519615        .594419
  Std. Err.:        .272336        .259808        .297209
   95% C.L.:        .866572        .826708         .94572


  S2 = .306668      S = .553776      P = 2

  A.9 Table value for 2 treatments and 9 d.f. =  2.61

  'DOSE1' vs. 'DOSE2':    A = 1.02202

  Mean of 'DOSE2' differs from the mean of 'DOSE1'
  by an amount between: -.0220205 and 2.02202.


  'DOSE1' vs. 'DOSE3':    A = 1.02202

  Mean of 'DOSE3' differs from the mean of 'DOSE1'
  by an amount between:  .22798 and 2.27202.
```

Procedure 45

Mann–Whitney Test

When two groups are drawn from populations that are normally distributed, the methods of Procedures 39 and 40 are used to determine whether the groups are drawn from the same or from different populations; in other words, is there a significant difference between the means of each group? When we have no knowledge of the distribution, different methods are used to determine whether the samples are drawn from the same or from different populations. In pharmacologic work the groups are usually a control group and a drug-treated group.

One of the most important of these *nonparametric* tests is the Mann–Whitney test. This test is particularly useful when behavioral effects are being studied.* The objective is to determine whether there is a significant difference in the distributions of the two groups based upon the ranking of scores from both groups.

For unequal sample sizes, we denote by n_1 the number of items in the smaller group and by n_2 the number of items in the larger. The values, or scores, from both groups are arranged in a sequence in increasing order. Ranks are assigned to each value—rank 1 to the smallest, rank 2 to the next, etc. For example, suppose the scores of the two groups are (1, 7, 9, 15) and (3, 8, 11, 18, 27). The combined array is shown below along with the ranks. The scores of group 1 are underlined for convenience.

$$\begin{array}{lcccccccccc} \text{Score:} & \underline{1} & 3 & \underline{7} & 8 & \underline{9} & 11 & \underline{15} & 18 & 27 \\ \text{Rank:} & 1 & 2 & 3 & 4 & 5 & 6 & 7 & 8 & 9 \end{array}$$

The sums of the ranks are denoted R_1 and R_2. Thus,

$$R_1 = 1 + 3 + 5 + 7 = 16$$

and

$$R_2 = 2 + 4 + 6 + 8 + 9 = 29.$$

The statistic U is computed as the smaller of U_1 and U_2, where

$$U_1 = n_1 n_2 + \frac{n_1(n_1 + 1)}{2} - R_1 \tag{45.1}$$

and

$$U_2 = n_1 n_2 + \frac{n_2(n_2 + 1)}{2} - R_2. \tag{45.2}$$

The significance of the difference of the distributions is determined from the values of n_1, n_2, and U by the use of tables. The choice of tables depends on the values of n_1 and n_2. Two cases are considered.

---

* For example, see Baldino, F., Cowan, A., Geller, E. B., and Adler, M. W. *J. Pharmacol. Exp. Therap.* **208**:63, 1979.

Case 1

Neither n_1 nor n_2 is larger than 8. Tables A.10a are used to determine the probability that both groups have the same distribution. The tables contain the probabilities p that the samples are drawn from populations with the same distribution. Thus, a small value of p, say $p < 0.05$, is required to show a difference.

Case 2

When n_2 is greater than 8, Tables A.10b are used. These give critical values of U for the various significance (p) levels. For a particular pair, n_1, n_2, if the computed U is less than or equal to the tabular value, the difference is significant.

Example 1

For the data given above, we have $n_1 = 4, n_2 = 5, R_1 = 16$, and $R_2 = 29$. Compute U and, thus, determine p.

From Equation (45.1), $U_1 = (4)(5) + (4)(5)/(2) - 16 = 14$. From Equation (45.2), $U_2 = (4)(5) + (5)(6)/(2) - 29 = 6$. Thus, $U = 6$. From Table A.10a, $p = 0.206$. Therefore, we cannot conclude that there is a significant difference.

When scores are tied these are assigned the average of the tied ranks. In such cases the value of U may not be an integer, and interpolation is necessary in using the tables.

Computer Screen

```
                    <45> Mann-Whitney U-Test
         Pharmacologic Calculation System - Version 4.0 - 03/13/86

Enter the sample with the smallest n first.

Input: <K>eyboard, <D>isk, or <E>xit this procedure? D

You may enter 2 'Y' data files. Press <ENTER> after last file name.
File name 1 ? GROUP1<ENTER>
File name 2 ? GROUP2<ENTER>

Data: <E>dit, <L>ist, <S>ave, or <ENTER> to continue? L

   File name:        GROUP1         GROUP2
   -----------    ------------   ------------
        # 1:            1             11
        # 2:            9              8
        # 3:            7              3
        # 4:           15             18
        # 5:                          27

Data: <E>dit, <L>ist, <S>ave, or <ENTER> to continue? <ENTER>
```

```
'GROUP1' Sorted:   1 7 9 15
'GROUP2' Sorted:   3 8 11 18 27

Sequence of ranks (members of 'GROUP1' are indicated with *)
 1* 2  3* 4  5* 6  7* 8  9

    File name:        GROUP1        GROUP2
  ------------  ------------  ------------
           N:         4             5
           R:        16            29
           U:        14             6

         N  =         5
         U  =         6

Report: <P>rint, <S>ave, or <V>iew? <ENTER>
```

Computer Report

```
                              <45> Mann-Whitney U-Test
                  Pharmacologic Calculation System - Version 4.0 - 03/13/86

    File name:        GROUP1        GROUP2
  ------------  ------------  ------------
        # 1:         1            11
        # 2:         9             8
        # 3:         7             3
        # 4:        15            18
        # 5:                      27

'GROUP1' Sorted:   1 7 9 15
'GROUP2' Sorted:   3 8 11 18 27

Sequence of ranks (members of 'GROUP1' are indicated with *)
 1* 2  3* 4  5* 6  7* 8  9

    File name:        GROUP1        GROUP2
  ------------  ------------  ------------
           N:         4             5
           R:        16            29
           U:        14             6

         N  =         5
         U  =         6
```

Example 2

Shaking behavior was studied in rats treated with 4 mg/kg of diazepam and gave the following scores: 3, 3, 4, 4, 5, 8, 9, 10, 12. Another group, receiving saline, gave the scores: 1, 2, 2, 3, 4, 5. Test for significance.

Using the average for tied ranks, we get the sequence of ranks

$$\underline{1} \quad \underline{2.5} \quad \underline{2.5} \quad \underline{5} \quad 5 \quad 5 \quad \underline{8} \quad 8 \quad 8 \quad \underline{10.5} \quad 10.5 \quad 12 \quad 13 \quad 14 \quad 15$$

in which the underlined items represent the ranks from the control (saline) group. Thus, $R_1 = 29.5$ and $R_2 = 90.5$. From Equations (45.1) and (45.2), $U_1 = 45.5$ and $U_2 = 8.5$; hence, $U = 8.5$. Since $n_2 = 9$, we must use Table A.10b. The critical value of U is seen to be 10. Thus, our computed $U = 8.5$ is indicative of significance in the two-tailed test at $p = 0.05$.

Computer Screen

```
                        <45> Mann-Whitney U-Test
              Pharmacologic Calculation System - Version 4.0 - 03/13/86

Enter the sample with the smallest n first.

Input: <K>eyboard, <D>isk, or <E>xit this procedure? D

You may enter 2 'Y' data files. Press <ENTER> after last file name.
File name 1 ? SALINE<ENTER>
File name 2 ? DIAZEPAM<ENTER>

Data: <E>dit, <L>ist, <S>ave, or <ENTER> to continue? L

    File name:        SALINE      DIAZEPAM
  ------------   ------------  ------------
        # 1:           2             8
        # 2:           5             9
        # 3:           1             3
        # 4:           3             4
        # 5:           4            12
        # 6:           2            10
        # 7:                         5
        # 8:                         4
        # 9:                         3
```

```
Data: <E>dit, <L>ist, <S>ave, or <ENTER> to continue? <ENTER>

'SALINE' Sorted:  1  2  2  3  4  5
'DIAZEPAM' Sorted:  3  3  4  4  5  8  9  10  12

Sequence of ranks (members of 'SALINE' are indicated with *)
 1* 2* 3* 5* 10   8* 16  10.5* 10.5  12  13  14  15

    File name:        SALINE      DIAZEPAM
  ------------   ------------  ------------
          N:           6             9
          R:          29.5          90.5
          U:          45.5           8.5

        N =           9
        U =          8.5

Report: <P>rint, <S>ave, or <V>iew? <ENTER>
```

Computer Report

```
                        <45> Mann-Whitney U-Test
              Pharmacologic Calculation System - Version 4.0 - 03/13/86

    File name:        SALINE      DIAZEPAM
  ------------   ------------  ------------
        # 1:           2             8
        # 2:           5             9
        # 3:           1             3
        # 4:           3             4
        # 5:           4            12
        # 6:           2            10
        # 7:                         5
        # 8:                         4
        # 9:                         3

'SALINE' Sorted:  1  2  2  3  4  5
'DIAZEPAM' Sorted:  3  3  4  4  5  8  9  10  12
```

```
Sequence of ranks (members of 'SALINE' are indicated with *)
  1* 2* 3* 5* 10  8* 16  10.5* 10.5  12  13  14  15

   File name:        SALINE      DIAZEPAM
  ------------    ------------  ------------
            N:            6             9
            R:         29.5          90.5
            U:         45.5           8.5

        N =            9
        U =          8.5
```

Procedure 46

Litchfield and Wilcoxon I: Confidence Limits of ED50

The use of the probit conversion for drawing smooth quantal log dose–effect curves was discussed in Procedure 9. Since there are no values of the probit corresponding to 0 and 100 % effects the method of Procedure 9 does not handle such *complete* log dose–effect curves. The problem of analyzing such complete curves was addressed by Litchfield and Wilcoxon* who gave a method for "correcting" the 0 and 100 % effects. Although their method preceded the widespread use of calculators and computers, it is still widely used for determining ED50 and its 95 % confidence limits.

Figure 46.1 illustrates the method of correction for 0 and 100 % effects. The upper panel shows a plot of the actual effect as percent of animals responding versus log dose. These values are plotted as circles: open circles for intermediate points, filled circles for the 0 and 100% points, and triangles for "corrected" values corresponding to 0 and 100%. These corrections are made as follows:

1. Convert the intermediate effects ($\bigcirc$) to probits from Table A.3.
2. Find the regression line of probits versus log dose, using only the intermediate points. These points are shown as squares in the bottom panel of the figure.
3. From the regression line locate the probit values (X) corresponding to log doses that produced each 0 or 100% effect.
4. Convert the probit values (X) to percent using Table A.3. These are the "expected" percent effects. If any values are greater than 99.99 % or less than 0.01 % delete them.
5. Use Table A.12 to convert these expected 0 and 100 % effects into "corrected" percent effects. The latter are then plotted as triangles in the upper panel and, together with the other observed points, constitute the observed effects for the remainder of the analysis. Not more than two 0 % points or two 100 % points are plotted.

---

* Litchfield, J. T. and Wilcoxon, F. *J. Pharmacol. Exp. Ther.* **96**:99, 1949.

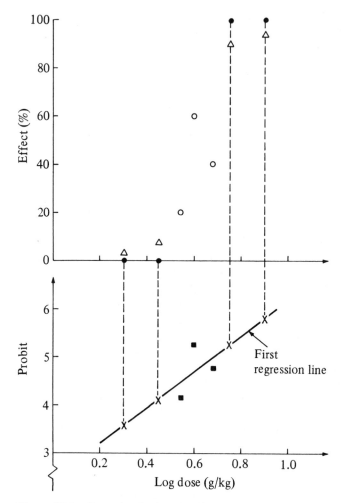

Figure 46.1   Correction for 0 and 100% effects.

Example

The graphs of Figure 46.1 were constructed from the dose–effect data shown in columns (1) and (2) of Table 46.1. The ratio of the number of animals responding to the number tested from which percent is computed is given in parenthesis in column (2). The items of column (3) and (4) in the box were used to compute the regression line of probit versus log dose from which the probit values of column (5) were determined. The "corrected" observed effects, given in parentheses in column (7), were obtained from the adjacent items in column (6) and Table A.12.

It is then necessary to compute χ^2. To do this, the observed (or corrected) effect (column 7) versus log doses (column 3) is plotted and smoothed using probits, as described in Procedure 9. Thus, each entry in column (7) is converted to probits and a

Table 46.1

(1)	(2)	(3)	(4)	(5)	(6)	(7)
					Expected	
			Probit		effect	Observed effect
Dose	Effect		from col. (2)	Probit	from col. (5)	or
(g/kg)	(%)	log dose	and Table A.3	from line	and Table A.3	(corrected effect)
2.0	0 (0/5)	0.301		3.59	8	(2.6)
2.8	0 (0/5)	0.447		4.13	19	(5.7)
3.5	20 (1/5)	0.544	4.16	4.48	30	20
4.0	60 (3/5)	0.602	5.25	4.69	38	60
4.8	40 (2/5)	0.681	4.75	4.98	49	40
5.6	100 (5/5)	0.748		5.23	59	(90.0)
8.0	100 (5/5)	0.903		5.79	79	(93.8)

second regression line is obtained. This is illustrated in Table 46.2 below which begins with column (7) of the previous table and contains the values of log dose again in column (8). The entries of column (7) are converted to probits and listed in column (9). Linear regression of probit (9) against log dose (8) yields the values of the corrected probit listed in column (10). The regression line is shown in Figure 46.2a. The probits of column (10) are converted to percent effect and listed in column (11) as expected effect and plotted as the curve of Figure 46.2b. Column (12) lists the contribution to χ^2 for each dose. There are denoted g_i, where $g_i = (o_i - e_i)^2/(e_i)(100 - e_i)$.

To determine χ^2 the g_i are summed and multiplied by the total number of animals/number of doses. In the example, this multiplier is $(35/7) = 5$. Thus,

$$\chi^2 = (5)(\textstyle\sum g_i) = 2.58.$$

Table 46.2

(7)	(8)	(9)	(10)	(11)	(12)
Observed effect				Expected	
(o_i) or			Corrected	effect	
(corrected effect)	log dose	Probit*	probit	(e_i)	g_i
(%)					
(2.6)	0.301	3.12	2.88	2	0.002
(5.7)	0.447	3.45	3.80	12	0.038
20	0.544	4.16	4.42	28	0.032
60	0.602	5.25	4.78	41	0.149
40	0.681	4.75	5.28	61	0.185
(90.0)	0.748	6.28	5.70	76	0.107
(93.8)	0.903	6.55	6.69	95	0.003
					$\sum g_i = 0.516$

* Probit derived from rounded values in column (7) and Table A.3.

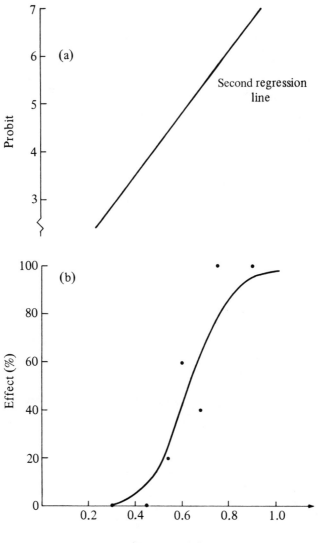

Figure 46.2   (a) Expected probit. (b) Expected percent effect curve is shown with original (uncorrected) observed points.

The degrees of freedom n for χ^2 is two less than the number of doses plotted; thus, $n = 7 - 2 = 5$. The computed value of χ^2 is compared to that given Table A.8. In the example, the tabular value is 11.07. When the computed χ^2 is less than the tabular value as in this example, the data are not heterogeneous, meaning that the curve is a good fit. On the other hand if χ^2 is greater than the tabular value, Student's t should be noted from Table A.2 for subsequent use.

A parameter called the slope function S is calculated from the doses that produce 16%, 50%, and 84% expected effects. These are denoted ED16, ED50, and ED84, respectively, and are determined from Figure 46.2b. The log doses for each of these is, in our example, 0.48, 0.64, 0.79. Thus, ED16 = 3.0, ED50 = 4.3, and ED84 = 6.2. S is defined by the equation

$$S = \frac{ED84/ED50 + ED50/ED16}{2}.$$
(46.1)

In our example,

$$S = \frac{6.2/4.3 + 4.3/3.0}{2} = 1.44.$$

In order to determine the 95% confidence limits of the ED50 it is necessary to determine a factor f_{ED50}. This value is determined by either of two formulas, depending on the results of the χ^2-test determined previously.

1. If χ^2 computed $< \chi^2$ tabular, then

$$f_{ED50} = S^{2.77/\sqrt{N'}},$$
(46.2)

where N' = total number of animals used between 16 and 84% expected effects (see column 11).
2. If χ^2 computed $> \chi^2$ tabular, then

$$f_{ED50} = S^{1.4t\sqrt{\chi^2/nN'}},$$
(46.3)

where t is the value of student's distribution for n degrees of freedom determined from Table A.2. In the example, Equation (46.2) is used and $N' = 20$; thus

$$f_{ED50} = 1.44^{2.77/\sqrt{20}} = 1.25.$$

The upper and lower 95% limits of the ED50 are given by

$$\text{upper} = ED50 \times f_{ED50}$$
(46.4)

and

$$\text{lower} = ED50/f_{ED50}.$$
(46.5)

In our example, these values are

$$\text{upper} = 4.3 \times 1.25 = 5.4 \text{ g/kg}$$

and

$$\text{lower} = 4.3/1.25 = 3.5 \text{ g/kg}.$$

Therefore, the ED50 and 95% confidence limits are 4.3 (3.5–5.4) g/kg.

The computation is lengthy. In their original paper the authors used nomographs to aid in the calculation, and they relied on approximate methods for fitting the regression lines. The nomographs are not needed if one uses an electronic calculator for the computations and for finding the regression lines. The computer program is particularly useful in this analysis.

Computer Screen

```
              <46> Litchfield & Wilcoxon I: Confidence Limits of ED50
              Pharmacologic Calculation System - Version 4.0 - 03/12/86

  You will be entering # Responding and # in Group, not percent responding.

  Do not enter more than two 0% and two 100% points for each curve.

  Input: <K>eyboard, <D>isk, or <E>xit this procedure? D

  File name: ? LINE1<ENTER>

  Data: <E>dit, <L>ist, <S>ave, or <ENTER> to continue? L

      File name:          LINE1
       Variable:          Dose # Responding   # in Group
      ------------   ------------ ------------ ------------
          # 1:            2             0            5
          # 2:            2.8           0            5
          # 3:            3.5           1            5
          # 4:            4             3            5
          # 5:            4.8           2            5
          # 6:            5.6           5            5
          # 7:            8             5            5

  Data: <E>dit, <L>ist, <S>ave, or <ENTER> to continue? <ENTER>
```

```
  Do you want to show intermediate results (Y/N) ? N

  (1) Probit =  3.66044 * Log(Dose) + 2.48986

  (2) Probit =  6.40096 * Log(Dose) + .914091

  Total number of animals used = 35
  Animals between ED16 & ED84  = 20

  Chi-Square for 5 d.f.      = 11.07
  Chi-Square, calculated     = 2.56221

          LINE1          Value    95% Limits:   Lower C.L.   Upper C.L.
      ------------   ------------             ------------ ------------
          ED50        4.34838                    3.48413      5.42702


       Log(ED50)      .638328                     .542095      .734561

  Report: <P>rint, <S>ave, or <V>iew? <ENTER>
```

Computer Report

```
              <46> Litchfield & Wilcoxon I: Confidence Limits of ED50
              Pharmacologic Calculation System - Version 4.0 - 03/12/86

      File name:          LINE1
       Variable:          Dose # Responding   # in Group
      ------------   ------------ ------------ ------------
          # 1:            2             0            5
          # 2:            2.8           0            5
          # 3:            3.5           1            5
          # 4:            4             3            5
          # 5:            4.8           2            5
          # 6:            5.6           5            5
          # 7:            8             5            5

  (1) Probit =  3.66044 * Log(Dose) + 2.48986

  (2) Probit =  6.40096 * Log(Dose) + .914091
```

```
Total number of animals used = 35
Animals between ED16 & ED84  = 20

Chi-Square for 5 d.f.        = 11.07
Chi-Square, calculated       = 2.56221
```

	LINE1	Value	95% Limits:	Lower C.L.	Upper C.L.
	ED50	4.34838		3.48413	5.42702
	Log(ED50)	.638328		.542095	.734561

Procedure 47
Litchfield and Wilcoxon II

Procedure 46 presented the methodology for estimating confidence limits of an ED50 from quantal dose-effect data. Discussed here is the computational technique used by Litchfield and Wilcoxon for (1) determining confidence limits for ED16 and ED84 doses and (2) determining the potency ratio (ED50$_1$/ED50$_2$) and confidence limits for drugs 1 and 2 from the quantal dose-effect data of each.

ED16 and ED84.

As in Procedure 46 the computation of confidence limits requires values of the slope function, S, and x^2 from the regression line. Additionally, we must compute a factor f_s that depends on the value of x^2 and other parameters as described below.

1. Let R = largest dose/smallest dose
2. Compute A from the equation

$$A = 10^\beta, \tag{47.1}$$

where

$$\beta = 1.1(\log S)^2/(\log R) \tag{47.2}$$

3. Compute f_s according to either of the following, depending on x^2 (all symbols are the same as in Procedure 46 and K = number of doses plotted.)

$$f_s = \begin{cases} A^{10(k-1)/k\sqrt{N'}} & \text{if } x^2 \leq x_{table}^2 \\ \text{or} \\ A^{[5.1t(k-1)\sqrt{x^2/nN'}]/k} & \text{if } x^2 > x_{table}^2 \end{cases} \tag{47.3}$$

4. Compute f_{ED84} from

$$\log(f_{ED84}) = (\log f_s)^2 + (\log f_{ED50})^2 \tag{47.4}$$

5. Obtain upper and lower confidence limits of ED84 from

$$\text{upper} = \text{ED84} \times f_{\text{ED84}}$$
$$\text{lower} = \text{ED84}/f_{\text{ED84}} \tag{47.5}$$

6. Obtain upper and lower confidence limits of ED16 using a factor f_{ED16} that *is also equal to* f_{ED84}:

$$\text{upper} = \text{ED16} \times f_{\text{ED16}}$$
$$\text{lower} = \text{ED16}/f_{\text{ED16}} \tag{47.6}$$

The potency ratio for drugs 1 and 2 is the ratio of their ED50 values:

$$\text{PR} = \text{ED50}_{(1)}/\text{ED50}_{(2)} \tag{47.7}$$

Calculates a factor f_{PR} as follows:

$$f_{PR} = 10^{\gamma} \tag{47.8}$$

where

$$\gamma = \sqrt{(\log f_{\text{ED50}_1})^2 + (\log f_{\text{ED50}_2})^2}. \tag{47.9}$$

Confidence limits of the potency ratio are denoted $(PR)_{\text{upper}}$ and $(PR)_{\text{lower}}$, where

$$(PR)_{\text{upper}} = PR \times f_{PR}$$
$$(PR)_{\text{lower}} = PR/f_{PR} \tag{47.10}$$

When $(PR)_{\text{lower}}$ is greater than one, the ratio is significant.

Example

The percentage of animals showing a response to test doses of two drugs are given below along with values calculated from Procedure 46. It is desired to obtain confidence limits for the ED16 and ED84 doses of each and for the potency ratio.

	DRUG #1			DRUG #2	
Dose	Percent responders	(Fraction responding)	Dose	Percent responders	(Fraction responding)
1	0	(0/5)	0.01	0	(0/5)
2	20	(1/5)	0.05	20	(1/5)
4	25	(2/8)	0.10	20	(1/5)
8	60	(3/5)	0.25	60	(3/5)
16	75	(6/8)	0.50	80	(4/5)
32	100	(5/5)	1.00	100	(5/5)

$$x^2_{(calculated)} = 0.801 \qquad x^2_{(calculated)} = 0.720$$
$$x^2_{4,95\%} = 9.49 \qquad x^2_{4,95\%} = 9.49$$
$$ED16 = 2.449 \qquad ED16 = 0.0615$$
$$ED50 = 6.477 \qquad ED50 = 0.1746$$
$$ED84 = 17.13 \qquad ED84 = 0.4955$$
$$S = 2.64 \qquad S = 2.84$$
$$N' = 21 \qquad N' = 10$$
$$K = 6 \qquad K = 6$$
$$f_{ED50} = 1.80 \qquad f_{ED50} = 2.49$$

conf. limits of ED50: 3.60 to 11.7   conf. limits of ED50: 0.070 to 0.435

For drug #1 we compute confidence limits (95%) for ED16 and ED84:

$$R = 32/1 = 32$$

and $\beta = 1.1(\log\ 2.64)^2/\log\ 32 = 1.1 \times (0.422)^2/1.51 = 0.130$, so that $A = 10^{0.130} = 1.35$.

The quantity f_s is computed using A, determined above, and $K = 6$, $N' = 21$, according to

$$f_s = 1.35^{(10)(5)/6\sqrt{21}} = 1.35^{1.82} = 1.73.$$

These permit the computation of $\log(f_{ED84})$:

$$\log(f_{ED84}) = [\log(1.73)]^2 + [\log(1.80)]^2$$
$$= 0.0567 + 0.0651$$
$$= 0.122,$$

so that $f_{ED84} = 1.32$ (which is also f_{ED16}).

The upper and lower confidence limits for ED84 are 13.0 to 22.6, while for ED16, these are 1.86 to 3.23.

For drug #2

$R = 1/0.01 = 100$ and $\beta = 1.1[\log(2.84)]^2/\log(100) = 0.113$ so that $A = 10^\beta = 10^{0.113} = 1.30$. Also,

$$f_s = A^{(10)(5)/6\sqrt{10}} = A^{2.64} = (1.30)^{2.64} = 2.00.$$

Thus, $\log(f_{ED84}) = (\log 2.00)^2 + (\log 2.494)^2$
$$= 0.0906 + 0.158 = 0.249$$

and

$$f_{ED84} = 10^{0.249} = 1.77. \text{ (Also } = f_{ED16}).$$

From ED84 = 0.496, we get confidence limits 0.280 to 0.873.
From ED16 = 0.0615, confidence limits are 0.0347 to 0.109.

The potency ratio, $PR = 6.477/0.1746 = 37.1$. Confidence limits require computation of $f_{PR} = 10^\gamma$, where

$$\gamma = \sqrt{(\log 1.80)^2 + (\log 2.49)^2}$$
$$= 0.471$$

Thus $f_{PR} = 10^{0.471} = 2.96$, so that confidence limits of *PR* are 12.5 to 110!

Computer Screen

```
                    <47> Litchfield & Wilcoxon II
              Pharmacologic Calculation System - Version 4.0 - 03/12/86

This procedure takes a quantal d-r curve and calculates ED16, ED50, and ED85,
and associated confidence limits.  You may then enter a 2nd curve to get a
potency ratio with confidence limits.

You will be entering # Responding and # in Group, not percent responding.

Do not enter more than two 0% and two 100% points for each curve.

Input: <K>eyboard, <D>isk, or <E>xit this procedure? D

File name: ? DRUG1<ENTER>

Data: <E>dit, <L>ist, <S>ave, or <ENTER> to continue? L

       File name:          DRUG1
       Variable:          Dose # Responding   # in Group
      ------------ ------------- ------------- ------------
         # 1:           1             0             5
         # 2:           2             1             5
         # 3:           4             2             8
         # 4:           8             3             5
         # 5:          16             6             8
         # 6:          32             5             5
```

```
Data: <E>dit, <L>ist, <S>ave, or <ENTER> to continue? <ENTER>

Do you want to show intermediate results (Y/N) ? N

 (1) Probit =  1.81845 * Log(Dose) + 3.48435

 (2) Probit =  2.35445 * Log(Dose) + 3.0897

Total number of animals used = 36
Animals between ED16 & ED84  = 21

Chi-Square for 4 d.f.        = 9.488
Chi-Square, calculated       = .800609

          DRUG1        Value  95% Limits:   Lower C.L.   Upper C.L.
      ------------ ------------- ------------ ------------
          ED16       2.44886                  1.85163      3.23874
          ED50       6.47675                  3.59779      11.6594
          ED84      17.1297                   12.952       22.6548

       Log(ED16)     .388965                  .267554      .510376
       Log(ED50)     .811357                  .556036      1.06668
       Log(ED84)    1.23375                   1.11234      1.35516

Do you want to compare the potency of 'DRUG1' with another quantal
dose-response curve (Y/N)? Y
```

```
Input: <K>eyboard, <D>isk, or <E>xit this procedure? D

File name: ? DRUG2<ENTER>

Data: <E>dit, <L>ist, <S>ave, or <ENTER> to continue? L

    File name:        DRUG2
    Variable:         Dose # Responding  # in Group
  ------------  ------------  ------------  ------------
        # 1:         .01           0             5
        # 2:         .05           1             5
        # 3:         .1            1             5
        # 4:         .25           3             5
        # 5:         .5            4             5
        # 6:         1             5             5

Data: <E>dit, <L>ist, <S>ave, or <ENTER> to continue? <ENTER>

Do you want to show intermediate results (Y/N) ? N

 (1) Probit =  1.82881 * Log(Dose) + 6.3178

 (2) Probit =  2.19512 * Log(Dose) + 6.66385
```

```
Total number of animals used = 30
Animals between ED16 & ED84  = 10

Chi-Square for 4 d.f.          = 9.488
Chi-Square, calculated         = .720339


          DRUG2        Value  95% Limits:  Lower C.L.   Upper C.L.
     ------------  ------------              ------------  ------------
          ED16       .0615137                .0349124      .108384
          ED50       .174591                 .070012       .435385
          ED84       .495534                 .281243       .873103

      Log(ED16)     -1.21103               -1.45702       -.965037
      Log(ED50)      -.757978              -1.15483        -.361127
      Log(ED84)      -.304926               -.550918       -.0589346

   Pot. Ratio:      37.0966                 12.5154        109.957

The Potency Ratio of DRUG1 versus DRUG2 is significant.

Do you want to compare the potency of 'DRUG1' with another quantal
dose-response curve (Y/N)? N


Report: <P>rint, <S>ave, or <V>iew? <ENTER>
```

Computer Report

```
                        <47> Litchfield & Wilcoxon II
             Pharmacologic Calculation System - Version 4.0 - 03/12/86

    File name:        DRUG1
    Variable:         Dose # Responding  # in Group
  ------------+-----  ------------  ------------  ------------
        # 1:          1             0             5
        # 2:          2             1             5
        # 3:          4             2             8
        # 4:          8             3             5
        # 5:         16             6             8
        # 6:         32             5             5

 (1) Probit =  1.81845 * Log(Dose) + 3.48435

 (2) Probit =  2.35445 * Log(Dose) + 3.0897
```

```
Total number of animals used = 36
Animals between ED16 & ED84   = 21

Chi-Square for 4 d.f.         = 9.488
Chi-Square, calculated        = .800609
```

DRUG1	Value	95% Limits:	Lower C.L.	Upper C.L.
ED16	2.44886		1.85163	3.23874
ED50	6.47675		3.59779	11.6594
ED84	17.1297		12.952	22.6548
Log(ED16)	.388965		.267554	.510376
Log(ED50)	.811357		.556036	1.06668
Log(ED84)	1.23375		1.11234	1.35516

File name:	DRUG2		
Variable:	Dose	# Responding	# in Group
# 1:	.01	0	5
# 2:	.05	1	5
# 3:	.1	1	5
# 4:	.25	3	5
# 5:	.5	4	5
# 6:	1	5	5

(1) Probit = 1.82881 * Log(Dose) + 6.3178

(2) Probit = 2.19512 * Log(Dose) + 6.66385

```
Total number of animals used = 30
Animals between ED16 & ED84   = 10

Chi-Square for 4 d.f.         = 9.488
Chi-Square, calculated        = .720339
```

DRUG2	Value	95% Limits:	Lower C.L.	Upper C.L.
ED16	.0615137		.0349124	.108384
ED50	.174591		.070012	.435385
ED84	.495534		.281243	.873103
Log(ED16)	-1.21103		-1.45702	-.965037
Log(ED50)	-.757978		-1.15483	-.361127
Log(ED84)	-.304926		-.550918	-.0589346
Pot. Ratio:	37.0966		12.5154	109.957

The Potency Ratio of DRUG1 versus DRUG2 is significant.

Procedure 48

Differential Equations

Differential equations arise frequently in the analysis of dose response and pharmacokinetic data. Given a differential equation

$$dy/dx = f(x, y)$$

and a value $y = y_0$ at $x = x_0$, one may obtain approximate solutions at $x_1 = x_0 + h$, $x_2 = x_1 + h$, etc., where h is the increment in x-values. Thus, the approximate solution is the set (x_0, y_0), $(x_1, y_1), \ldots, (x_n, y_n)$. The procedure employed in obtaining the values $y_1, y_2, \ldots, y_n$ is a one-step process that uses an algorithm known as the Runge–Kutta method. By "one-step" we mean that each value (y_{i+1}) uses the previously found value y_i:

$$y_{i+1} = y_i + \tfrac{1}{6}(k_1 + 2k_2 + 2k_3 + k_4)$$

where

$$k_1 = h \cdot f(x_i, y_i)$$

$$k_2 = h \cdot f\left(x_i + \frac{h}{2}, y_i + \frac{k_1}{2}\right)$$

$$k_3 = h \cdot f\left(x_i + \frac{h}{2}, y_i + \frac{k_2}{2}\right)$$

and

$$k_4 = h \cdot f(x_i + h, y_i + k_3).$$

Example

Solve $dy/dx = x + y$, given $x_1 = 0$, $y_1 = 1$, taking increments $h = 0.1$. It is seen that

$$k_1 = (0.1)(0 + 1) = 0.1$$
$$k_2 = (0.1)f(0.05, 1.05) = (0.1)(1.1) = 0.11$$
$$k_3 = (0.1)f(0.05, 1.055) = (0.1)(1.105) = 0.1105$$
$$k_4 = (0.1)f(0.1, 1.1105) = (0.1)(1.2105) = 0.12105$$

Thus, the value y_2 corresponding to $x_2 = 0.1$ is

$$y_2 = y_1 + \tfrac{1}{6}(k_1 + 2k_2 + 2k_3 + k_4)$$
$$= 1 + \tfrac{1}{6}(0.1 + 0.22 + 0.2210 + 0.12105)$$
$$= 1.110.$$

From the values x_2 and y_2, the value of y_3 corresponding to $x_3 = 0.2$ is similarly computed.

Computer Screen

```
                    <48> Differential Equations
         Pharmacologic Calculation System - Version 4.0 - 03/16/86

This procedure solves 1st order differential equations using the Runge-Kutta
approximation.   You will be prompted for the equation, initial values, and
increment in x.

For example, the equation, dY/dX = X - 2Y, must be entered as: dY/dX = X - 2*Y.
Be sure to use parenthesis when needed.

Equation currently in memory: dY/dX = X + Y

Press <ENTER> to retain this equation or enter new equation (right side only,
no '=').

        dy/dx = ?  <ENTER>

Enter initial conditions:
        X = ?  0<ENTER>
        Y = ?  1<ENTER>
  Increment = ?  .1<ENTER>
      X max = ?  2<ENTER>
```

```
Equation: dy/dx = X + Y

        Xo = 0
        Yo = 1
      Xmax = 2
 Increment = .1

Press <ESC> to abort printout.

         Xi              Yi
    ------------    ------------
          0               1
         .1          1.11034
         .2          1.24281
         .3          1.39972
         .4          1.58365
         .5          1.79744
         .6          2.04424
         .7           2.3275
         .8          2.65108
         .9           3.0192
          1          3.43656
        1.1          3.90833
        1.2          4.44023
        1.3          5.03859
        1.4          5.71039
        1.5          6.46337
        1.6          7.30605
        1.7          8.24788
        1.8          9.29928
        1.9          10.4718
          2          11.7781

Report: <P>rint, <S>ave, or <V>iew? <ENTER>
```

Computer Report

```
                        <48> Differential Equations
            Pharmacologic Calculation System - Version 4.0 - 03/16/86

Equation: dy/dx = X + Y

        Xo = 0
        Yo = 1
      Xmax = 2
 Increment = .1

         Xi              Yi
    ------------    ------------
          0               1
         .1          1.11034
         .2          1.24281
         .3          1.39972
         .4          1.58365
         .5          1.79744
         .6          2.04424
         .7           2.3275
         .8          2.65108
         .9           3.0192
          1          3.43656
        1.1          3.90833
        1.2          4.44023
        1.3          5.03859
        1.4          5.71039
        1.5          6.46337
        1.6          7.30605
        1.7          8.24788
        1.8          9.29928
        1.9          10.4718
          2          11.7781
```

Appendix A

Mathematical Tables

Table A.1
Areas Under the Standard Normal Curve

z	0.00	0.01	0.02	0.03	0.04	0.05	0.06	0.07	0.08	0.09
0.0	0.0000	0.0040	0.0080	0.0120	0.0160	0.0199	0.0239	0.0279	0.0319	0.0359
0.1	0.0398	0.0438	0.0478	0.0517	0.0557	0.0596	0.0636	0.0675	0.0714	0.0753
0.2	0.0793	0.0832	0.0871	0.0910	0.0948	0.0987	0.1026	0.1064	0.1103	0.1141
0.3	0.1179	0.1217	0.1255	0.1293	0.1331	0.1368	0.1406	0.1443	0.1480	0.1517
0.4	0.1554	0.1591	0.1628	0.1664	0.1700	0.1736	0.1772	0.1808	0.1844	0.1879
0.5	0.1915	0.1950	0.1985	0.2019	0.2054	0.2088	0.2123	0.2157	0.2190	0.2224
0.6	0.2257	0.2291	0.2324	0.2357	0.2389	0.2422	0.2454	0.2486	0.2517	0.2549
0.7	0.2580	0.2611	0.2642	0.2673	0.2704	0.2734	0.2764	0.2794	0.2823	0.2852
0.8	0.2881	0.2910	0.2939	0.2967	0.2995	0.3023	0.3051	0.3078	0.3106	0.3133
0.9	0.3159	0.3186	0.3212	0.3238	0.3264	0.3289	0.3315	0.3340	0.3365	0.3389
1.0	0.3413	0.3438	0.3461	0.3485	0.3508	0.3531	0.3554	0.3577	0.3599	0.3621
1.1	0.3643	0.3665	0.3686	0.3708	0.3729	0.3749	0.3770	0.3790	0.3810	0.3830
1.2	0.3849	0.3869	0.3888	0.3907	0.3925	0.3944	0.3962	0.3980	0.3997	0.4015
1.3	0.4032	0.4049	0.4066	0.4082	0.4099	0.4115	0.4131	0.4147	0.4162	0.4177
1.4	0.4192	0.4207	0.4222	0.4236	0.4251	0.4265	0.4279	0.4292	0.4306	0.4319
1.5	0.4332	0.4345	0.4357	0.4370	0.4382	0.4394	0.4406	0.4418	0.4429	0.4441
1.6	0.4452	0.4463	0.4474	0.4484	0.4495	0.4505	0.4515	0.4525	0.4535	0.4545
1.7	0.4554	0.4564	0.4573	0.4582	0.4591	0.4599	0.4608	0.4616	0.4625	0.4633
1.8	0.4641	0.4649	0.4656	0.4664	0.4671	0.4678	0.4686	0.4693	0.4699	0.4706
1.9	0.4713	0.4719	0.4726	0.4732	0.4738	0.4744	0.4750	0.4756	0.4761	0.4767
2.0	0.4772	0.4778	0.4783	0.4788	0.4793	0.4798	0.4803	0.4808	0.4812	0.4817
2.1	0.4821	0.4826	0.4830	0.4834	0.4838	0.4842	0.4846	0.4850	0.4854	0.4857
2.2	0.4861	0.4864	0.4868	0.4871	0.4875	0.4878	0.4881	0.4884	0.4887	0.4890
2.3	0.4893	0.4896	0.4898	0.4901	0.4904	0.4906	0.4909	0.4911	0.4913	0.4916
2.4	0.4918	0.4920	0.4922	0.4925	0.4927	0.4929	0.4931	0.4932	0.4934	0.4936
2.5	0.4938	0.4940	0.4941	0.4943	0.4945	0.4946	0.4948	0.4949	0.4951	0.4952
2.6	0.4953	0.4955	0.4956	0.4957	0.4959	0.4960	0.4961	0.4962	0.4963	0.4964
2.7	0.4965	0.4966	0.4967	0.4968	0.4969	0.4970	0.4971	0.4972	0.4973	0.4974
2.8	0.4974	0.4975	0.4976	0.4977	0.4977	0.4978	0.4979	0.4979	0.4980	0.4981
2.9	0.4981	0.4982	0.4982	0.4983	0.4984	0.4984	0.4985	0.4985	0.4986	0.4986
3.0	0.4987	0.4987	0.4987	0.4988	0.4988	0.4989	0.4989	0.4989	0.4990	0.4990

Table A.2
t Distribution

deg. freedom, ν	90% ($P = 0.1$)	95% ($P = 0.05$)	99% ($P = 0.01$)
1	6.314	12.706	63.657
2	2.920	4.303	9.925
3	2.353	3.182	5.841
4	2.132	2.776	4.604
5	2.015	2.571	4.032
6	1.943	2.447	3.707
7	1.895	2.365	3.499
8	1.860	2.306	3.355
9	1.833	2.262	3.250
10	1.812	2.228	3.169
11	1.796	2.201	3.106
12	1.782	2.179	3.055
13	1.771	2.160	3.012
14	1.761	2.145	2.977
15	1.753	2.131	2.947
16	1.746	2.120	2.921
17	1.740	2.110	2.898
18	1.734	2.101	2.878
19	1.729	2.093	2.861
20	1.725	2.086	2.845
21	1.721	2.080	2.831
22	1.717	2.074	2.819
23	1.714	2.069	2.807
24	1.711	2.064	2.797
25	1.708	2.060	2.787
26	1.706	2.056	2.779
27	1.703	2.052	2.771
28	1.701	2.048	2.763
29	1.699	2.045	2.756
inf.	1.645	1.960	2.576

Table A.3
Probit Transformation[a]

%		%		%		%		%	
0		20	4.1584	40	4.7467	60	5.2533	80	5.8416
1	2.6737	21	4.1936	41	4.7725	61	5.2793	81	5.8779
2	2.9463	22	4.2278	42	4.7981	62	5.3055	82	5.9154
3	3.1192	23	4.2612	43	4.8236	63	5.3319	83	5.9542
4	3.2493	24	4.2937	44	4.8490	64	5.3585	84	5.9945
5	3.3551	25	4.3255	45	4.8743	65	5.3853	85	6.0364
6	3.4452	26	4.3567	46	4.8996	66	5.4125	86	6.0803
7	3.5242	27	4.3872	47	4.9247	67	5.4399	87	6.1264
8	3.5949	28	4.4172	48	4.9498	68	5.4677	88	6.1750
9	3.6592	29	4.4466	49	4.9749	69	5.4959	89	6.2265
10	3.7184	30	4.4756	50	5.0000	70	5.5244	90	6.2816
11	3.7735	31	4.5041	51	5.0251	71	5.5534	91	6.3408
12	3.8250	32	4.5323	52	5.0502	72	5.5828	92	6.4051
13	3.8736	33	4.5601	53	5.0753	73	5.6128	93	6.4758
14	3.9197	34	4.5875	54	5.1004	74	5.6433	94	6.5548
15	3.9636	35	4.6147	55	5.1257	75	5.6745	95	6.6449
16	4.0055	36	4.6415	56	5.1510	76	5.7063	96	6.7507
17	4.0458	37	4.6681	57	5.1764	77	5.7388	97	6.8808
18	4.0846	38	4.6945	58	5.2019	78	5.7722	98	7.0537
19	4.1221	39	4.7207	59	5.2275	79	5.8064	99	7.3263

[a] The percentages of the area under the normal distribution curve from negative infinity and the corresponding probits. The computer programs contain a subroutine that calculates probit values directly, thus avoiding interpolation of tabular values.

Table A.4
Common Logarithms

n	0	1	2	3	4	5	6	7	8	9
1.0	0.0000	0.0043	0.0086	0.0128	0.0170	0.0212	0.0253	0.0294	0.0334	0.0374
1.1	0.0414	0.0453	0.0492	0.0531	0.0569	0.0607	0.0645	0.0682	0.0719	0.0755
1.2	0.0792	0.0828	0.0864	0.0899	0.0934	0.0969	0.1004	0.1038	0.1072	0.1106
1.3	0.1139	0.1173	0.1206	0.1239	0.1271	0.1303	0.1335	0.1367	0.1399	0.1430
1.4	0.1461	0.1492	0.1523	0.1553	0.1584	0.1614	0.1644	0.1673	0.1703	0.1732
1.5	0.1761	0.1790	0.1818	0.1847	0.1875	0.1903	0.1931	0.1959	0.1987	0.2014
1.6	0.2041	0.2068	0.2095	0.2122	0.2148	0.2175	0.2201	0.2227	0.2253	0.2279
1.7	0.2304	0.2330	0.2355	0.2380	0.2405	0.2430	0.2455	0.2480	0.2504	0.2529
1.8	0.2553	0.2577	0.2601	0.2625	0.2648	0.2672	0.2695	0.2718	0.2742	0.2765
1.9	0.2788	0.2810	0.2833	0.2856	0.2878	0.2900	0.2923	0.2945	0.2967	0.2989

(*Continued*)

Table A.4   (*Continued*)

n	0	1	2	3	4	5	6	7	8	9
2.0	0.3010	0.3032	0.3054	0.3075	0.3096	0.3118	0.3139	0.3160	0.3181	0.3201
2.1	0.3222	0.3243	0.3263	0.3284	0.3304	0.3324	0.3345	0.3365	0.3385	0.3404
2.2	0.3424	0.3444	0.3464	0.3483	0.3502	0.3522	0.3541	0.3560	0.3579	0.3598
2.3	0.3617	0.3636	0.3655	0.3674	0.3692	0.3711	0.3729	0.3747	0.3766	0.3784
2.4	0.3802	0.3820	0.3838	0.3856	0.3874	0.3892	0.3909	0.3927	0.3945	0.3962
2.5	0.3979	0.3997	0.4014	0.4031	0.4048	0.4065	0.4082	0.4099	0.4116	0.4133
2.6	0.4150	0.4166	0.4183	0.4200	0.4216	0.4232	0.4249	0.4265	0.4281	0.4298
2.7	0.4314	0.4330	0.4346	0.4362	0.4378	0.4393	0.4409	0.4425	0.4440	0.4456
2.8	0.4472	0.4487	0.4502	0.4518	0.4533	0.4548	0.4564	0.4579	0.4594	0.4609
2.9	0.4624	0.4639	0.4654	0.4669	0.4683	0.4698	0.4713	0.4728	0.4742	0.4757
3.0	0.4771	0.4786	0.4800	0.4814	0.4829	0.4843	0.4857	0.4871	0.4886	0.4900
3.1	0.4914	0.4928	0.4942	0.4955	0.4969	0.4983	0.4997	0.5011	0.5024	0.5038
3.2	0.5051	0.5065	0.5079	0.5092	0.5105	0.5119	0.5132	0.5145	0.5159	0.5172
3.3	0.5185	0.5198	0.5211	0.5224	0.5237	0.5250	0.5263	0.5276	0.5289	0.5302
3.4	0.5315	0.5328	0.5340	0.5353	0.5366	0.5378	0.5391	0.5403	0.5416	0.5428
3.5	0.5441	0.5453	0.5465	0.5478	0.5490	0.5502	0.5514	0.5527	0.5539	0.5551
3.6	0.5563	0.5575	0.5587	0.5599	0.5611	0.5623	0.5635	0.5647	0.5658	0.5670
3.7	0.5682	0.5694	0.5705	0.5717	0.5729	0.5740	0.5752	0.5763	0.5775	0.5786
3.8	0.5798	0.5809	0.5821	0.5832	0.5843	0.5855	0.5866	0.5877	0.5888	0.5899
3.9	0.5911	0.5922	0.5933	0.5944	0.5955	0.5966	0.5977	0.5988	0.5999	0.6010
4.0	0.6021	0.6031	0.6042	0.6053	0.6064	0.6075	0.6085	0.6096	0.6107	0.6117
4.1	0.6128	0.6138	0.6149	0.6160	0.6170	0.6180	0.6191	0.6201	0.6212	0.6222
4.2	0.6232	0.6243	0.6253	0.6263	0.6274	0.6284	0.6294	0.6304	0.6314	0.6325
4.3	0.6335	0.6345	0.6355	0.6365	0.6375	0.6385	0.6395	0.6405	0.6415	0.6425
4.4	0.6435	0.6444	0.6454	0.6464	0.6474	0.6484	0.6493	0.6503	0.6513	0.6522
4.5	0.6532	0.6542	0.6551	0.6561	0.6571	0.6580	0.6590	0.6599	0.6609	0.6618
4.6	0.6628	0.6637	0.6646	0.6656	0.6665	0.6675	0.6684	0.6693	0.6702	0.6712
4.7	0.6721	0.6730	0.6739	0.6749	0.6758	0.6767	0.6776	0.6785	0.6794	0.6803
4.8	0.6812	0.6821	0.6830	0.6839	0.6848	0.6857	0.6866	0.6875	0.6884	0.6893
4.9	0.6902	0.6911	0.6920	0.6928	0.6937	0.6946	0.6955	0.6964	0.6972	0.6981
5.0	0.6990	0.6998	0.7007	0.7016	0.7024	0.7033	0.7042	0.7050	0.7059	0.7067
5.1	0.7076	0.7084	0.7093	0.7101	0.7110	0.7118	0.7126	0.7135	0.7143	0.7152
5.2	0.7160	0.7168	0.7177	0.7185	0.7193	0.7202	0.7210	0.7218	0.7226	0.7235
5.3	0.7243	0.7251	0.7259	0.7267	0.7275	0.7284	0.7292	0.7300	0.7308	0.7316
5.4	0.7324	0.7332	0.7340	0.7348	0.7356	0.7364	0.7372	0.7380	0.7388	0.7396
5.5	0.7404	0.7412	0.7419	0.7427	0.7435	0.7443	0.7451	0.7459	0.7466	0.7474
5.6	0.7482	0.7490	0.7497	0.7505	0.7513	0.7520	0.7528	0.7536	0.7543	0.7551
5.7	0.7559	0.7566	0.7574	0.7582	0.7589	0.7597	0.7604	0.7612	0.7619	0.7627
5.8	0.7634	0.7642	0.7649	0.7657	0.7664	0.7672	0.7679	0.7686	0.7694	0.7701
5.9	0.7709	0.7716	0.7723	0.7731	0.7738	0.7745	0.7752	0.7760	0.7767	0.7774

Table A.4   (*Continued*)

n	0	1	2	3	4	5	6	7	8	9
6.0	0.7782	0.7789	0.7796	0.7803	0.7810	0.7818	0.7825	0.7832	0.7839	0.7846
6.1	0.7853	0.7860	0.7868	0.7875	0.7882	0.7889	0.7896	0.7903	0.7910	0.7917
6.2	0.7924	0.7931	0.7938	0.7945	0.7952	0.7959	0.7966	0.7973	0.7980	0.7987
6.3	0.7993	0.8000	0.8007	0.8014	0.8021	0.8028	0.8035	0.8041	0.8048	0.8055
6.4	0.8062	0.8069	0.8075	0.8082	0.8089	0.8096	0.8102	0.8109	0.8116	0.8122
6.5	0.8129	0.8136	0.8142	0.8149	0.8156	0.8162	0.8169	0.8176	0.8182	0.8189
6.6	0.8195	0.8202	0.8209	0.8215	0.8222	0.8228	0.8235	0.8241	0.8248	0.8254
6.7	0.8261	0.8267	0.8274	0.8280	0.8287	0.8293	0.8299	0.8306	0.8312	0.8319
6.8	0.8325	0.8331	0.8338	0.8344	0.8351	0.8357	0.8363	0.8370	0.8376	0.8382
6.9	0.8388	0.8395	0.8401	0.8407	0.8414	0.8420	0.8426	0.8432	0.8439	0.8445
7.0	0.8451	0.8457	0.8463	0.8470	0.8476	0.8482	0.8488	0.8494	0.8500	0.8506
7.1	0.8513	0.8519	0.8525	0.8531	0.8537	0.8543	0.8549	0.8555	0.8561	0.8567
7.2	0.8573	0.8579	0.8585	0.8591	0.8597	0.8603	0.8609	0.8615	0.8621	0.8627
7.3	0.8633	0.8639	0.8645	0.8651	0.8657	0.8663	0.8669	0.8675	0.8681	0.8686
7.4	0.8692	0.8698	0.8704	0.8710	0.8716	0.8722	0.8727	0.8733	0.8739	0.8745
7.5	0.8751	0.8756	0.8762	0.8768	0.8774	0.8779	0.8785	0.8791	0.8797	0.8802
7.6	0.8808	0.8814	0.8820	0.8825	0.8831	0.8837	0.8842	0.8848	0.8854	0.8859
7.7	0.8865	0.8871	0.8876	0.8882	0.8887	0.8893	0.8899	0.8904	0.8910	0.8915
7.8	0.8921	0.8927	0.8932	0.8938	0.8943	0.8949	0.8954	0.8960	0.8965	0.8971
7.9	0.8976	0.8982	0.8987	0.8993	0.8998	0.9004	0.9009	0.9015	0.9020	0.9025
8.0	0.9031	0.9036	0.9042	0.9047	0.9053	0.9058	0.9063	0.9069	0.9074	0.9079
8.1	0.9085	0.9090	0.9096	0.9101	0.9106	0.9112	0.9117	0.9122	0.9128	0.9133
8.2	0.9138	0.9143	0.9149	0.9154	0.9159	0.9165	0.9170	0.9175	0.9180	0.9186
8.3	0.9191	0.9196	0.9201	0.9206	0.9212	0.9217	0.9222	0.9227	0.9232	0.9238
8.4	0.9243	0.9248	0.9253	0.9258	0.9263	0.9269	0.9274	0.9279	0.9284	0.9289
8.5	0.9294	0.9299	0.9304	0.9309	0.9315	0.9320	0.9325	0.9330	0.9335	0.9340
8.6	0.9345	0.9350	0.9355	0.9360	0.9365	0.9370	0.9375	0.9380	0.9385	0.9390
8.7	0.9395	0.9400	0.9405	0.9410	0.9415	0.9420	0.9425	0.9430	0.9435	0.9440
8.8	0.9445	0.9450	0.9455	0.9460	0.9465	0.9469	0.9474	0.9479	0.9484	0.9489
8.9	0.9494	0.9499	0.9504	0.9509	0.9513	0.9518	0.9523	0.9528	0.9533	0.9538
9.0	0.9542	0.9547	0.9552	0.9557	0.9562	0.9566	0.9571	0.9576	0.9581	0.9586
9.1	0.9590	0.9595	0.9600	0.9605	0.9609	0.9614	0.9619	0.9624	0.9628	0.9633
9.2	0.9638	0.9643	0.9647	0.9652	0.9657	0.9661	0.9666	0.9671	0.9675	0.9680
9.3	0.9685	0.9689	0.9694	0.9699	0.9703	0.9708	0.9713	0.9717	0.9722	0.9727
9.4	0.9731	0.9736	0.9741	0.9745	0.9750	0.9754	0.9759	0.9763	0.9768	0.9773
9.5	0.9777	0.9782	0.9786	0.9791	0.9795	0.9800	0.9805	0.9809	0.9814	0.9818
9.6	0.9823	0.9827	0.9832	0.9836	0.9841	0.9845	0.9850	0.9854	0.9859	0.9863
9.7	0.9868	0.9872	0.9877	0.9881	0.9886	0.9890	0.9894	0.9899	0.9903	0.9908
9.8	0.9912	0.9917	0.9921	0.9926	0.9930	0.9934	0.9939	0.9943	0.9948	0.9952
9.9	0.9956	0.9961	0.9965	0.9969	0.9974	0.9978	0.9983	0.9987	0.9991	0.9996

Table A.5
Natural Logarithms

x	$\ln x$	x	$\ln x$	x	$\ln x$
		4.5	1.5041	9.0	2.1972
0.1	$7.6974 - 10$	4.6	1.5261	9.1	2.2083
0.2	$8.3906 - 10$	4.7	1.5476	9.2	2.2192
0.3	$8.7960 - 10$	4.8	1.5686	9.3	2.2300
0.4	$9.0837 - 10$	4.9	1.5892	9.4	2.2407
0.5	$9.3069 - 10$	5.0	1.6094	9.5	2.2513
0.6	$9.4892 - 10$	5.1	1.6292	9.6	2.2618
0.7	$9.6433 - 10$	5.2	1.6487	9.7	2.2721
0.8	$9.7769 - 10$	5.3	1.6677	9.8	2.2824
0.9	$9.8946 - 10$	5.4	1.6864	9.9	2.2925
1.0	0.0000	5.5	1.7047	10	2.3026
1.1	0.0953	5.6	1.7228	11	2.3979
1.2	0.1823	5.7	1.7405	12	2.4849
1.3	0.2624	5.8	1.7579	13	2.5649
1.4	0.3365	5.9	1.7750	14	2.6391
1.5	0.4055	6.0	1.7918	15	2.7081
1.6	0.4700	6.1	1.8083	16	2.7726
1.7	0.5306	6.2	1.8245	17	2.8332
1.8	0.5878	6.3	1.8405	18	2.8904
1.9	0.6419	6.4	1.8563	19	2.9444
2.0	0.6931	6.5	1.8718	20	2.9957
2.1	0.7419	6.6	1.8871		
2.2	0.7885	6.7	1.9021	25	3.2189
2.3	0.8329	6.8	1.9169	30	3.4012
2.4	0.8755	6.9	1.9315	35	3.5553
				40	3.6889
2.5	0.9163	7.0	1.9459		
2.6	0.9555	7.1	1.9601	45	3.8067
2.7	0.9933	7.2	1.9741	50	3.9120
2.8	1.0296	7.3	1.9879		
2.9	1.0647	7.4	2.0015	55	4.0073
				60	4.0943
3.0	1.0986	7.5	2.0149	65	4.1744
3.1	1.1314	7.6	2.0281		
3.2	1.1632	7.7	2.0412	70	4.2485
3.3	1.1939	7.8	2.0541	75	4.3175
3.4	1.2238	7.9	2.0669	80	4.3820
				85	4.4427
3.5	1.2528	8.0	2.0794	90	4.4998
3.6	1.2809	8.1	2.0919		
3.7	1.2083	8.2	2.1041	95	4.5539
3.8	1.3350	8.3	2.1163	100	4.6052
3.9	1.3610	8.4	2.1281		
4.0	1.3863	8.5	2.1401		
4.1	1.4110	8.6	2.1518		
4.2	1.4351	8.7	2.1633		
4.3	1.4586	8.8	2.1748		
4.4	1.4816	8.9	2.1861		

Table A.6
Powers of e: $\exp(x)$ and $\exp(-x)$

x	e^x	e^{-x}	x	e^x	e^{-x}
0.00	1.00000	1.00000	1.60	4.95302	0.20189
0.01	1.01005	0.99004	1.70	5.47394	0.18268
0.02	1.02020	0.98019	1.80	6.04964	0.16529
0.03	1.03045	0.97044	1.90	6.68589	0.14956
0.04	1.04081	0.96078	2.00	7.38905	0.13533
0.05	1.05127	0.95122			
0.06	1.06183	0.94176	2.10	8.16616	0.12245
0.07	1.07250	0.93239	2.20	9.02500	0.11080
0.08	1.08328	0.92311	2.30	9.97417	0.10025
0.09	1.09417	0.91393	2.40	11.02316	0.09071
0.10	1.10517	0.90483	2.50	12.18248	0.08208
			2.60	13.46372	0.07427
0.11	1.11628	0.89583	2.70	14.87971	0.06720
0.12	1.12750	0.88692	2.80	16.44463	0.06081
0.13	1.13883	0.87810	2.90	18.17412	0.05502
0.14	1.15027	0.86936	3.00	20.08551	0.04978
0.15	1.16183	0.86071			
0.16	1.17351	0.85214	3.50	33.11545	0.03020
0.17	1.18530	0.84366			
0.18	1.19722	0.83527	4.00	54.95815	0.01832
0.19	1.20925	0.82696	4.50	90.01713	0.01111
0.20	1.22140	0.81873	5.00	148.41316	0.00674
0.30	1.34985	0.74081	5.50	224.69193	0.00409
0.40	1.49182	0.67032			
0.50	1.64872	0.60653	6.00	403.42879	0.00248
0.60	1.82211	0.54881	6.50	665.14163	0.00150
0.70	2.01375	0.49658			
0.80	2.22554	0.44932	7.00	1096.63316	0.00091
0.90	2.45960	0.40656	7.50	1808.04241	0.00055
1.00	2.71828	0.36787			
			8.00	2980.95799	0.00034
			8.50	4914.76884	0.00020
1.10	3.00416	0.33287			
1.20	3.32011	0.30119	9.00	8130.08393	0.00012
1.30	3.66929	0.27253	9.50	13359.72683	0.00007
1.40	4.05519	0.24659			
1.50	4.48168	0.22313	10.00	22026.46579	0.00005

Table A.7
Squares and Square Roots

n	n^2	$\sqrt{n}$	$\sqrt{10n}$	n	n^2	$\sqrt{n}$	$\sqrt{10n}$
1	1	1.000	3.162	41	1681	6.403	20.248
2	4	1.414	4.472	42	1764	6.481	20.494
3	9	1.732	5.477	43	1849	6.557	20.736
4	16	2.000	6.325	44	1936	6.633	20.976
5	25	2.236	7.071	45	2025	6.708	21.213
6	36	2.449	7.746	46	2116	6.782	21.448
7	49	2.646	8.367	47	2209	6.856	21.679
8	64	2.828	8.944	48	2304	6.928	21.909
9	81	3.000	9.487	49	2401	7.000	22.136
10	100	3.162	10.000	50	2500	7.071	22.361
11	121	3.317	10.488	51	2601	7.141	22.583
12	144	3.464	10.954	52	2704	7.211	22.804
13	169	3.606	11.402	53	2809	7.280	23.022
14	196	3.742	11.832	54	2916	7.348	23.238
15	225	3.873	12.247	55	3025	7.416	23.452
16	256	4.000	12.649	56	3136	7.483	23.664
17	289	4.123	13.038	57	3249	7.550	23.875
18	324	4.243	13.416	58	3364	7.616	24.083
19	361	4.359	13.784	59	3481	7.681	24.290
20	400	4.472	14.142	60	3600	7.746	24.495
21	441	4.583	14.491	61	3721	7.810	24.698
22	484	4.690	14.832	62	3844	7.874	24.900
23	529	4.796	15.166	63	3969	7.937	25.100
24	576	4.899	15.492	64	4096	8.000	25.298
25	625	5.000	15.811	65	4225	8.062	25.495
26	676	5.099	16.125	66	4356	8.124	25.690
27	729	5.196	16.432	67	4489	8.185	25.884
28	784	5.292	16.733	68	4624	8.246	26.077
29	841	5.385	17.029	69	4761	8.307	26.268
30	900	5.477	17.321	70	4900	8.367	26.458
31	961	5.568	17.607	71	5041	8.426	26.646
32	1024	5.657	17.889	72	5184	8.485	26.833
33	1089	5.745	18.166	73	5329	8.544	27.019
34	1156	5.831	18.439	74	5476	8.602	27.203
35	1225	5.916	18.708	75	5625	8.660	27.386
36	1296	6.000	18.974	76	5776	8.718	27.568
37	1369	6.083	19.235	77	5929	8.775	27.749
38	1444	6.164	19.494	78	6084	8.832	27.928
39	1521	6.245	19.748	79	6241	8.888	28.107
40	1600	6.325	20.000	80	6400	8.944	28.284

(*Continued*)

Table A.7   (*Continued*)

n	n^2	$\sqrt{n}$	$\sqrt{10n}$	n	n^2	$\sqrt{n}$	$\sqrt{10n}$
81	6561	9.000	28.460	91	8281	9.539	30.166
82	6724	9.055	28.636	92	8464	9.592	30.332
83	6889	9.110	28.810	93	8649	9.644	30.496
84	7056	9.165	28.983	94	8836	9.695	30.659
85	7225	9.220	29.155	95	9025	9.747	30.822
86	7396	9.274	29.326	96	9216	9.798	30.984
87	7569	9.327	29.496	97	9409	9.849	31.145
88	7744	9.381	29.665	98	9604	9.899	31.305
89	7921	9.434	29.833	99	9801	9.950	31.464
90	8100	9.487	30.000	100	10000	10.000	31.623

Table A.8
x^2 distribution

v	0.05	0.025	0.01	0.005
1	3.841	5.024	6.635	7.879
2	5.991	7.378	9.210	10.597
3	7.815	9.348	11.345	12.838
4	9.488	11.143	13.277	14.860
5	11.070	12.832	15.086	16.750
6	12.592	14.449	16.812	18.548
7	14.067	16.013	18.475	20.278
8	15.507	17.535	20.090	21.955
9	16.919	19.023	21.666	23.589
10	18.307	20.483	23.209	25.188
11	19.675	21.920	24.725	26.757
12	21.026	23.337	26.217	28.300
13	22.362	24.736	27.688	29.819
14	23.685	26.119	29.141	31.319
15	24.996	27.488	30.578	32.801
16	26.296	28.845	32.000	34.267
17	27.587	30.191	33.409	35.718
18	28.869	31.526	34.805	37.156
19	30.144	32.852	36.191	38.582
20	31.410	34.170	37.566	39.997
21	32.671	35.479	38.932	41.401
22	33.924	36.781	40.289	42.796
23	35.172	38.076	41.638	44.181
24	36.415	39.364	42.980	45.558
25	37.652	40.646	44.314	46.928
26	38.885	41.923	45.642	48.290
27	40.113	43.194	46.963	49.645
28	41.337	44.461	48.278	50.993
29	42.557	45.722	49.588	52.336
30	43.773	46.979	50.892	53.672

Reprinted from: John E. Freund and Frank J. Williams, *Elementary Business Statistics: The Modern Approach*, Second Edition, © 1972. By permission of Prentice-Hall, Inc., Englewood Cliffs, N.J.

Table A.9a

t for Two-Sided Comparisons Between p Treatments and a Control for a Joint Confidence Coefficient of P = 95%

					p = number of treatment means (excluding the control)									
d.f.	1	2	3	4	5	6	7	8	9	10	11	12	15	20
5	2.57	3.03	3.29	3.48	3.62	3.73	3.82	3.90	3.97	4.03	4.09	4.14	4.26	4.42
6	2.45	2.86	3.10	3.26	3.39	3.49	3.57	3.64	3.71	3.76	3.81	3.86	3.97	4.11
7	2.36	2.75	2.97	3.12	3.24	3.33	3.41	3.47	3.53	3.58	3.63	3.67	3.78	3.91
8	2.31	2.67	2.88	3.02	3.13	3.22	3.29	3.35	3.41	3.46	3.50	3.54	3.64	3.76
9	2.26	2.61	2.81	2.95	3.05	3.14	3.20	3.26	3.32	3.36	3.40	3.44	3.53	3.65
10	2.23	2.57	2.76	2.89	2.99	3.07	3.14	3.19	3.24	3.29	3.33	3.36	3.45	3.57
11	2.20	2.53	2.72	2.84	2.94	3.02	3.08	3.14	3.19	3.23	3.27	3.30	3.39	3.50
12	2.18	2.50	2.68	2.81	2.90	2.98	3.04	3.09	3.14	3.18	3.22	3.25	3.34	3.45
13	2.16	2.48	2.65	2.78	2.87	2.94	3.00	3.06	3.10	3.14	3.18	3.21	3.29	3.40
14	2.14	2.46	2.63	2.75	2.84	2.91	2.97	3.02	3.07	3.11	3.14	3.18	3.26	3.36
15	2.13	2.44	2.61	2.73	2.82	2.89	2.95	3.00	3.04	3.08	3.12	3.15	3.23	3.33
16	2.12	2.42	2.59	2.71	2.80	2.87	2.92	2.97	3.02	3.06	3.09	3.12	3.20	3.30
17	2.11	2.41	2.58	2.69	2.78	2.85	2.90	2.95	3.00	3.03	3.07	3.10	3.18	3.27
18	2.10	2.40	2.56	2.68	2.76	2.83	2.89	2.94	2.98	3.01	3.05	3.08	3.16	3.25
19	2.09	2.39	2.55	2.66	2.75	2.81	2.87	2.92	2.96	3.00	3.03	3.06	3.14	3.23
20	2.09	2.38	2.54	2.65	2.73	2.80	2.86	2.90	2.95	2.98	3.02	3.05	3.12	3.22
24	2.06	2.35	2.51	2.61	2.70	2.76	2.81	2.86	2.90	2.94	2.97	3.00	3.07	3.16
30	2.04	2.32	2.47	2.58	2.66	2.72	2.77	2.82	2.86	2.89	2.92	2.95	3.02	3.11
40	2.02	2.29	2.44	2.54	2.62	2.68	2.73	2.77	2.81	2.85	2.87	2.90	2.97	3.06
60	2.00	2.27	2.41	2.51	2.58	2.64	2.69	2.73	2.77	2.80	2.83	2.86	2.92	3.00
120	1.98	2.24	2.38	2.47	2.55	2.60	2.65	2.69	2.73	2.76	2.79	2.81	2.87	2.95
∞	1.96	2.21	2.35	2.44	2.51	2.57	2.61	2.65	2.69	2.72	2.74	2.77	2.83	2.91

Table A.9b
t for Two-Sided Comparisons Between *p* Treatments and a Control for a Joint
Confidence Coefficient of *P* = 99%

d.f.	\multicolumn{14}{c}{*p* = number of treatment means (excluding the control)}

d.f.	1	2	3	4	5	6	7	8	9	10	11	12	15	20
5	4.03	4.63	4.98	5.22	5.41	5.56	5.69	5.80	5.89	5.98	6.05	6.12	6.30	6.52
6	3.71	4.21	4.51	4.71	4.87	5.00	5.10	5.20	5.28	5.35	5.41	5.47	5.62	5.81
7	3.50	3.95	4.21	4.39	4.53	4.64	4.74	4.82	4.89	4.95	5.01	5.06	5.19	5.36
8	3.36	3.77	4.00	4.17	4.29	4.40	4.48	4.56	4.62	4.68	4.73	4.78	4.90	5.05
9	3.25	3.63	3.85	4.01	4.12	4.22	4.30	4.37	4.43	4.48	4.53	4.57	4.68	4.82
10	3.17	3.53	3.74	3.88	3.99	4.08	4.16	4.22	4.28	4.33	4.37	4.42	4.52	4.65
11	3.11	3.45	3.65	3.79	3.89	3.98	4.05	4.11	4.16	4.21	4.25	4.29	4.39	4.52
12	3.05	3.39	3.58	3.71	3.81	3.89	3.96	4.02	4.07	4.12	4.16	4.19	4.29	4.41
13	3.01	3.33	3.52	3.65	3.74	3.82	3.89	3.94	3.99	4.04	4.08	4.11	4.20	4.32
14	2.98	3.29	3.47	3.59	3.69	3.76	3.83	3.88	3.93	3.97	4.01	4.05	4.13	4.24
15	2.95	3.25	3.43	3.55	3.64	3.71	3.78	3.83	3.88	3.92	3.95	3.99	4.07	4.18
16	2.92	3.22	3.39	3.51	3.60	3.67	3.73	3.78	3.83	3.87	3.91	3.94	4.02	4.13
17	2.90	3.19	3.36	3.47	3.56	3.63	3.69	3.74	3.79	3.83	3.86	3.90	3.98	4.08
18	2.88	3.17	3.33	3.44	3.53	3.60	3.66	3.71	3.75	3.79	3.83	3.86	3.94	4.04
19	2.86	3.15	3.31	3.42	3.50	3.57	3.63	3.68	3.72	3.76	3.79	3.83	3.90	4.00
20	2.85	3.13	3.29	3.40	3.48	3.55	3.60	3.65	3.69	3.73	3.77	3.80	3.87	3.97
24	2.80	3.07	3.22	3.32	3.40	3.47	3.52	3.57	3.61	3.64	3.68	3.70	3.78	3.87
30	2.75	3.01	3.15	3.25	3.33	3.39	3.44	3.49	3.52	3.56	3.59	3.62	3.69	3.78
40	2.70	2.95	3.09	3.19	3.26	3.32	3.37	3.41	3.44	3.48	3.51	3.53	3.60	3.68
60	2.66	2.90	3.03	3.12	3.19	3.25	3.29	3.33	3.37	3.40	3.42	3.45	3.51	3.59
120	2.62	2.85	2.97	3.06	3.12	3.18	3.22	3.26	3.29	3.32	3.35	3.37	3.43	3.51
∞	2.58	2.79	2.92	3.00	3.06	3.11	3.15	3.19	3.22	3.25	3.27	3.29	3.35	3.42

Table A.10a
Probabilities Associated with Values as Small as Observed Values of U in the Mann–Whitney Test[a]

	$n_2 = 3$				$n_2 = 4$			
		n_1				n_1		
U	1	2	3	U	1	2	3	4
0	0.250	0.100	0.050	0	0.200	0.067	0.028	0.014
1	0.500	0.200	0.100	1	0.400	0.133	0.057	0.029
2	0.750	0.400	0.200	2	0.600	0.267	0.114	0.057
3		0.600	0.350	3		0.400	0.200	0.100
4			0.500	4		0.600	0.314	0.171
5			0.650	5			0.429	0.243
				6			0.571	0.343
				7				0.443
				8				0.557

	$n_2 = 5$						$n_2 = 6$					
			n_1						n_1			
U	1	2	3	4	5	U	1	2	3	4	5	6
0	0.167	0.047	0.018	0.008	0.004	0	0.143	0.036	0.012	0.005	0.002	0.001
1	0.333	0.095	0.036	0.016	0.008	1	0.286	0.071	0.024	0.010	0.004	0.002
2	0.500	0.190	0.071	0.032	0.016	2	0.428	0.143	0.048	0.019	0.009	0.004
3	0.667	0.286	0.125	0.056	0.028	3	0.571	0.214	0.083	0.033	0.015	0.008
4		0.429	0.196	0.095	0.048	4		0.321	0.131	0.057	0.026	0.013
5		0.571	0.286	0.143	0.075	5		0.429	0.190	0.086	0.041	0.021
6			0.393	0.206	0.111	6		0.571	0.274	0.129	0.063	0.032
7			0.500	0.278	0.155	7			0.357	0.176	0.089	0.047
8			0.607	0.365	0.210	8			0.452	0.238	0.123	0.066
9				0.452	0.274	9			0.548	0.305	0.165	0.090
10				0.548	0.345	10				0.381	0.214	0.120
11					0.421	11				0.457	0.268	0.155
12					0.500	12				0.545	0.331	0.197
13					0.579	13					0.396	0.242
						14					0.465	0.294
						15					0.535	0.350
						16						0.409
						17						0.469
						18						0.531

[a] Reproduced from Mann, H. B., and Whitney, D. R. 1947. On a test of whether one of two random variables is stochastically larger than the other. *Ann. Math. Statist.*, **18**, 52–54, with the kind permission of the authors and the publisher.

Table A.10a   (*Continued*)

				$n_2 = 7$			
				n_1			
U	1	2	3	4	5	6	7
0	0.125	0.028	0.008	0.003	0.001	0.001	0.000
1	0.250	0.056	0.017	0.006	0.003	0.001	0.001
2	0.375	0.111	0.033	0.012	0.005	0.002	0.001
3	0.500	0.167	0.058	0.021	0.009	0.004	0.002
4	0.625	0.250	0.092	0.036	0.015	0.007	0.003
5		0.333	0.133	0.055	0.024	0.011	0.006
6		0.444	0.192	0.082	0.037	0.017	0.009
7		0.556	0.258	0.115	0.053	0.026	0.013
8			0.333	0.158	0.074	0.037	0.019
9			0.417	0.206	0.101	0.051	0.027
10			0.500	0.264	0.134	0.069	0.036
11			0.583	0.324	0.172	0.090	0.049
12				0.394	0.216	0.117	0.064
13				0.464	0.265	0.147	0.082
14				0.538	0.319	0.183	0.104
15					0.378	0.223	0.130
16					0.438	0.267	0.159
17					0.500	0.314	0.191
18					0.562	0.365	0.228
19						0.418	0.267
20						0.473	0.310
21						0.527	0.355
22							0.402
23							0.451
24							0.500
25							0.549

Table A.10a   (*Continued*)

						$n_2 = 8$					
						n_1					
U	1	2	3	4	5	6	7	8	t	Normal
0	0.111	0.022	0.006	0.002	0.001	0.000	0.000	0.000	3.308	0.001
1	0.222	0.044	0.012	0.004	0.002	0.001	0.000	0.000	3.203	0.001
2	0.333	0.089	0.024	0.008	0.003	0.001	0.001	0.000	3.098	0.001
3	0.444	0.133	0.042	0.014	0.005	0.002	0.001	0.001	2.993	0.001
4	0.556	0.200	0.067	0.024	0.009	0.004	0.002	0.001	2.888	0.002
5		0.267	0.097	0.036	0.015	0.006	0.003	0.001	2.783	0.003
6		0.356	0.139	0.055	0.023	0.010	0.005	0.002	2.678	0.004
7		0.444	0.188	0.077	0.033	0.015	0.007	0.003	2.573	0.005
8		0.556	0.248	0.107	0.047	0.021	0.010	0.005	2.468	0.007
9			0.315	0.141	0.064	0.030	0.014	0.007	2.363	0.009
10			0.387	0.184	0.085	0.041	0.020	0.010	2.258	0.012
11			0.461	0.230	0.111	0.054	0.027	0.014	2.153	0.016
12			0.539	0.285	0.142	0.071	0.036	0.019	2.048	0.020
13				0.341	0.177	0.091	0.047	0.025	1.943	0.026
14				0.404	0.217	0.114	0.060	0.032	1.838	0.033
15				0.467	0.262	0.141	0.076	0.041	1.733	0.041
16				0.533	0.311	0.172	0.095	0.052	1.628	0.052
17					0.362	0.207	0.116	0.065	1.523	0.064
18					0.416	0.245	0.140	0.080	1.418	0.078
19					0.472	0.286	0.168	0.097	1.313	0.094
20					0.528	0.331	0.198	0.117	1.208	0.113
21						0.377	0.232	0.139	1.102	0.135
22						0.426	0.268	0.164	0.998	0.159
23						0.475	0.306	0.191	0.893	0.185
24						0.525	0.347	0.221	0.788	0.215
25							0.389	0.253	0.683	0.247
26							0.433	0.287	0.578	0.282
27							0.478	0.323	0.473	0.318
28							0.522	0.360	0.368	0.356
29								0.399	0.263	0.396
30								0.439	0.158	0.437
31								0.480	0.052	0.481
32								0.520		

Table A.10b
Critical Values of U in the Mann–Whitney Test[a]

Critical Values of U for a One-Tailed Test at $\alpha = 0.001$ or for a Two-Tailed Test at $\alpha = 0.002$

n_1	\multicolumn{12}{c}{n_2}
	9	10	11	12	13	14	15	16	17	18	19	20
1												
2												
3									0	0	0	0
4		0	0	0	1	1	1	2	2	3	3	3
5	1	1	2	2	3	3	4	5	5	6	7	7
6	2	3	4	4	5	6	7	8	9	10	11	12
7	3	5	6	7	8	9	10	11	13	14	15	16
8	5	6	8	9	11	12	14	15	17	18	20	21
9	7	8	10	12	14	15	17	19	21	23	25	26
10	8	10	12	14	17	19	21	23	25	27	29	32
11	10	12	15	17	20	22	24	27	29	32	34	37
12	12	14	17	20	23	25	28	31	34	37	40	42
13	14	17	20	23	26	29	32	35	38	42	45	48
14	15	19	22	25	29	32	36	39	43	46	50	54
15	17	21	24	28	32	36	40	43	47	51	55	59
16	19	23	27	31	35	39	43	48	52	56	60	65
17	21	25	29	34	38	43	47	52	57	61	66	70
18	23	27	32	37	42	46	51	56	61	66	71	76
19	25	29	34	40	45	50	55	60	66	71	77	82
20	26	32	37	42	48	54	59	65	70	76	82	88

[a] Adapted and abridged from Tables 1, 3, 5, and 7 of Auble, D. 1953. Extended tables for the Mann-Whitney statistic. *Bulletin of the Institute of Educational Research at Indiana University*, 1, No. 2, with the kind permission of the author and the publisher.

Table A.10b   (*Continued*)
Critical Values of *U* for a One-Tailed Test at $\alpha = 0.01$
or for a Two-Tailed Test at $\alpha = 0.02$

n_1	9	10	11	12	13	14	15	16	17	18	19	20
1												
2					0	0	0	0	0	0	1	1
3	1	1	1	2	2	2	3	3	4	4	4	5
4	3	3	4	5	5	6	7	7	8	9	9	10
5	5	6	7	8	9	10	11	12	13	14	15	16
6	7	8	9	11	12	13	15	16	18	19	20	22
7	9	11	12	14	16	17	19	21	23	24	26	28
8	11	13	15	17	20	22	24	26	28	30	32	34
9	14	16	18	21	23	26	28	31	33	36	38	40
10	16	19	22	24	27	30	33	36	38	41	44	47
11	18	22	25	28	31	34	37	41	44	47	50	53
12	21	24	28	31	35	38	42	46	49	53	56	60
13	23	27	31	35	39	43	47	51	55	59	63	67
14	26	30	34	38	43	47	51	56	60	65	69	73
15	28	33	37	42	47	51	56	61	66	70	75	80
16	31	36	41	46	51	56	61	66	71	76	82	87
17	33	38	44	49	55	60	66	71	77	82	88	93
18	36	41	47	53	59	65	70	76	82	88	94	100
19	38	44	50	56	63	69	75	82	88	94	101	107
20	40	47	53	60	67	73	80	87	93	100	107	114

Table A.10b   (*Continued*)
Critical Values of *U* for a One-Tailed Test at $\alpha = 0.025$
or for a Two-Tailed Test at $\alpha = 0.05$

							n_2					
n_1	9	10	11	12	13	14	15	16	17	18	19	20
1												
2	0	0	0	1	1	1	1	1	2	2	2	2
3	2	3	3	4	4	5	5	6	6	7	7	8
4	4	5	6	7	8	9	10	11	11	12	13	13
5	7	8	9	11	12	13	14	15	17	18	19	20
6	10	11	13	14	16	17	19	21	22	24	25	27
7	12	14	16	18	20	22	24	26	28	30	32	34
8	15	17	19	22	24	26	29	31	34	36	38	41
9	17	20	23	26	28	31	34	37	39	42	45	48
10	20	23	26	29	33	36	39	42	45	48	52	55
11	23	26	30	33	37	40	44	47	51	55	58	62
12	26	29	33	37	41	45	49	53	57	61	65	69
13	28	33	37	41	45	50	54	59	63	67	72	76
14	31	36	40	45	50	55	59	64	67	74	78	83
15	34	39	44	49	54	59	64	70	75	80	85	90
16	37	42	47	53	59	64	70	75	81	86	92	98
17	39	45	51	57	63	67	75	81	87	93	99	105
18	42	48	55	61	67	74	80	86	93	99	106	112
19	45	52	58	65	72	78	85	92	99	106	113	119
20	48	55	62	69	76	83	90	98	105	112	119	127

Table A.10b (*Continued*)
Critical Values of *U* for a One-Tailed Test at $\alpha = 0.05$ or
for a Two-Tailed Test at $\alpha = 0.10$

n_2	n_1											
	9	10	11	12	13	14	15	16	17	18	19	20
1											0	0
2	1	1	1	2	2	2	3	3	3	4	4	4
3	3	4	5	5	6	7	7	8	9	9	10	11
4	6	7	8	9	10	11	12	14	15	16	17	18
5	9	11	12	13	15	16	18	19	20	22	23	25
6	12	14	16	17	19	21	23	25	26	28	30	32
7	15	17	19	21	24	26	28	30	33	35	37	39
8	18	20	23	26	28	31	33	36	39	41	44	47
9	21	24	27	30	33	36	39	42	45	48	51	54
10	24	27	31	34	37	41	44	48	51	55	58	62
11	27	31	34	38	42	46	50	54	57	61	65	69
12	30	34	38.	42	47	51	55	60	64	68	72	77
13	33	37	42	47	51	56	61	65	70	75	80	84
14	36	41	46	51	56	61	66	71	77	82	87	92
15	39	44	50	55	61	66	72	77	83	88	94	100
16	42	48	54	60	65	71	77	83	89	95	101	107
17	45	51	57	64	70	77	83	89	96	102	109	115
18	48	55	61	68	75	82	88	95	102	109	116	123
19	51	58	65	72	80	87	94	101	109	116	123	130
20	54	62	69	77	84	92	100	107	115	123	130	138

Table A.11
Variance Ratio[a]

					$F(95\%)$[b]					
						n_1				
n_2	1	2	3	4	5	6	8	12	24	∞
1	161.4	199.5	215.7	224.6	230.2	234.0	238.9	243.9	249.0	254.3
2	18.51	19.00	19.16	19.25	19.30	19.33	19.37	19.41	19.45	19.50
3	10.13	9.55	9.28	9.12	9.01	8.94	8.84	8.74	8.64	8.53
4	7.71	6.94	6.59	6.39	6.26	6.16	6.04	5.91	5.77	5.63
5	6.61	5.79	5.41	5.19	5.05	4.95	4.82	4.68	4.53	4.36
6	5.99	5.14	4.76	4.53	4.39	4.28	4.15	4.00	3.84	3.67
7	5.59	4.74	4.35	4.12	3.97	3.87	3.73	3.57	3.41	3.23
8	5.32	4.46	4.07	3.84	3.69	3.58	3.44	3.28	3.12	2.93
9	5.12	4.26	3.86	3.63	3.48	3.37	3.23	3.07	2.90	2.71
10	4.96	4.10	3.71	3.48	3.33	3.22	3.07	2.91	2.74	2.54
11	4.84	3.98	3.59	3.36	3.20	3.09	2.95	2.79	2.61	2.40
12	4.75	3.88	3.49	3.26	3.11	3.00	2.85	2.69	2.50	2.30
13	4.67	3.80	3.41	3.18	3.02	2.92	2.77	2.60	2.42	2.21
14	4.60	3.74	3.34	3.11	2.96	2.85	2.70	2.53	2.35	2.13
15	4.54	3.68	3.29	3.06	2.90	2.79	2.64	2.48	2.29	2.07
16	4.49	3.63	3.24	3.01	2.85	2.74	2.59	2.42	2.24	2.01
17	4.45	3.59	3.20	2.96	2.81	2.70	2.55	2.38	2.19	1.96
18	4.41	3.55	3.16	2.93	2.77	2.66	2.51	2.34	2.15	1.92
19	4.38	3.52	3.13	2.90	2.74	2.63	2.48	2.31	2.11	1.88
20	4.35	3.49	3.10	2.87	2.71	2.60	2.45	2.28	2.08	1.84
21	4.32	3.47	3.07	2.84	2.68	2.57	2.42	2.25	2.05	1.81
22	4.30	3.44	3.05	2.82	2.66	2.55	2.40	2.23	2.03	1.78
23	4.28	3.42	3.03	2.80	2.64	2.53	2.38	2.20	2.00	1.76
24	4.26	3.40	3.01	2.78	2.62	2.51	2.36	2.18	1.98	1.73
25	4.24	3.38	2.99	2.76	2.60	2.49	2.34	2.16	1.96	1.71
26	4.22	3.37	2.98	2.74	2.59	2.47	2.32	2.15	1.95	1.69
27	4.21	3.35	2.96	2.73	2.57	2.46	2.30	2.13	1.93	1.67
28	4.20	3.34	2.95	2.71	2.56	2.44	2.29	2.12	1.91	1.65
29	4.18	3.33	2.93	2.70	2.54	2.43	2.28	2.10	1.90	1.64
30	4.17	3.32	2.92	2.69	2.53	2.42	2.27	2.09	1.89	1.62
40	4.08	3.23	2.84	2.61	2.45	2.34	2.18	2.00	1.79	1.51
60	4.00	3.15	2.76	2.52	2.37	2.25	2.10	1.92	1.70	1.39
120	3.92	3.07	2.68	2.45	2.29	2.17	2.02	1.83	1.61	1.25
∞	3.84	2.99	2.60	2.37	2.21	2.10	1.94	1.75	1.52	1.00

[a] From R. A. Fisher and F. Yates, *Statistical Tables for Biological, Agricultural and Medical Research*. Oliver & Boyd, London, 1957, pp. 51 and 53, Table V. By permission of the authors and publishers.
[b] Five percent points of F. Lower 5% points are found by interchange of n_1 and n_2—that is, n_1 must always correspond with the greater mean square, where n_1 and n_2 are appropriate degrees of freedom.
[c] One percent points of F. Lower 1% points are found by interchange of n_1 and n_2—that is, n_1 must always correspond with the greater mean square, where n_1 and n_2 are appropriate degrees of freedom.

Table A.11   (*Continued*)

					$F(99\%)^b$					
					n_1					
n_2	1	2	3	4	5	6	8	12	24	∞
1	4,052	4,999	5,403	5,625	5,764	5,859	5,982	6,106	6,234	6,366
2	98.50	99.00	99.17	99.25	99.30	99.33	99.37	99.42	99.46	99.50
3	34.12	30.82	29.46	28.71	28.24	27.91	27.49	27.05	26.60	26.12
4	21.20	18.00	16.69	15.98	15.52	15.21	14.80	14.37	13.93	13.46
5	16.26	13.27	12.06	11.39	10.97	10.67	10.29	9.89	9.47	9.02
6	13.74	10.92	9.78	9.15	8.75	8.47	8.10	7.72	7.31	6.88
7	12.25	9.55	8.45	7.85	7.46	7.19	6.84	6.47	6.07	5.65
8	11.26	8.65	7.59	7.01	6.63	6.37	6.03	5.67	5.28	4.86
9	10.56	8.02	6.99	6.42	6.06	5.80	5.47	5.11	4.73	4.31
10	10.04	7.56	6.55	5.99	5.64	5.39	5.06	4.71	4.33	3.91
11	9.65	7.20	6.22	5.67	5.32	5.07	4.74	4.40	4.02	3.60
12	9.33	6.93	5.95	5.41	5.06	4.82	4.50	4.16	3.78	3.36
13	9.07	6.70	5.74	5.20	4.86	4.62	4.30	3.96	3.59	3.16
14	8.86	6.51	5.56	5.03	4.69	4.46	4.14	3.80	3.43	3.00
15	8.68	6.36	5.42	4.89	4.56	4.32	4.00	3.67	3.29	2.87
16	8.53	6.23	5.29	4.77	4.44	4.20	3.89	3.55	3.18	2.75
17	8.40	6.11	5.18	4.67	4.34	4.10	3.79	3.45	3.08	2.65
18	8.28	6.01	5.09	4.58	4.25	4.01	3.71	3.37	3.00	2.57
19	8.18	5.93	5.01	4.50	4.17	3.94	3.63	3.30	2.92	2.49
20	8.10	5.85	4.94	4.43	4.10	3.87	3.56	3.23	2.86	2.42
21	8.02	5.78	4.87	4.37	4.04	3.81	3.51	3.17	2.80	2.36
22	7.94	5.72	4.82	4.31	3.99	3.76	3.45	3.12	2.75	2.31
23	7.88	5.66	4.76	4.26	3.94	3.71	3.41	3.07	2.70	2.26
24	7.82	5.61	4.72	4.22	3.90	3.67	3.36	3.03	2.66	2.21
25	7.77	5.57	4.68	4.18	3.86	3.63	3.32	2.99	2.62	2.17
26	7.72	5.53	4.64	4.14	3.82	3.59	3.29	2.96	2.58	2.13
27	7.68	5.49	4.60	4.11	3.78	3.56	3.26	2.93	2.55	2.10
28	7.64	5.45	4.57	4.07	3.75	3.53	3.23	2.90	2.52	2.06
29	7.60	5.42	4.54	4.04	3.73	3.50	3.20	2.87	2.49	2.03
30	7.56	5.39	4.51	4.02	3.70	3.47	3.17	2.84	2.47	2.01
40	7.31	5.18	4.31	3.83	3.51	3.29	2.99	2.66	2.29	1.80
60	7.08	4.98	4.13	3.65	3.34	3.12	2.82	2.50	2.12	1.60
120	6.85	4.79	3.95	3.48	3.17	2.96	2.66	2.34	1.95	1.38
∞	6.64	4.60	3.78	3.32	3.02	2.80	2.51	2.18	1.79	1.00

Table A.12

Corrected Values[a] of 0 or 100% Effect (Body of Table) Corresponding to Expected Values (Margins)

Expected	0	1	2	3	4	5	6	7	8	9
0	—	0.3	0.7	1.0	1.3	1.6	2.0	2.3	2.6	2.9
10	3.2	3.5	3.8	4.1	4.4	4.7	4.9	5.2	5.5	5.7
20	6.0	6.2	6.5	6.7	7.0	7.2	7.4	7.6	7.8	8.1
30	8.3	8.4	8.6	8.8	9.0	9.2	9.3	9.4	9.6	9.8
40	9.9	10.0	10.1	10.2	10.3	10.3	10.4	10.4	10.4	10.5
50	—	89.5	89.6	89.6	89.6	89.7	89.7	89.8	89.9	90.0
60	90.1	90.2	90.4	90.5	90.7	90.8	91.0	91.2	91.4	91.6
70	91.7	91.9	92.2	92.4	92.6	92.8	93.0	93.3	93.5	93.8
80	94.0	94.3	94.5	94.8	95.1	95.3	95.6	95.9	96.2	96.5
90	96.8	97.1	97.4	97.7	98.0	98.4	98.7	99.0	99.3	99.7

[a] These values are derived from the maximal and minimal corrected probits of Bliss, C. I. *Quart. J. Pharm. Pharmacol.* **11**:192, 1938.

Table A.13
Critical Values of the q Distribution

				$\alpha = 0.05$					
ν	$w = 2$	3	4	5	6	7	8	9	10
1	17.97	26.98	32.82	37.08	40.41	43.12	45.40	47.36	49.07
2	6.085	8.331	9.798	10.88	11.74	12.44	13.03	13.54	13.99
3	4.501	5.910	6.825	7.502	8.037	8.478	8.853	9.177	9.462
4	3.927	5.040	5.757	6.287	6.707	7.053	7.347	7.602	7.826
5	3.635	4.602	5.218	5.673	6.033	6.330	6.582	6.802	6.995
6	3.461	4.339	4.896	5.305	5.628	5.895	6.122	6.319	6.493
7	3.344	4.165	4.681	5.060	5.359	5.606	5.815	5.998	6.158
8	3.261	4.041	4.529	4.886	5.167	5.399	5.597	5.767	5.918
9	3.199	3.949	4.415	4.756	5.024	5.244	5.432	5.595	5.739
10	3.151	3.877	4.327	4.654	4.912	5.124	5.305	5.461	5.599
11	3.113	3.820	4.256	4.574	4.823	5.028	5.202	5.353	5.487
12	3.082	3.773	4.199	4.508	4.751	4.950	5.119	5.265	5.395
13	3.055	3.735	4.151	4.453	4.690	4.885	5.049	5.192	5.318
14	3.033	3.702	4.111	4.407	4.639	4.829	4.990	5.131	5.254
15	3.014	3.674	4.076	4.367	4.595	4.782	4.940	5.077	5.198
16	2.998	3.649	4.046	4.333	4.557	4.741	4.897	5.031	5.150
17	2.984	3.628	4.020	4.303	4.524	4.705	4.858	4.991	5.108
18	2.971	3.609	3.997	4.277	4.495	4.673	4.824	4.956	5.071
19	2.960	3.593	3.977	4.253	4.469	4.645	4.794	4.924	5.038
20	2.950	3.578	3.958	4.232	4.445	4.620	4.768	4.896	5.008
24	2.919	3.532	3.901	4.166	4.373	4.541	4.684	4.807	4.915
30	2.888	3.486	3.845	4.102	4.302	4.464	4.602	4.720	4.824
40	2.858	3.442	3.791	4.039	4.232	4.389	4.521	4.635	4.735
60	2.829	3.399	3.737	3.977	4.163	4.314	4.441	4.550	4.646
120	2.800	3.356	3.685	3.917	4.096	4.241	4.363	4.468	4.560
∞	2.772	3.314	3.633	3.858	4.030	4.170	4.286	4.387	3.474

ν	$w = 11$	12	13	14	15	16	17	18	19
1	50.59	51.96	53.20	54.33	55.36	56.32	57.22	58.04	58.83
2	14.39	14.75	15.08	15.38	15.65	15.91	16.14	16.37	16.57
3	9.717	9.946	10.15	10.35	10.53	10.69	10.84	10.98	11.11
4	8.027	8.208	8.373	8.525	8.664	8.794	8.914	9.028	9.134
5	7.168	7.324	7.466	7.596	7.717	7.828	7.932	8.030	8.122
6	6.649	6.789	6.917	7.034	7.143	7.244	7.338	7.426	7.508
7	6.302	6.431	6.550	6.658	6.759	6.852	6.939	7.020	7.097
8	6.054	6.175	6.287	6.389	6.483	6.571	6.653	6.729	6.802
9	5.867	5.983	6.089	6.186	6.276	6.359	6.437	6.510	6.579
10	5.722	5.833	5.935	6.028	6.114	6.194	6.269	6.339	6.405
11	5.605	5.713	5.811	5.901	5.984	6.062	6.134	6.202	6.265
12	5.511	5.615	5.710	5.798	5.878	5.953	6.023	6.089	6.151
13	5.431	5.533	5.625	5.711	5.789	5.862	5.931	5.995	6.055
14	5.364	5.463	5.554	5.637	5.714	5.786	5.852	5.915	5.974
15	5.306	5.404	5.493	5.574	5.649	5.720	5.785	5.846	5.904
16	5.256	5.352	5.439	5.520	5.593	5.662	5.727	5.786	5.843
17	5.212	5.307	5.392	5.471	5.544	5.612	5.675	5.734	5.790
18	5.174	5.267	5.352	5.429	5.501	5.568	5.630	5.688	5.743
19	5.140	5.231	5.315	5.391	5.462	5.528	5.589	5.647	5.701
20	5.108	5.199	5.282	5.357	5.427	5.493	5.553	5.610	5.663
24	5.012	5.099	5.179	5.251	5.319	5.381	5.439	5.494	5.545
30	4.917	5.001	5.077	5.147	5.211	5.271	5.327	5.379	5.429
40	4.824	4.904	4.977	5.044	5.106	5.163	5.216	5.266	5.313
60	4.732	4.808	4.878	4.942	5.001	5.056	5.107	5.154	5.199
120	4.641	4.714	4.781	4.842	4.898	4.950	4.998	5.044	5.086
∞	4.552	4.622	4.685	4.743	4.796	4.845	4.891	4.934	4.974

Table A.13 (*Continued*)
Critical Values of the *q* Distribution

					$\alpha = 0.05$				
v	*w* = 20	22	24	26	28	30	32	34	36
1	59.56	60.91	62.12	63.22	64.23	65.15	66.01	66.81	67.56
2	16.77	17.13	17.45	17.75	18.02	18.27	18.50	18.72	18.92
3	11.24	11.47	11.68	11.87	12.05	12.21	12.36	12.50	12.63
4	9.233	9.418	9.584	9.736	9.875	10.00	10.12	10.23	10.34
5	8.208	8.368	8.512	8.643	8.764	8.875	8.979	9.075	9.165
6	7.587	7.730	7.861	7.979	8.088	8.189	8.283	8.370	8.452
7	7.170	7.303	7.423	7.533	7.634	7.728	7.814	7.895	7.972
8	6.870	6.995	7.109	7.212	7.307	7.395	7.477	7.554	7.625
9	6.644	6.763	6.871	6.970	7.061	7.145	7.222	7.295	7.363
10	6.467	6.582	6.686	6.781	6.868	6.948	7.023	7.093	7.159
11	6.326	6.436	6.536	6.628	6.712	6.790	6.863	6.930	6.994
12	6.209	6.317	6.414	6.503	6.585	6.660	6.731	6.796	6.858
13	6.112	6.217	6.312	6.398	6.478	6.551	6.620	6.684	6.744
14	6.029	6.132	6.224	6.309	6.387	6.459	6.526	6.588	6.647
15	5.958	6.059	6.149	6.233	6.309	6.379	6.445	6.506	6.564
16	5.897	5.995	6.084	6.166	6.241	6.310	6.374	6.434	6.491
17	5.842	5.940	6.027	6.107	6.181	6.249	6.313	6.372	6.427
18	5.794	5.890	5.977	6.055	6.128	6.195	6.258	6.316	6.371
19	5.752	5.846	5.932	6.009	6.081	6.147	6.209	6.267	6.321
20	5.714	5.807	5.891	5.968	6.039	6.104	6.165	6.222	6.275
24	5.594	5.683	5.764	5.838	5.906	5.968	6.027	6.081	6.132
30	5.475	5.561	5.638	5.709	5.774	5.833	5.889	5.941	5.990
40	5.358	5.439	5.513	5.581	5.642	5.700	5.753	5.803	5.849
60	5.241	5.319	5.389	5.453	5.512	5.566	5.617	5.664	5.708
120	5.126	5.200	5.266	5.327	5.382	5.434	5.481	5.526	5.568
∞	5.012	5.081	5.144	5.201	5.253	5.301	5.346	5.388	5.427

v	*w* = 38	40	50	60	70	80	90	100
1	68.26	68.92	71.73	73.97	75.82	77.40	78.77	78.98
2	19.11	19.28	20.05	20.66	21.16	21.59	21.96	22.29
3	12.75	12.87	13.36	13.76	14.08	14.36	14.61	14.82
4	10.44	10.53	10.93	11.24	11.51	11.73	11.92	12.09
5	9.250	9.330	9.674	9.949	10.18	10.38	10.54	10.69
6	8.529	8.601	8.913	9.163	9.370	9.548	9.702	9.839
7	8.043	8.110	8.400	8.632	8.824	8.989	9.133	9.261
8	7.693	7.756	8.029	8.248	8.430	8.586	8.722	8.843
9	7.428	7.488	7.749	7.958	8.132	8.281	8.410	8.526
10	7.220	7.279	7.529	7.730	7.897	8.041	8.166	8.276
11	7.053	7.110	7.352	7.546	7.708	7.847	7.968	8.075
12	6.916	6.970	7.205	7.394	7.552	7.687	7.804	7.909
13	6.800	6.854	7.083	7.267	7.421	7.552	7.667	7.769
14	6.702	6.754	6.979	7.159	7.309	7.438	7.550	7.650
15	6.618	6.669	6.888	7.065	7.212	7.339	7.449	7.546
16	6.544	6.594	6.810	6.984	7.128	7.252	7.360	7.457
17	6.479	6.529	6.741	6.912	7.054	7.176	7.283	7.377
18	6.422	6.471	6.680	6.848	6.989	7.109	7.213	7.307
19	6.371	6.419	6.626	6.792	6.930	7.048	7.152	7.244
20	6.325	6.373	6.576	6.740	6.877	6.994	7.097	7.187
24	6.181	6.226	6.421	6.579	6.710	6.822	6.920	7.008
30	6.037	6.080	6.267	6.417	6.543	6.650	6.744	6.827
40	5.893	5.934	6.112	6.255	6.375	6.477	6.566	6.645
60	5.750	5.789	5.958	6.093	6.206	6.303	6.387	6.462
120	5.607	5.644	5.802	5.929	6.035	6.126	6.205	6.275
∞	5.463	5.498	5.646	5.764	5.863	5.947	6.020	6.085

Table A.13 (*Continued*)
Critical Values of the q Distribution

				$\alpha = 0.01$					
v	$w = 2$	3	4	5	6	7	8	9	10
1	90.03	135.0	164.3	185.6	202.2	215.8	227.2	237.0	245.6
2	14.04	19.02	22.29	24.72	26.63	28.20	29.53	30.68	31.69
3	8.261	10.62	12.17	13.33	14.24	15.00	15.64	16.20	16.69
4	6.512	8.120	9.173	9.958	10.58	11.10	11.55	11.93	12.27
5	5.702	6.976	7.804	8.421	8.913	9.321	9.669	9.972	10.24
6	5.243	6.331	7.033	7.556	7.973	8.318	8.613	8.869	9.097
7	4.949	5.919	6.543	7.005	7.373	7.679	7.939	8.166	8.368
8	4.746	5.635	6.204	6.625	6.960	7.237	7.474	7.681	7.863
9	4.596	5.428	5.957	6.348	6.658	6.915	7.134	7.325	7.495
10	4.482	5.270	5.769	6.136	6.428	6.669	6.875	7.055	7.213
11	4.392	5.146	5.621	5.970	6.247	6.476	6.672	6.842	6.992
12	4.320	5.046	5.502	5.836	6.101	6.321	6.507	6.670	6.814
13	4.260	4.964	5.404	5.727	5.981	6.192	6.372	6.528	6.667
14	4.210	4.895	5.322	5.634	5.881	6.085	6.258	6.409	6.543
15	4.168	4.836	5.252	5.556	5.796	5.994	6.162	6.309	6.439
16	4.131	4.786	5.192	5.489	5.722	5.915	6.079	6.222	6.349
17	4.099	4.742	5.140	5.430	5.659	5.847	6.007	6.147	6.270
18	4.071	4.703	5.094	5.379	5.603	5.788	5.944	6.081	6.201
19	4.046	4.670	5.054	5.334	5.554	5.735	5.889	6.022	6.141
20	4.024	4.639	5.018	5.294	5.510	5.688	5.839	5.970	6.087
24	3.956	4.546	4.907	5.168	5.374	5.542	5.685	5.809	5.919
30	3.889	4.455	4.799	5.048	5.242	5.401	5.536	5.653	5.756
40	3.825	4.367	4.696	4.931	5.114	5.265	5.392	5.502	5.559
60	3.762	4.282	4.595	4.818	4.991	5.133	5.253	5.356	5.447
120	3.702	4.200	4.497	4.709	4.872	5.005	5.118	5.214	5.299
∞	3.643	4.120	4.403	4.603	4.757	4.882	4.987	5.078	5.157

v	$w = 11$	12	13	14	15	16	17	18	19
1	253.2	260.0	266.2	271.8	277.0	281.8	286.3	290.4	294.3
2	32.59	33.40	34.13	34.81	35.43	36.00	36.53	37.03	37.50
3	17.13	17.53	17.89	18.22	18.52	18.81	19.07	19.32	19.55
4	12.57	12.84	13.09	13.32	13.53	13.73	13.91	14.08	14.24
5	10.48	10.70	10.89	11.08	11.24	11.40	11.55	11.68	11.81
6	9.301	9.485	9.653	9.808	9.951	10.08	10.21	10.32	10.43
7	8.548	8.711	8.860	8.997	9.124	9.242	9.353	9.456	9.554
8	8.027	8.176	8.312	8.436	8.552	8.659	8.760	8.854	8.943
9	7.647	7.784	7.910	8.025	8.132	8.232	8.325	8.412	8.495
10	7.356	7.485	7.603	7.712	7.812	7.906	7.993	8.076	8.153
11	7.128	7.250	7.362	7.465	7.560	7.649	7.732	7.809	7.883
12	6.943	7.060	7.167	7.265	7.356	7.441	7.520	7.594	7.665
13	6.791	6.903	7.006	7.101	7.188	7.269	7.345	7.417	7.485
14	6.664	6.772	6.871	6.962	7.047	7.126	7.199	7.268	7.333
15	6.555	6.660	6.757	6.845	6.927	7.003	7.074	7.142	7.204
16	6.462	6.564	6.658	6.744	6.823	6.898	6.967	7.032	7.093
17	6.381	6.480	6.572	6.656	6.734	6.806	6.873	6.937	6.997
18	6.310	6.407	6.497	6.579	6.655	6.725	6.792	6.854	6.912
19	6.247	6.342	6.430	6.510	6.585	6.654	6.719	6.780	6.837
20	6.191	6.285	6.371	6.450	6.523	6.591	6.654	6.714	6.771
24	6.017	6.106	6.186	6.261	6.330	6.394	6.453	6.510	6.563
30	5.849	5.932	6.008	6.078	6.143	6.203	6.259	6.311	6.361
40	5.686	5.764	5.835	5.900	5.961	6.017	6.069	6.119	6.165
60	5.528	5.601	5.667	5.728	5.785	5.837	5.886	5.931	5.974
120	5.375	5.443	5.505	5.562	5.614	5.662	5.708	5.750	5.790
∞	5.227	5.290	5.348	5.400	5.448	5.493	5.535	5.574	5.611

Table A.13 (*Continued*)
Critical Values of the q Distribution

					$\alpha = 0.01$				
v	$w = 20$	22	24	26	28	30	32	34	36
1	298.0	304.7	310.8	316.3	321.3	326.0	330.3	334.3	338.0
2	37.95	38.76	39.49	40.15	40.76	41.32	41.84	42.33	42.78
3	19.77	20.17	20.53	20.86	21.16	21.44	21.70	21.95	22.17
4	14.40	14.68	14.93	15.16	15.37	15.57	15.75	15.92	16.08
5	11.93	12.16	12.36	12.54	12.71	12.87	13.02	13.15	13.28
6	10.54	10.73	10.91	11.06	11.21	11.34	11.47	11.58	11.69
7	9.646	9.815	9.970	10.11	10.24	10.36	10.47	10.58	10.67
8	9.027	9.182	9.322	9.450	9.569	9.678	9.779	9.874	9.964
9	8.573	8.717	8.847	8.966	9.075	9.177	9.271	9.360	9.443
10	8.226	8.361	8.483	8.595	8.698	8.794	8.883	8.966	9.044
11	7.952	8.080	8.196	8.303	8.400	8.491	8.575	8.654	8.728
12	7.731	7.853	7.964	8.066	8.159	8.246	8.327	8.402	8.473
13	7.548	7.665	7.772	7.870	7.960	8.043	8.121	8.193	8.262
14	7.395	7.508	7.611	7.705	7.792	7.873	7.948	8.018	8.084
15	7.264	7.374	7.474	7.566	7.650	7.728	7.800	7.869	7.932
16	7.152	7.258	7.356	7.445	7.527	7.602	7.673	7.739	7.802
17	7.053	7.158	7.253	7.340	7.420	7.493	7.563	7.627	7.687
18	6.968	7.070	7.163	7.247	7.325	7.398	7.465	7.528	7.587
19	6.891	6.992	7.082	7.166	7.242	7.313	7.379	7.440	7.498
20	6.823	6.922	7.011	7.092	7.168	7.237	7.302	7.362	7.419
24	6.612	6.705	6.789	6.865	6.936	7.001	7.062	7.119	7.173
30	6.407	6.494	6.572	6.644	6.710	6.772	6.828	6.881	6.932
40	6.209	6.289	6.362	6.429	6.490	6.547	6.600	6.650	6.697
60	6.015	6.090	6.158	6.220	6.277	6.330	6.378	6.424	6.467
120	5.827	5.897	5.959	6.016	6.069	6.117	6.162	6.204	6.244
∞	5.645	5.709	5.766	5.818	5.866	5.911	5.952	5.990	6.026

v	$w = 38$	40	50	60	70	80	90	100
1	341.5	344.8	358.9	370.1	379.4	387.3	394.1	400.1
2	43.21	43.61	45.33	46.70	47.83	48.80	49.64	50.38
3	22.39	22.59	23.45	24.13	24.71	25.19	25.62	25.99
4	16.23	16.37	16.98	17.46	17.86	18.02	18.50	18.77
5	13.40	13.52	14.00	14.39	14.72	14.99	15.23	15.45
6	11.80	11.90	12.31	12.65	12.92	13.16	13.37	13.55
7	10.77	10.85	11.23	11.52	11.77	11.99	12.17	12.34
8	10.05	10.13	10.47	10.75	10.97	11.17	11.34	11.49
9	9.521	9.594	9.912	10.17	10.38	10.57	10.73	10.87
10	9.117	9.187	9.486	9.726	9.927	10.10	10.25	10.39
11	8.798	8.864	9.148	9.377	9.568	9.732	9.875	10.00
12	8.539	8.603	8.875	9.094	9.277	9.434	9.571	9.693
13	8.326	8.387	8.648	8.859	9.035	9.187	9.318	9.436
14	8.146	8.204	8.457	8.661	8.832	8.978	9.106	9.219
15	7.992	8.049	8.295	8.492	8.658	8.800	8.924	9.035
16	7.860	7.916	8.154	8.347	8.507	8.646	8.767	8.874
17	7.745	7.799	8.031	8.219	8.377	8.511	8.630	8.735
18	7.643	7.696	7.924	8.107	8.261	8.393	8.508	8.611
19	7.553	7.605	7.828	8.008	8.159	8.288	8.401	8.502
20	7.473	7.523	7.742	7.919	8.067	8.194	8.305	8.404
24	7.223	7.270	7.476	7.642	7.780	7.900	8.004	8.097
30	6.978	7.023	7.215	7.370	7.500	7.611	7.709	7.796
40	6.740	6.782	6.960	7.104	7.225	7.328	7.419	7.500
60	6.507	6.546	6.710	6.843	6.954	7.050	7.133	7.207
120	6.281	6.316	6.467	6.588	6.689	6.776	6.852	6.919
∞	6.060	6.092	6.228	6.338	6.429	6.507	6.575	6.636

Table A.14

Duncan's Multiple Ranges (5 % Level)[a]

	p = number of means within range being tested											
d.f.	2	3	4	5	6	7	8	9	10	20	50	100
1	18.00	18.00	18.00	18.00	18.00	18.00	18.00	18.00	18.00	18.00	18.00	18.00
2	6.08	6.08	6.08	6.08	6.08	6.08	6.08	6.08	6.08	6.08	6.08	6.08
3	4.50	4.52	4.52	4.52	4.52	4.52	4.52	4.52	4.52	4.52	4.52	4.52
4	3.93	4.01	4.03	4.03	4.03	4.03	4.03	4.03	4.03	4.03	4.03	4.03
5	3.64	3.75	3.80	3.81	3.81	3.81	3.81	3.81	3.81	3.81	3.81	3.81
6	3.46	3.59	3.65	3.68	3.69	3.70	3.70	3.70	3.70	3.70	3.70	3.70
7	3.34	3.48	3.55	3.59	3.61	3.62	3.63	3.63	3.63	3.63	3.63	3.63
8	3.26	3.40	3.48	3.52	3.55	3.57	3.58	3.58	3.58	3.58	3.58	3.58
9	3.20	3.34	3.42	3.47	3.50	3.52	3.54	3.54	3.55	3.55	3.55	3.55
10	3.15	3.29	3.38	3.43	3.46	3.49	3.50	3.52	3.52	3.53	3.53	3.53
11	3.11	3.26	3.34	3.40	3.44	3.46	3.48	3.49	3.50	3.51	3.51	3.51
12	3.08	3.22	3.31	3.37	3.41	3.44	3.46	3.47	3.48	3.50	3.50	3.50
13	3.06	3.20	3.29	3.35	3.39	3.42	3.44	3.46	3.47	3.49	3.49	3.49
14	3.03	3.18	3.27	3.33	3.37	3.40	3.43	3.44	3.46	3.48	3.48	3.48
15	3.01	3.16	3.25	3.31	3.36	3.39	3.41	3.43	3.45	3.48	3.48	3.48
16	3.00	3.14	3.24	3.30	3.34	3.38	3.40	3.42	3.44	3.48	3.48	3.48
17	2.98	3.13	3.22	3.28	3.33	3.37	3.39	3.41	3.43	3.48	3.48	3.48
18	2.97	3.12	3.21	3.27	3.32	3.36	3.38	3.40	3.42	3.47	3.47	3.47
19	2.96	3.11	3.20	3.26	3.31	3.35	3.38	3.40	3.42	3.47	3.47	3.47
20	2.95	3.10	3.19	3.26	3.30	3.34	3.37	3.39	3.41	3.47	3.47	3.47
30	2.89	3.04	3.13	3.20	3.25	3.29	3.32	3.35	3.37	3.47	3.49	3.49
40	2.86	3.01	3.10	3.17	3.22	3.27	3.30	3.33	3.35	3.47	3.50	3.50
60	2.83	2.98	3.07	3.14	3.20	3.24	3.28	3.31	3.33	3.47	3.54	3.54
120	2.80	2.95	3.04	3.12	3.17	3.22	3.25	3.29	3.31	3.47	3.58	3.60
∞	2.77	2.92	3.02	3.09	3.15	3.19	3.23	3.26	3.29	3.47	3.64	3.74

[a] The numbers given in this table are the values of Q_p used to find $R_p = Q_p s_{\bar{x}}$. The value of R_p, then, is the shortest significant range for comparing the largest and smallest of p means arranged in order of magnitude.

Table A.14 (*Continued*)
Duncan's Multiple Ranges (1 % Level)

d.f.	p = number of means within range being tested											
	2	3	4	5	6	7	8	9	10	20	50	100
1	90.00	90.00	90.00	90.00	90.00	90.00	90.00	90.00	90.00	90.00	90.00	90.00
2	14.00	14.00	14.00	14.00	14.00	14.00	14.00	14.00	14.00	14.00	14.00	14.00
3	8.26	8.32	8.32	8.32	8.32	8.32	8.32	8.32	8.32	8.32	8.32	8.32
4	6.51	6.68	6.74	6.76	6.76	6.76	6.76	6.76	6.76	6.76	6.76	6.76
5	5.70	5.89	6.00	6.04	6.06	6.07	6.07	6.07	6.07	6.07	6.07	6.07
6	5.25	5.44	5.55	5.61	5.66	5.68	5.69	5.70	5.70	5.70	5.70	5.70
7	4.95	5.14	5.26	5.33	5.38	5.42	5.44	5.45	5.46	5.47	5.47	5.47
8	4.75	4.94	5.06	5.14	5.19	5.23	5.26	5.28	5.29	5.32	5.32	5.32
9	4.60	4.79	4.91	4.99	5.04	5.09	5.12	5.14	5.16	5.21	5.21	5.21
10	4.48	4.67	4.79	4.87	4.93	4.98	5.01	5.04	5.06	5.12	5.12	5.12
11	4.39	4.58	4.70	4.78	4.84	4.89	4.92	4.95	4.98	5.06	5.06	5.06
12	4.32	4.50	4.62	4.71	4.77	4.82	4.85	4.88	4.91	5.01	5.01	5.01
13	4.26	4.44	4.56	4.64	4.71	4.76	4.79	4.82	4.85	4.96	4.97	4.97
14	4.21	4.39	4.51	4.59	4.65	4.70	4.74	4.78	4.80	4.92	4.94	4.94
15	4.17	4.35	4.46	4.55	4.61	4.66	4.70	4.73	4.76	4.89	4.91	4.91
16	4.13	4.31	4.42	4.51	4.57	4.62	4.66	4.70	4.72	4.86	4.89	4.89
17	4.10	4.28	4.39	4.48	4.54	4.59	4.63	4.66	4.69	4.83	4.87	4.87
18	4.07	4.25	4.36	4.44	4.51	4.56	4.60	4.64	4.66	4.81	4.86	4.86
19	4.05	4.22	4.34	4.42	4.48	4.53	4.58	4.61	4.64	4.79	4.84	4.84
20	4.02	4.20	4.31	4.40	4.46	4.51	4.55	4.59	4.62	4.77	4.83	4.83
30	3.89	4.06	4.17	4.25	4.31	4.37	4.41	4.44	4.48	4.65	4.77	4.78
40	3.82	3.99	4.10	4.18	4.24	4.30	4.34	4.38	4.41	4.59	4.74	4.76
60	3.76	3.92	4.03	4.11	4.17	4.23	4.27	4.31	4.34	4.53	4.71	4.76
120	3.70	3.86	3.96	4.04	4.11	4.16	4.20	4.24	4.27	4.47	4.67	4.77
∞	3.64	3.80	3.90	3.98	4.04	4.09	4.14	4.17	4.20	4.41	4.64	4.78

Appendix B

PHARM/PCS User's Guide

Contents

A. Diskette versus Source Code Listing

PHARM/PCS is available on diskette to run without modification on most popular microcomputers. Ordering information can be found on the last page of this book or by writing directly to:

> MicroComputer Specialists
> P.O. Box 40346
> Philadelphia, PA 19106

The inclusion of a program listing at the end of this appendix is intended for use by experienced programmers who may wish to modify or add to PHARM/PCS for their own use, or for owners of computers for which a diskette version is not available. Certain features of the diskette version are not possible to duplicate if the listing form is typed in. For example, the diskette version contains several files that contain statistical tables that are automatically used by PHARM/PCS. Also, the "HELP" screens, shown below, are on the diskette for easy access.

The source code was written in Microsoft BASIC as implemented under the TRSDOS[1] operating system on the TRS-80[1] Model III. The use of this computer and language reflects the evolution of PHARM/PCS from the time of the first edition of this book. (In 1979, the TRS-80 Model I and Apple II[2] were the most popular personal computers available at a modest cost and preceded the introduction of the IBM-PC[3] and other MS-DOS[4] computers.)

Throughout this appendix, specific instructions will be given for the use of PHARM/PCS under the MS-DOS (same as PC-DOS[3]) and the TRSDOS disk operating systems.

B. Installation

B-1. Create a working diskette with DOS and BASIC

You must first create a working diskette containing your DOS and BASIC. Referring to your computer's user manual, format a new system diskette with BASIC on it. This is most easily accomplished with a 2-drive system. Insert your

---

[1] TRSDOS and TRS-80 are trademarks of Tandy Corporation/Radio Shack.

[2] Apple II is a trademark of Apple Computer, Inc.

[3] IBM-PC and PC-DOS are trademarks of International Business Machines.

[4] MS-DOS is a trademark of Microsoft Corporation.

System diskette (or a backup) in the primary drive and a new blank diskette in the secondary drive.

NOTE: If you have a hard disk system, you may skip this step and install PHARM/PCS directly on your hard disk (go to Sec. B-2 paragraph b or c, below).

For MS-DOS, where Drive A: contains your DOS diskette type:

```
A>FORMAT B: /S

A>COPY BASIC.* B:
```

or for TRSDOS, format your blank diskette in Drive 1, and then make a backup:

```
TRSDOS Ready
FORMAT :1

TRSDOS Ready
BACKUP :0 :1
```

Delete any unnecessary files from your newly formatted TRSDOS diskette in order to retain as much space as possible for PHARM/PCS. PHARM/PCS runtime files leave only about 5K on a 180K disk drive (the TRS-80 Model 4D has 360K disks, as do most MS-DOS computers). Of course, you may save your data and report files on a data diskette in Drive 1.

B-2. Installation from <u>DISKETTE</u>

a. Floppy Disk Systems

Label your newly formatted DOS diskette (with BASIC) with "PHARM/PCS Runtime Diskette," and put it in your primary drive (A: or 0). Put the PHARM/PCS Master diskette into your secondary drive (B: or 1).

For MS-DOS, execute the installation program by typing the following, assuming "A" is your destination drive:

```
A>B:

B>INSTALL B: A:
```

or for TRSDOS type:

```
TRSDOS Ready
DO INSTALL
```

A number of messages will appear on your screen, after which PHARM/PCS will automatically load. You have now installed PHARM/PCS. You will still need your PHARM/PCS Master diskette in order to customize your system (see Section C.2). After customizing your "Runtime" diskette, put your PHARM/PCS Master diskette away in a safe place.

b. MS-DOS Hard Disk Installations (e.g. IBM-PC XT)

The following assumes that your hard disk is configured as drive C: and you have a single floppy disk drive, A:. Put the PHARM/PCS Master diskette into Drive A:.

Execute the install program, specifying A: as the source and C: as the destination, assuming that C: is your current default drive.

```
C>A:

A>INSTALL A: C:
```

A number of messages will appear on your screen. The above procedure installs the runtime programs and library files on drive C:, creating the necessary subdirectories (requires MS-DOS/PC-DOS 2.0 or later).

Now you may execute PHARM/PCS (already on Hard Drive C), for customizing, by entering:

```
C> PCS
```

c. TRSDOS Hard Disk Installation

Since TRSDOS Hard Disk Systems may split the hard disk into 4 or more "logical" drives (i.e., Drive 0, 1, 2, and 3), we will assume that the source floppy disk is configured as Drive 4. Drive 0 is the "System" destination disk on the hard drive.

Place your PHARM/PCS Master disk in drive 4, and type:

```
TRSDOS Ready
DO HINSTALL
```

A number of messages will appear on your screen, after which PHARM/PCS will automatically load. You have now installed PHARM/PCS runtime programs on drive 0 and library files on drive 1.

To execute PHARM/PCS at the TRSDOS prompt, type:

```
TRSDOS Ready
BASIC PCS
```

B-3. Installation from SOURCE CODE LISTING

Type in the following ASCII text files at the end of this appendix using your text editor or word processor. Type everything *between* the dotted line and the end of file marker, "EOF." Do not forget to type blank lines (press ⟨ENTER⟩ where needed). The file names are listed below followed by the length of the file in characters (bytes). Each blank line uses only byte. Use a period instead of a slash "/" if you have an MS-DOS computer. The "HELP" files are optional.

```
HELP1/PCS      1845
HELP2/PCS       353
HELP3/PCS      1005
HELP4/PCS       782
HELP5/PCS       657
SYS2/PCS        439
SYS3/PCS       1971
```

Using your computer's BASIC language, type in the following programs. Save them in compressed format, not in ASCII format (i.e., SAVE "SYS1/PCS"). These programs are not optional.

```
PCS              512
SYS1/PCS        4000
PHARM/LIB      21667
```

Using your computer's BASIC language (or a text editor), type in the following program modules. Save them in ASCII format (i.e., in BASIC, type SAVE "PCS01/LIB", A).

```
PCS01/LIB       1515
PCS03/LIB        959
PCS04/LIB        391
PCS05/LIB       1945
PCS06/LIB        606
PCS07/LIB        650
PCS08/LIB       3056
PCS09/LIB       2406
PCS10/LIB       2044
PCS11/LIB        190
PCS12/LIB        632
PCS13/LIB        581
PCS14/LIB        566
PCS15/LIB       1251
PCS16/LIB        942
PCS17/LIB        661
PCS18/LIB        520
PCS19/LIB        741
PCS20/LIB        368
PCS21/LIB        721
PCS22/LIB        588
PCS23/LIB        770
PCS24/LIB        757
PCS25/LIB       1621
PCS26/LIB       2187
PCS27/LIB       1961
PCS28/LIB       1263
PCS29/LIB       1934
PCS30/LIB       1285
PCS31/LIB       1001
PCS32/LIB       2466
PCS33/LIB       2928
PCS34/LIB        215
PCS35/LIB       2292
PCS36/LIB       2543
PCS37/LIB       1226
PCS38/LIB        745
PCS39/LIB        508
PCS40/LIB        625
PCS41/LIB        581
PCS42/LIB       1750
PCS43/LIB       1011
PCS44/LIB        982
PCS45/LIB       2001
PCS46/LIB       4915
PCS47/LIB        173
PCS48/LIB       1960
```

C. Operation

C-1. Starting PHARM/PCS

If you have just installed PHARM/PCS, it should already be running. To start PHARM/PCS after you have exited the program, first place the PHARM/PCS Runtime Diskette in your primary disk drive (Drive A: for MS-DOS, Drive 0 for

TRSDOS). (NOTE: You must have already installed PHARM/PCS, see Section B.)

To execute PHARM/PCS at the MS-DOS prompt, type:

```
A> PCS
```

To execute PHARM/PCS at the TRSDOS prompt, type:

```
TRSDOS Ready
BASIC PCS
```

PHARM/PCS will load, and you will see the Copyright Screen...

```
PHARM/PCS Version 4.0 (04/15/86) TRS-80 Model III

Pharmacologic Calculation System
(C) 1986 Rodney B. Murray.
All Rights Reserved.

Reproduction without written
permission from MicroComputer
Specialists, of any portion of
this program, is prohibited.

Initializing, Please Stand By ...
```

After initialization, you will see the Title Screen...

```
                 Pharmacologic Calculation System

                      PHARM/PCS - Version 4

                            based on

               "Manual of Pharmacologic Calculations
                     with Computer Programs"
                           2nd Edition

                  by R.J. Tallarida and R.B. Murray
                  Springer-Verlag, New York, 1986




Procedure: <##>, <E>xit, <?>, or <ENTER> for next screen ?
```

C-2. Procedure Menu

The "Procedure Menu" of PHARM/PCS is the last line on your video display. The flashing cursor at the end of the line is your signal that PHARM/PCS is waiting for your input. Several choices await you. Valid keystrokes are surrounded by brackets (⟨⟩).

a. ⟨?⟩ Help—Onlines User's Guide

The first option you may want to try at the Procedure Menu prompt is to ask for help! Should you forget what some of your options are, press ⟨?⟩ for Help at ANY Menu. After the first Help Screen appears, you may press ⟨ENTER⟩ to continue to the next Help Screen. Pressing ⟨ENTER⟩ after the last Help Screen will return you to the Table of Contents screen (see below).

NOTE: All Help screens are duplicated later in this appendix.

b. ⟨ENTER⟩—Table of Contents Screen

Pressing ⟨ENTER⟩ at the Procedure Menu prompt will cause the Table of Contents to be displayed. You will have to press ⟨ENTER⟩ more than once to view the entire Table of Contents.

```
        Pharmacologic Calculation System - Version 4.0
--- ----------------------------------------------------------
      Data space: 10 groups @ 20 items each. 39040 Bytes Free.

<  1> Dosage & Concentration: Drug Stock Solutions
<  2>*Mean, Standard Deviation & Confidence Limits
<  3> Linear Regression I
<  4> Linear Regression II: Lines Through Origin
<  5> Analysis of the Regression Line
<  6> Parallel Lines I: Test for Parallelism
<  7> Parallel Lines II: Construction of Parallel Lines
<  8> Graded Dose-Response
<  9> Quantal Dose-Response: Probits
<10> Relative Potency I

Procedure: <##>, <E>xit, <?>, or <ENTER> for next screen ?
```

The asterisk (*) associated with Procedure 2 on the Table of Contents screen above means that Procedure 2 is currently resident in memory. In order to make enough room for data in memory, and because different users have different needs, only those procedures actually required to perform a particular analysis are actually resident in memory. When you select a Procedure, it is loaded into memory automatically from your Master diskette in your secondary disk drive or hard disk.

The message "Data Space: 10 groups @ 20 items each" at the top of the Table of Contents indicates the dimensions of memory reserved for your data. You may change the data space to your specifications (see Sec. D-4).

The message "39040 Bytes Free" shows the remaining RAM memory (not diskette space) available to load additional procedures. If this number falls below 1000 and you want to select a procedure that is not currently resident in memory, you will have to select the ⟨V⟩ersion Maintanence option (see Sec. D-4).

c. ⟨##⟩—Selecting Procedure

You may select any of the 48 procedures by entering a one or two-digit procedure number, Two-digit numbers may be entered without pressing ⟨ENTER⟩. Procedures 1 through 9, however, require that you type the digit followed by ⟨ENTER⟩, or type a leading zero.

For example, to select Procedure 2 (Mean, Standard Deviation and Confidence Limits) you may type either...

02   or   2⟨ENTER⟩.

NOTE: Not all procedures are resident in memory at one time. Selecting a non-resident procedure will cause it to be automatically loaded from the PHARM/PCS Master Diskette, which must be in your secondary disk drive, or else an error message will result (see Sec. C-2b, above). Of course, if you have installed PHARM/PCS on a hard disk system, you will not need your Master diskette.

Selecting Procedure 5 (Analysis of the Regression Line) when Procedure 2 is the only procedure that is currently in memory will automatically cause Procedure 5 to be loaded. Since Procedure 5 also requires Procedure 3, you will see the following display...

```
Pharmacologic Calculation System - Version 4.0 - 07/30/86
----------------------------------------------------------
    Data space: 10 groups @ 20 items each. 39040 Bytes Free.

Merging PCS05/LIB ...
Merging PCS03/LIB ...
```

Procedure 5 will then begin. Since both procedures are now loaded, pressing ⟨ENTER⟩ at the Procedure Menu will display the following Table of Contents (note the new asterisks). You should save this particular configuration of PHARM/PCS if you will be using Procedure 5 often or other procedures that require it (use ⟨S⟩ave Configuration command, see Sec. D-3).

```
      Pharmacologic Calculation System - Version 4.0
  ----------------------------------------------------------
     Data space: 10 groups @ 20 items each. 39040 Bytes Free.

 < 1> Dosage & Concentration: Drug Stock Solutions
 < 2>*Mean, Standard Deviation & Confidence Limits
 < 3>*Linear Regression I
 < 4> Linear Regression II: Lines Through Origin
 < 5>*Analysis of the Regression Line
 < 6> Parallel Lines I: Test for Parallelism
 < 7> Parallel Lines II: Construction of Parallel Lines
 < 8> Graded Dose-Response
 < 9> Quantal Dose-Response: Probits
 <10> Relative Potency I

 Procedure: <##>, <E>xit, <?>, or <ENTER> for next screen ?
```

d. ⟨E⟩xit PHARM/PCS

After your data analysis session, you must exit PHARM/PCS properly, Pressing ⟨E⟩ will close all open files and return to DOS.

C-3. Data File Preparation

a. Input: ⟨K⟩eyboard, ⟨D⟩isk, or ⟨E⟩xit this procedure?

Procedures in PHARM/PCS require input of either a single variable (Y), paired variables (XY), or 3-variable (XYZ) data. The "Computer Screens" shown after each worked example in the text of each Procedure are used to illustrate data entry. The computer screens at the end of Procedure 2 (page 9) are used to illustrate keyboard data entry of Y-type data. Procedure 3, Linear Regress I, is used to illustrate keyboard data entry of XY-type data (see Computer Screen, p. 12).

After selecting a procedure, e.g. 2, from the Procedure Menu you will see...

```
        <2> Mean, Standard Deviation & Confidence Limits
    Pharmacologic Calculation System - Version 4.0 - 08/02/86

Input: <K>eyboard, <D>isk, or <E>xit this procedure? K
```

The first prompt asks you to specify the input mode of your data, or allows you to abort the procedure by pressing ⟨E⟩ to exit to the Procedure Menu. If you are entering data for the first time, press ⟨K⟩ for keyboard data entry, otherwise press ⟨D⟩ to enter data that you have already stored on diskette.

Next, you will be asked for a "filespec"...

```
You may enter 10 'Y' data files. Type 'END' after last file.
Enter file name or <ENTER> for default name:
'FILE1/Y' (or 'END') ? <ENTER>
```

Here you are asked to enter the filespec (see Glossary for discussion of valid filespecs) for the data you are about to enter. In this case you may enter up to 10 data files.

NOTE: This number (10) is dependent on your available memory and the settings of your system parameters (see Sec. D-4).

Here we have pressed the ⟨ENTER⟩ key, thereby keeping the default filespec of "FILE/Y" (or the equivalent filespec of "FILE.Y" for MS-DOS). If you plan to keep your data for future analysis, you may want to give a more meaningful name at this point.

Now, you can actually enter your data...

```
You may enter up to 20 observations. Press <ENTER> after the
last entry.

   File name:     FILE1/Y
   -----------   -----------
      # 1: 130<ENTER>
      # 2: 141<ENTER>
      # 3: 120<ENTER>
      # 4: 110<ENTER>
      # 5: 118<ENTER>
      # 6: 124<ENTER>
      # 7: 165<ENTER>
      # 8: 128<ENTER>
      # 9: <ENTER>

FILE2/Y' (or 'END') ? END<ENTER>
```

Here we have entered 8 items of data (130, ..., 128) to be analyzed. Press the ⟨ENTER⟩ key after the last entry in a particular file, and type "END" when asked for the next filespec, if you are finished entering data files.

NOTE: Scientific notation may be used to enter data values. Enter the mantissa followed by the letter "E" and the exponent. For example, "1,250,000" may be entered as "1.25E6."

Next we use Procedure 5, "Analysis of the Regression Line," to illustrate data entry from a disk file that was previously entered from the keyboard.

```
              <5> Analysis of the Regression Line
   Pharmacologic Calculation System - Version 4.0 - 08/08/86

 Input: <K>eyboard, <D>isk, or <E>xit this procedure? D
```

In the above sample screen, we requested that a previously created data file will be loaded, instead of entering data from the keyboard. The file is named "FILE5/XY". Although we can run Procedure 5 with as many as 10 data files, below we load only "FILE5/XY".

```
 You may enter 10 'XY' data files. Press <ENTER> after last
 file name.
 File name 1 ? FILE5/XY
 File name 2 ? <ENTER>

 Data: <E>dit, <L>ist, <S>ave, or <ENTER> to continue?
```

NOTE: When entering XY or XYZ data types from the keyboard, you may assign your own variable names in certain procedures. Before you are prompted for the file name you will be asked...

```
 Enter new variable name(s), or <ENTER> for default(s):
 Variable X: 'X' ? X Value<ENTER>
 Variable Y: 'Y' ? Y Value<ENTER>
```

b. Data: ⟨E⟩dit, ⟨L⟩ist, ⟨S⟩ave, or ⟨ENTER⟩ to continue?

After entering all of your data from either the keyboard or the disk, you are presented with a new menu, which will be called the "Data" menu. Here, you will usually want to ⟨L⟩ist the data before continuing with the computation.

NOTE: You must ⟨L⟩ist the data file at this Data Menu in order that the data appear on the final report.

⟨L⟩ist

```
 Data: <E>dit, <L>ist, <S>ave, or <ENTER> to continue? L

   File name:      FILE5/XY
    Variable:      X Value      Y Value
   ----------    ----------    ----------
       # 1:           -5           -4
       # 2:           -1           -2
       # 3:            3            4
       # 4:            5            6
       # 5:            8            7
       # 6:           10           10
       # 7:           15           12

 Data: <E>dit, <L>ist, <S>ave, or <ENTER> to continue?
```

Your data are listed in column format with adjacent "index" numbers. Index numbers may be used later to pinpoint data to be edited.

If you had just entered your data from the keyboard, you should get into the habit of saving it immediately...

⟨S⟩ave

```
Data: <E>dit, <L>ist, <S>ave, or <ENTER> to continue? S


Saving 'FILE5/XY' ...


Data: <E>dit, <L>ist, <S>ave, or <ENTER> to continue?
```

The next section illustrates various ways to edit your data file.

c. Edit: ⟨C⟩hange, ⟨D⟩elete, ⟨I⟩nsert, ⟨L⟩ist, or ⟨R⟩ename? ⟨C⟩hange Data

In the first prompt, shown below, we elected to edit our data. We could also have continued with the computation by pressing ⟨ENTER⟩ or ⟨S⟩aved our data. After choosing ⟨E⟩dit, we are presented with the "Edit" menu. Let us change our 7th data values from (15, 12) to (20, 15). We have to enter ⟨C⟩ for "Change" and "7" at the next prompt. The remainder of the screen illustrates the change...

```
Data: <E>dit, <L>ist, <S>ave, or <ENTER> to continue? E

Edit: <C>hange, <D>elete, <I>nsert, <L>ist, or <R>ename ? C

Change which entry (1 - 7) in 'FILE5/XY' ? 7

  File name:    FILE5/XY
   Variable:     X Value      Y Value
 ----------- ----------- -----------
       # 7:         15          12
       # 7: 20<ENTER>    15<ENTER>

<ENTER> to continue, or
Change which entry (1 - 7) in 'FILE5/XY' ? <ENTER>

Edit: <C>hange, <D>elete, <I>nsert, <L>ist, or <R>ename ?
```

NOTE: If you had loaded more than one data file, you would first be asked which data file to edit.

At the Edit Menu we could also have ⟨D⟩eleted or ⟨I⟩nserted one or more values. First enter your editing subcommand and then give the "index" number (referring to the above listing) of the value where you want to delete or insert.

⟨D⟩elete Data

This time we will illustrate how to delete data from our file. First select ⟨D⟩ to delete...

```
Edit: <C>hange, <D>elete, <I>nsert, <L>ist, or <R>ename ? D

Delete which entry (1 - 7) in 'FILE5/XY' ? 1

Delete which entry (1 - 6) in 'FILE5/XY' ? <ENTER>

Edit: <C>hange, <D>elete, <I>nsert, <L>ist, or <R>ename ?
```

We decided to delete the first data pair by replying "1" to the "which entry" prompt. The range of possible indices is listed within parenthesis. After we delete one data pair, this range is decreased by one. Since we want to delete only one pair at this time, we pressed ⟨ENTER⟩ to return to the previous ⟨E⟩dit Menu.

NOTE: After deleting data, indices larger than the index of the deletion point are decreased by one. For example, to delete three data points starting at the 5th position, you would delete the data point at index number 5 THREE times!

Now that we have deleted a data pair, let us insert a different pair...

⟨I⟩nsert Data

```
Edit: <C>hange, <D>elete, <I>nsert, <L>ist, or <R>ename ? I

Insert at which entry (1 - 7) in 'FILE5/XY' ? 7

You may enter up to 14 x,y data pairs. Press <ENTER> after the
last entry.

   File name:     FILE5/XY
   Variable:      X Value      Y Value
  -----------   -----------  -----------
       # 7: 30<ENTER>    20<ENTER>
       # 8: <ENTER>
```

Although we could have inserted data at any point in our file, here we elected to add new data to the end of our list (index #7). Since we have 6 pairs of data, we are reminded that we may only insert up to 14 more pairs. Remember, the total of 20 pairs is a function of the dimensions of memory reserved for our data, and can be altered only by selecting ⟨V⟩ at the Procedure Menu.

⟨R⟩ename

The last option we have at the Edit Menu is ⟨R⟩ename. This option allows us to change the names of our data files and variables.

```
Edit: <C>hange, <D>elete, <I>nsert, <L>ist, or <R>ename? R

Enter new filename or press <ENTER> for no change:
File name: FILE5/XY ? DATA5/XY<ENTER>

Enter new variable name(s), or <ENTER> for default(s):
Variable X: 'X Value' ? GROUP-1<ENTER>
Variable Y: 'Y Value' ? GROUP-2<ENTER>
```

NOTE: Variable names are available only for XY and XYZ data types. The filename alone is sufficient to identify Y-type data.

Since we are now finished editing our data, we want to be sure to save the altered data file to disk. We shall try to save it as "DATA5/XY"...

```
Data: <E>dit, <L>ist, <S>ave, or <ENTER> to continue? S

Saving 'DATA5/XY' ...

'DATA5/XY' already exists!
<R>eplace, <C>hange name, or <S>kip? C

File name: ? DATA5B/XY

Saving 'DATA5B/XY' ...

Data: <E>dit, <L>ist, <S>ave, or <ENTER> to continue?
```

We are reminded that our data file, "DATA5/XY", already exists. Here, we chose not to erase the original file. PHARM/PCS allows us to save our newly edited data file under a different filespec by selecting ⟨C⟩hange. We took the option and chose "DATA5B/XY". We could have also chosen to ⟨R⟩eplace the original file or to ⟨S⟩kip the save command all together.

Now that we have edited our file and saved the changes, it is advisable to list the file for a final check before continuing with the computation...

```
Data: <E>dit, <L>ist, <S>ave, or <ENTER> to continue? L

  File name: DATA5B/XY:1
   Variable:      GROUP-1      GROUP-2
  -----------  -----------  -----------
      # 1:           -1           -2
      # 2:            3            4
      # 3:            5            6
      # 4:            8            7
      # 5:           10           10
      # 6:           20           15
      # 7:           30           20
```

NOTE: Or newly edited data file is shown labeled with the new filespec and variable names that we gave to it.

Finally, we may continue the Procedure 5 computation by pressing ⟨ENTER⟩.

```
Data: <E>dit, <L>ist, <S>ave, or <ENTER> to continue? <ENTER>

  GROUP-2 =  .657354 * GROUP-1 + 1.52834

  etc...
```

After all computation is completed you will see the Report Menu (see C-4).

C-4. Report: ⟨P⟩rint, ⟨S⟩ave, or ⟨V⟩iew

Each time you list data at the Data Menu and each time that the results of computation are shown on the screen, the text is automatically saved in an ASCII text file called "REPORT/TXT". This text file is created anew every time a procedure is run. At the end of a procedure you will see the following Report Menu...

```
Report: <P>rint, <S>ave, or <V>iew? S
File name: ? RESULTS5/TXT<ENTER>
```

Selecting ⟨V⟩iew will just re-display the results of the procedure just completed (i.e., the file REPORT/TXT). You will have to press ⟨ENTER⟩ each time the screen fills. This is useful for quickly reviewing a procedure you may have missed because it scrolled by too fast.

Pressing ⟨P⟩rint will send the results file, REPORT/TXT, directly to your printer. NOTE: Be sure that the printer is connected and turned on, or you may have to reset your computer and lose the results file just created!

Selecting ⟨S⟩ave at the Report Menu, as in the above example, actually renames the results file, REPORT/TXT, to a file name of your own choosing. Remember that if you do not select ⟨S⟩ave, the REPORT/TXT file will be overwritten, the next time you run any procedure.

NOTE 1: You may ⟨V⟩iew and/or ⟨P⟩rint the REPORT/TXT file or your own ⟨S⟩aved results file at the Procedure Menu by selecting ⟨R⟩eport (see D-2).

NOTE 2: ⟨S⟩aving the results of your computation will allow you to incorporate them into a manuscript or report using most word processors. See your word processor's manual for instructions on merging ASCII text files into documents.

D. Utility Programs

Several Utility Programs are available from the Procedure Menu even though they are not listed. In case you forget what they do, the following utilities are described on the Help screen at the Procedure Menu (press ⟨?⟩ key). Each of the utilities are described below, along with sample screens illustrating their use.

D-1. ⟨D⟩irectory—View Disk Directory

The directory on your diskette may be listed on the video display without leaving PHARM/PCS. The optional use of a "wildcard" allows groups of related files to be displayed. The wildcard character is specific for your computer (usually "$" or "*"). In the example below, we illustrate how to display the files on Drive 0 (or A:) that contain the "/PCS" extension.

```
Procedure:  <##>,  <E>xit,  <?>,  or  <ENTER>  for  next  screen  ?  D


                     <D>irectory Utility
   Pharmacologic Calculation System - Version 4.0 - 08/02/86

 Enter directory wildcard, or press <ENTER> for entire directory
 ? $/PCS:0


 Listing '$/PCS:0' directory ...

  F99/PCS          T95/PCS          SYS3/PCS         Q99/PCS
  Q95/PCS          C95/PCS          A12/PCS          F95/PCS
  SYS0/PCS         SYS1/PCS         PHARM/PCS

 Procedure:  <##>,  <E>xit,  <?>,  or  <ENTER>  for  next  screen  ?
```

For MS-DOS, the equivalent wildcard construction would be:

```
A:*.PCS
```

D-2. ⟨R⟩eport—Text File Utility

Most word processing programs allow the use of ASCII text files. PHARM/PCS saves all results of computation for later incorporation into your final reports (see C-4).

Here we illustrate retrieval of the ASCII text file that we created when we ran Procedure 15. Sending the output to the printer, by selecting ⟨P⟩, also causes a non-stop display to appear on the screen; otherwise you must press ⟨ENTER⟩ to continue when the screen fills.

```
Procedure:  <##>,  <E>xit,  <?>,  or  <ENTER>  for  next  screen  ?  R


                     <R>eport File Utility
   Pharmacologic Calculation System - Version 4.0 - 08/02/86

 Output:  <P>rinter  or  <V>ideo  only?  V

 File name 1 ? S15/TXT:1
```

For MS-DOS, you would have asked for:

```
B:S15.TXT
```

The screen clears and your "TXT" file is displayed...

```
                  <15> pA2 Analysis I: Schild Plot
      Pharmacologic Calculation System - Version 4.0 - 08/01/86

   File name:        S15/XY
     Variable:          B          A'/A
   ------------ ----------- -----------
        # 1:      3.16E-07       4.16
        # 2:       .000001      18.78

     etc...
```

Your complete "TXT" file would be displayed on one or more screens.

D-3. ⟨S⟩ave—Save Configuration Utility

Once you select a procedure that is not resident in memory, it will automatically load into memory along with any additional procedures it may require. Since this "merging" takes some time, you may not want to do this each and every time you want to run a frequently-used procedure such as the "t-Test". The ⟨S⟩ave command at the Procedure Menu allows you the convenience of saving your "custom configuration" without leaving PHARM/PCS. If you press ⟨ENTER⟩ at the prompt, the configuration will be saved as "PHARM/PCS", and will automatically load the next time. In the following example the configuration is saved as "STATS/PCS".

```
Procedure: <##>, <E>xit, <?>, or <ENTER> for next screen ? S

                  <S>ave PHARM/PCS Utility
    Pharmacologic Calculation System - Version 4.0 - 08/02/86

Save current program configuration as 'PHARM/PCS' or enter
filespec ? STATS/PCS<ENTER>

Saving 'STATS/PCS' ...

Procedure: <##>, <E>xit, <?>, or <ENTER> for next screen ?
```

NOTE: If you give your own name to a configuration, you will have to run it after loading BASIC, e.g., with MS-DOS type

```
A>BASIC STATS.PCS
```

or with TRSDOS type

```
TRSDOS Ready
BASIC STATS/PCS
```

D-4. ⟨V⟩ersion—Change System Parameters

There are certain "system" parameters that you wish to change for your particular needs. The parameters that you may change are presented one at a time, along with the minimum and maximum acceptable values. The changes remain in place until you change them again by typing "V" at the Procedure

Menu. The ⟨V⟩ersion screen appears below followed by an explanation of each parameter. The number of files is changed to 4; the number of items to 100 and the left margin is left unchanged.

NOTE: The default parameters and acceptable ranges may be different for your particular hardware/DOS combination.

```
Procedure: <##>, <E>xit, <?>, or <ENTER> for next screen ? V

              <V>ersion Maintenance Utility
   Pharmacologic Calculation System - Version 4.0 - 08/02/86

Enter new variable or press <ENTER> to leave current value
unchanged. Enter 'M' to return to menu. See 'Manual' for
explanation of of variables.

Description          (Min,Max)     Default    New Value
-----------------------------------------------------------
Number of Files      (2,25)          10       ? 4<ENTER>
Number of Items/File (5,1024)        20       ? 100<ENTER>
Left Margin          (0,20)           5       ? <ENTER>
```

a. Number of Files

Enter the maximum number of data files that you will be analyzing. This number will be shown on the "Table of Contents" screen. This variable, along with the next, determine the dimensions of "data space" set aside for your data. The amount of RAM memory in your computer and the number of resident procedures will determine the maximum number of data files PHARM/PCS can hold. Here we reduced the number of files to 4 in order to accommodate larger data sets.

b. Number of Items/File

Enter the maximum number of data items, "n", that will occur in any of your data files. This number will also be listed on the "Table of Contents" screen. In the above sample display screen, we are increasing our "n" to 100 in order to accommodate a larger data set.

c. Left Margin

Enter the number of spaces that you want the printed output to be offset from the left margin. If you want to center 64 column video display on an 80 column printer, you may want to change this variable to 8 in order to center the printout (assuming 10 characters per inch and 8.5 inch wide paper, i.e., $80 = 8 + 64 + 8$).

After filling in the desired values, you are given a chance to make corrections. Since we have entered the desired responses we answer ⟨Y⟩es to the next prompt...

```
Are these values correct (Y/N) ? Y

Do you want to clear all procedures from memory (Y/N)? N
```

The next prompt, "Do you want to clear all procedures from memory (Y/N)?", allows one to start with a clean slate. Answer ⟨Y⟩es to this prompt when you wish to start building a custom configuration of PHARM/PCS allowing the maximum memory for data. Only Procedure 2 will be loaded into memory (the file PHARM/LIB from the Master Diskette is loaded).

NOTE: Users of floppy disk systems who answer ⟨Y⟩es must have the Master diskette inserted into the secondary drive (B: or 1).

Answering ⟨N⟩o, as in the above example causes the next prompt to appear...

```
Enter your custom PCS filespec or press <ENTER> to return to
'PHARM/PCS'? <ENTER>

Loading PHARM/PCS please standby ...
```

Enter the filespec for your custom configuration of PHARM/PCS, if you have created one (see D-3, above) that you wish to load. Pressing ⟨ENTER⟩ at the prompt, as in this example, will cause the default program PHARM/PCS to load. Now you may continue computation with the new data dimensions you have requested. These new dimensions of data space will be indicated at the top of the "Table of Contents" screen.

NOTE: This configration will continue to be used until you change it again. The BASIC language requires that the dimensions of any data arrays be determined in advance of executing a program, and cannot be redimensioned within a running program.

E. Glossary

DOS

"DOS" stands for Disk Operating System. PHARM/PCS runs on MS-DOS, PC-DOS, and TRSDOS.

filespec

Refers to the standard file name specification for your particular DOS. Filespecs usually have a filename and an extension, and may contain the disk drive on which the file is located. When PHARM/PCS asks for a "filename", you may use a full "filespec".

A valid filespec or "pathname" in MS-DOS would be:

drive:filename,extension

while in TRSDOS it would be:

filename/extension:drive

If you have more than one disk drive in use, you may specify the drive where a file is to be found or stored. In a filespec, the drive may be indicated by a letter

(A: or B:) in MS-DOS or by a number (0 or 1) in TRSDOS. Throughout this manual "primary drive" will indicate drive A: (or 0) and "secondary drive" will indicate drive B: (or 1).

filename

A filename is comprised of 1 to 8 alphanumeric characters, the first of which must be a letter. Since you will use filespecs to save data files, you should choose a filename that you will remember. For example try "EXP0730" to indicate an experiment you did on July 30, instead of just "DATA".

extension

The extension is comprised of 1 to 3 alphanumeric characters, the first of which must be a letter. The extension must be preceded with a slash "/" in TRSDOS or a period "." in MS-DOS. When saving data, it is recommended that you use the extension "XY" to refer to paired (e.g. dose-response) data, and "Y" to refer to single variable data. Each part of a filespec must conform to the rules of your DOS. An example of a valid filespec under MS-DOS is

```
B:TEST1234.XYZ
```

and under TRSDOS

```
TEST1234/XYZ:1
```

F. Source Code Listings

F.1. "PCS" Files

```
File name: HELP1/PCS
-------------------------------------------------------------------

Options at the 'PROCEDURE:' menu:

    <##> - Where '##' is any single or double digit Procedure number. If you type
a single digit, you must press <ENTER> after entering the digit.  For example,
to run Procedure 2, type '02' or '2<ENTER>'.

    <E>xit - Ends PHARM/PCS and returns to the disk operating system (DOS).

    <?> Help - Prints this help screen.  <?> may be pressed at ANY menu prompt
to help review your options.

    <ENTER> - Indicates the 'ENTER' or 'RETURN' key. Press this key to go to
the next screen to view the 'Table of Contents'. On the 'Table of Contents'
screens, an asterisk after a procedure number indicates that a procedure is
currently in memory.  Note - Procedure 2 is always in memory, as indicated by
'< 2>*'.

Several other options are available.  These are <D>, <R>, <S>, and <V>:

    <D>irectory - Prints directory of disk on screen.  You may enter a drive
number, pathname or wildcard - consult your DOS manual for valid directory
choices.

    <R>eport - Prints a report (ASCII text file) on the screen or printer. Text
files of program results are automatically saved to disk.  The last report is
stored under the file name 'REPORT/TXT'.  At the end of each procedure you
also have the option to save the report under a file name of your choice.
```

<S>ave - Saves custom configuration of PHARM. All procedure modules
currently merged are saved. Save as 'PHARM/PCS' (default) or enter your own
program name. Next time you run that configuration, you will not have to wait
for each procedure to load.

<V>ersion - Allows modificaton of certain system variables and options.
Use this option to increase the dimension of data space so that you can
analyse larger data sets, or to shrink data space so that you can load more
procedures into memory at one time.

EOF

File name: HELP2/PCS

Options at the 'INPUT:' menu:

<K>eyboard - Data will be entered via the keyboard. You will be prompted for
a file name so that you may save the data for later analysis.

<D>isk - Data will be loaded from a disk file that was saved during a
previous session.

<E>xit - Abort this procedure and return to the main 'Procedure:' menu.

EOF

File name: HELP3/PCS

Options at the 'DATA:' menu:

<E>dit - Goes to 'Edit:' sub-menu. Data may be edited, i.e., you may
change, delete, or insert individual data values. You may also change the
name of the data file, and the labels associated with the X and Y variables
(for the XY data type only).

<L>ist - The data file(s) will be listed on the screen and will appear on
the final report.

<S>ave - The data file(s) will be saved to disk. You will be prompted for
a name for each file, or you can use the default names that are supplied.
Use up to 8 characters for the name followed by an optional 'extension' of 3
characters. PHARM/PCS allows 3 different types of data. Try using 'Y',
'XY', or 'XYZ' as extensions to differentiate between data types. A disk
drive number or pathname may also be associated with the file name. Consult
your DOS manual for specifications of a valid file name.

<ENTER> - Continues with procedure. When in doubt, press <ENTER> to
continue.

EOF

File name: HELP4/PCS

Options at the 'EDIT:' sub-menu:

Each option below will present additional prompts to help select the particular
data to be edited.

<C>hange - Change an individual data point. Press <ENTER> to keep original
value.

<D>elete - Delete a particular data point.

<I>nsert - Insert new data anywhere within the file or append data to the end
of the file.

<L>ist - The data file(s) will be listed on the screen but will NOT appear on the final report. Use <L>ist at the 'Data:' menu to save listing with the final report.

<R>ename - You may also change the name of the data file, and the labels associated with the X and Y variables (for the XY data type only).

<ENTER> - Returns to 'Data:' menu. When in doubt, press <ENTER> to continue.

EOF

File name: HELP5/PCS

Options at the 'Report:' menu:

<P>rint - Send final report of procedure just completed to your printer. Make sure that the printer is turned on, or you may have to reset your computer.

<V>iew - Show the final report of the procedure just completed on your screen.

<ENTER> - Returns to 'Procedure:' menu. When in doubt, press <ENTER> to continue.

<S>ave - Save the final report of procedure just completed. You will be prompted for a file name. Do not confuse these file names with file names of your raw data. Use the 'TXT' extension. (Available only after completing a procedure, and not at the 'Procedure:' menu.

EOF

File name: SYS1/PCS

```
10 REM SYS1/PCS (C) R. Murray 1986 07/30/86
15 CLEAR 1000
20 DEFINT A-Z
25 ON ERROR GOTO 1270
30 ET$="/"
35 CW%=14
  :SW%=64
  :N=3
  :GOSUB 1000
  :REM MSDOS=14,80,6
40 CU$=CHR$(95)
  :RO$=CHR$(24)
  :REM MSDOS=29
45 P$="Enter new variable or press <ENTER> to leave "
50 P$=P$+"current value unchanged. Enter 'M' to return "
55 P$=P$+"to menu. See 'Manual' for explanation of "
60 P$=P$+"of variables."
  :GOSUB 402
65 PRINT"Description          (Min,Max)";TAB(35);"Default";TAB(46);
   "New Value"
67 PRINT STRING$(60,"-")
70 FOR I=1 TO N
75 PRINT M$(I);"(";MI$(I);",";MA$(I);")";TAB(35);C$(I);TAB(46);
  :Z1=ZZ(I)
  :GOSUB 200
  :PRINT
76 IF A$="N" THEN A$=""
  :C$(I)=A$
  :FL=1
  :GOTO 95
80 IF A$="M" THEN I=10
  :GOTO 100
85 IF A$="" THEN 95
90 IF VAL(A$)>=VAL(MI$(I)) AND VAL(A$)<=VAL(MA$(I)) THEN C$(I)=A$
  :FL=1
  :ELSE 75
```

```
95 NEXT I
100 PRINT
105 PRINT "Are these values correct (Y/N) ";
    :GOSUB 200
    :PRINT
    :PRINT
110 IF A$="Y" THEN 1080
115 IF A$="N" THEN 40
    :ELSE 105
120 END
200 SC%=0
    :PRINT "? ";
    :REM <-
202 A$=""
    :Z$=INKEY$
    :ZD=0
    :ZS=ZD
    :ZL%=ZD
    :IF Z1=ZD THEN Z1=1
204 PRINT STRING$(ABS(Z1),CU$);STRING$(ABS(Z1),RO$);
206 PRINT CU$;RO$;
    :Z%=1
208 Z$=INKEY$
    :IF Z$<>"" THEN 212
    :ELSE Z%=Z%+1
    :IF Z%<5 THEN 208
    :ELSE PRINT " ";RO$;
    :Z%=1
210 Z$=INKEY$
    :IF Z$<>"" THEN 212
    :ELSE Z%=Z%+1
    :IF Z%<5 THEN 210
    :ELSE 206
212 PRINT CU$;RO$;
    :IF ABS(Z1)=ZL% THEN 220
    :ELSE IF Z1>0 AND Z$>="*" AND Z$<="z" THEN 228
214 IF Z1<0 AND (Z$>"*" AND Z$<"
    ") OR (Z$="D" OR Z$="E") THEN 228
216 IF Z$="," THEN PRINT Z$;
    :ZL%=ZL%+1
    :GOTO 232
    :ELSE IF Z$="." AND ZD=0 THEN ZD=1
    :GOTO 228
218 IF (Z$="-" OR Z$="+") AND ZS=0 AND ZL%=0 THEN ZS=1
    :GOTO 228
220 IF Z$<>CHR$(8) THEN 224
    :ELSE IF ZL%=0 THEN 206
    :ELSE PRINT RO$;
    :IF Z1>0 THEN 222
222 A$=LEFT$(A$,LEN(A$)-1)
    :ZL%=ZL%-1
    :PRINT CU$;RO$;
    :GOTO 206
224 IF Z$=RO$ THEN PRINT STRING$(ZL%,RO$);
    :GOTO 202
    :ELSE IF Z$<>CHR$(13) THEN 206
226 PRINT STRING$(ABS(Z1)-ZL%,32);
    :GOTO 234
228 IF Z1=1 THEN IF ASC(Z$)>96 THEN Z$=CHR$(ASC(Z$)-32)
230 PRINT Z$;
    :A$=A$+Z$
    :ZL%=ZL%+1
232 IF ABS(Z1)<>1 THEN 206
234 Z1=1
236 RETURN
247 REM
248 REM            INPUT number
249 REM
250 GOSUB 310
    :GOSUB 200
    :GOSUB 300
    :RETURN
    :REM <- inkey$
260 GOSUB 310
    :Z1=CW%
    :GOSUB 200
```

```
        :GOSUB 300
        :RETURN
        :REM <- multi inkey$
270 REM
280 REM            Text Output Routines
290 REM
300 CR%=2
        :GOSUB 404
        :CR%=0
        :RETURN
        :REM <- PRINT w/CR
302 CR%=2
        :GOSUB 402
        :CR%=0
        :RETURN
        :REM <- PRINT w/2 CRs
310 CR%=1
        :GOSUB 404
        :CR%=0 .
        :RETURN
        :REM <- PRINT w/o CR
320 CR%=4
        :GOSUB 404
        :CR%=0
        :RETURN
        :REM <- PRINT w/centering
330 REM
340 REM            Adjust Text to Screen
350 REM
400 GOSUB 404
        :RETURN
        :REM <- LPRINT w/CR
402 GOSUB 404
        :GOSUB 404
        :RETURN
        :REM <- LPRINT w/2 CRs
404 IF LEN(P$)<=SW% THEN 430
        :ELSE II%=SW%
        :REM <- 400
405 IF MID$(P$,II%,1)<>" " THEN 420
410 PP$=LEFT$(P$,II%)
        :PR$=RIGHT$(P$,LEN(P$)-II%)
        :IF LEN(PP$)<SW% THEN PP$=PP$+CHR$(13)
412 GOSUB 465
415 P$=PR$
        :GOTO 400
420 II%=II%-1
        :IF II%>0 THEN 405
425 IF LEN(P$)>SW% THEN II%=SW%
        :GOTO 410
430 IF CR%=1 OR LEN(P$)=SW% THEN PP$=P$
        :ELSE PP$=P$+CHR$(13)
435 GOSUB 465
440 P$=""
445 RETURN
450 REM
455 REM            Output Text
457 REM
465 IF CR%>3 THEN PP$=FNS$(PP$)
        :REM center text?
467 PRINT PP$;
        :REM Screen
470 REM IF (LP=1 OR LP=3) AND (CR%=0 OR CR%=4) THEN LPRINT TAB(TB
        %);PP$;
        :REM Print
475 IF LP>1 AND (CR%=0 OR CR%=4) THEN PRINT #2,PP$;
        :REM File
480 SC%=SC%+1
        :REM Increment line counter
482 REM IF CR%>2 THEN IF SC%=SL%-1 THEN P$=""
        :GOSUB 510
        :RETURN
        :REM CR%=3
484 REM IF LP=0 AND CR%=0 THEN IF SC%=SL% THEN GOSUB 500
        :RETURN
485 RETURN
```

```
1000 OPEN "I",1,"SYS0"+ET$+"PCS"
1010 FOR I=1 TO N
1020 READ ZZ(I),MI$(I),MA$(I),D$(I),M$(I)
1030 IF ER=0 THEN INPUT #1,C$(I) ELSE C$(I)=D$(I)
1040 NEXT I
1050 IF ER=0 THEN INPUT #1,SN$
     :ELSE FL=1
1060 CLOSE
1070 RETURN
1080 PS$="PHARM"+ET$+"PCS"
1085 P$="Do you want to clear all procedures from memory (Y/N)"
     :GOSUB 250
     :IF A$<>"Y" AND A$<>"N" THEN 1085
1086 IF A$="Y" THEN PS$="PHARM"+ET$+"LIB"
     :GOTO 1100
1090 GOSUB 300
     :P$="Enter your custom PCS filespec or press <ENTER> to retur
      n to '"+PS$+"'"
     :GOSUB 260
     :PRINT
     :IF A$<>"" THEN PS$=A$
1100 CLS
     :PRINT STRING$(8,CHR$(13));"Loading ";PS$;" please standby ..
      ."
1110 IF FL=0 THEN 1170
1120 OPEN "O",1,"SYS0"+ET$+"PCS"
1130 FOR I=1 TO N
1140 PRINT #1,C$(I)
1150 NEXT I
1155 IF ER=1 THEN SN$="VER 4.0 "+TIME$
1160 PRINT #1,SN$
1170 CLOSE
1180 RUN PS$
1190 REM
1200 REM         Set Machine-Specific Variables
1210 REM
1240 DATA 2,2,25,10,"Number of Files      "
1250 DATA 4,5,1024,20,"Number of Items/File "
1260 DATA 2,0,20,10,"Left Margin          "
1270 IF ERL=1180 THEN PRINT
     :PRINT PS$;" not found!"
     :PRINT
     :RESUME 1080
1280 IF ERL=1000 THEN ER=1
     :RESUME 1010
1290 PRINT
     :PRINT"Unknown Error!"
     :PRINT ERL,ERR
1300 END
```

File name: SYS2/PCS

                    Pharmacologic Calculation System

                        PHARM/PCS - Version 4

                              based on

                  "Manual of Pharmacologic Calculations
                       with Computer Programs"
                            2nd Edition

                  by R.J. Tallarida and R.B. Murray
                    Springer-Verlag, New York, 1986

EOF

File name: SYS3/PCS

< 1> Dosage & Concentration: Drug Stock Solutions
< 2> Mean, Standard Deviation & Confidence Limits
< 3> Linear Regression I

< 4> Linear Regression II: Lines Through Origin
< 5> Analysis of the Regression Line
< 6> Parallel Lines I: Test for Parallelism
< 7> Parallel Lines II: Construction of Parallel Lines
< 8> Graded Dose-Response
< 9> Quantal Dose-Response: Probits
<10> Relative Potency I
<11> Relative Potency II: Statistical Analysis
<12> Dissociation Constant I: Agonists
<13> Dissociation Constant II: Partial Agonists
<14> Dissociation Constant III: Perturbation Methods
<15> pA2 Analysis I: Schild Plot
<16> pA2 Analysis II: Time-Dependent Method
<17> pA2 Analysis III: Constrained Plot
<18> Enzyme Kinetics I: Michaelis-Menten Equation
<19> Enzyme Kinetics II: Competitive Inhibition
<20> Enzyme Kinetics III: Noncompetitive Inhibition
<21> First Order Drug Decay
<22> Scatchard Plot
<23> Henderson-Hasselbalch Equation
<24> Exponential Growth & Decay
<25> Area Under a Curve: Trapezoidal & Simpson's Rules
<26> Pharmacokinetics I: Constant Infusion, 1st Order Elimination
<27> Pharmacokinetics II: Multiple Intravenous Injections
<28> Pharmacokinetics III: Volume of Distribution
<29> Pharmacokinetics IV: Plasma Concentration-Time Data
<30> Pharmacokinetics V: Renal Clearance
<31> Pharmacokinetics VI: Renal Excretion Data Following I.V. Administration
<32> Pharmacokinetics VII: Multiple Dosing from Absorptive Site
<33> Analysis of Variance I: One-way
<34> Analysis of Variance II: Two-way, Single Observation
<35> Analysis of Variance III: Two-way, with Replication
<36> Newman-Keuls Test
<37> Duncan Multiple Range Test
<38> Least Significant Difference Test
<39> t-Test I: Grouped Data
<40> t-Test II: Paired Data
<41> Ratio of Means
<42> Chi-Square Test
<43> Proportions: Confidence Limits
<44> Dunnett's Test
<45> Mann-Whitney U-Test
<46> Litchfield & Wilcoxon I: Confidence Limits of ED50
<47> Litchfield & Wilcoxon II
<48> Differential Equations

EOF

File name: PCS

```
1 CLS
 :PRINT"PHARM/PCS Version 4.0 (07/30/86) TRS-80 Model III"
2 REM Copyright (C) 1986 Rodney B. Murray / All Rights Reserved
3 PRINT
 :PRINT"Pharmacologic Calculation System"
 :PRINT"(C) 1986 Rodney B. Murray."
 :PRINT"All Rights Reserved."
 :PRINT
 :PRINT"Reproduction without written"
4 PRINT"permission from MicroComputer"
 :PRINT"Specialists, of any portion of"
 :PRINT"this program, is prohibited."
 :PRINT
 :PRINT
 :PRINT"Initializing, Please Stand By ...";
5 ON ERROR GOTO 10
6 RUN "PHARM/PCS"
7 ON ERROR GOTO 0
8 RUN "PHARM/LIB"
9 END
10 RESUME 7
```

F.2. "LIB" Files

```
File name: PHARM/LIB
-----------------------------------------------------------------------

1 REM Version 4.0 (07/30/86) TRS-80 Model III
2 REM PHARM/PCS Copyright (C) 1986 Rodney B. Murray
3 REM
4 REM            Initialize & Dimension Variables
5 REM
8 A$="0"
 :GOSUB 620
 :REM reset U%
9 CLS
 :CMD"LIST SYS2/PCS"
 :REM MSDOS,TR4
10 CLEAR 1000
12 DEFINT I,J,K,L,N
14 ON ERROR GOTO 60000
16 REM
18 REM            Dimension System Scalars
20 REM
22 DIM Z%,Z$,P$,CR%,RO$,I%,J%,X$,CU$,LP%,X!,Z1!,CW%,SC%,ZL%,Y!,A$
    ,ZD!,SW%,JJ%,II%,JP%,MX!,JS%,JL%,SX!,SY!,DS!
24 REM
26 REM            Dimension System Arrays
28 REM
29 GOSUB 58020
 :REM Get System Variables
30 DIM FI$(JZ)
 :REM Input Filespec
32 DIM N(JZ)
 :REM n for each group
34 DIM SR%(NZ)
 :SR%(0)=1
 :REM Subroutine flag
36 DIM X(IZ,JZ),Y(IZ,JZ)
 :REM main X,Y data matrix
38 I=IZ
 :IF JZ>I THEN I=JZ
40 DIM XA(I),YA(I),ZA(I)
 :REM temp X,Y,Z data array
42 DIM P$(JZ+2,JZ+2)
44 REM
46 REM            Define System Functions
48 REM
50 DEF FNF$(X$)=RIGHT$(STRING$(CW%," ")+X$,CW%)
52 DEF FNP$(X)=RIGHT$(STRING$(CW%," ")+STR$(X),CW%)
54 DEF FND$(X,Y)=STR$(INT(X*10[Y+.5)/10[Y)
 :REM MSDOS,TR4
56 DEF FNS$(X$)=STRING$(ABS(SW%-LEN(X$))/2," ")+X$
57 DEF FNX$(X$)=RIGHT$(STRING$(PW%," ")+LEFT$(X$,PW%),PW%)
58 REM
60 REM            Dimension Subroutine Arrays
62 REM
100 REM
102 DIM DE(JZ),DS(JZ),MX(JZ),MY(JZ),S1(JZ),S2(JZ),SE(JZ),SX(JZ),S
    Y(JZ),VA(JZ)
150 REM
155 REM            Read Subroutines
160 REM
170 GOSUB 58420
 :IF INKEY$=" " THEN P$=P$+" "+SN$
 :GOSUB 300
174 REM
176 REM          Skip to Menu
178 REM
185 GOSUB 630
 :U%=VAL(A$)
 :REM get U%
188 IF U%<>0 THEN A$="0"
 :GOSUB 620
 :REM reset U%
190 P$=""
 :GOTO 820
```

```
194 REM
196 REM             Inkey$ Routine
198 REM
200 SC%=0
   :PRINT "? ";
   :REM <-
202 A$=""
   :Z$=INKEY$
   :ZD=0
   :ZS=ZD
   :ZL%=ZD
   :IF Z1=ZD THEN Z1=1
204 PRINT STRING$(ABS(Z1),CU$);STRING$(ABS(Z1),RO$);
206 PRINT CU$;RO$;
   :Z%=1
208 Z$=INKEY$
   :IF Z$<>"" THEN 212
   :ELSE Z%=Z%+1
   :IF Z%<5 THEN 208
   :ELSE PRINT " ";RO$;
   :Z%=1
210 Z$=INKEY$
   :IF Z$<>"" THEN 212
   :ELSE Z%=Z%+1
   :IF Z%<5 THEN 210
   :ELSE 206
212 PRINT CU$;RO$;
   :IF ABS(Z1)=ZL% THEN 220
   :ELSE IF Z1>0 AND Z$>="*" AND Z$<="z" THEN 228
214 IF Z1<0 AND (Z$>"*" AND Z$<"
   :") OR (Z$="D" OR Z$="E") THEN 228
216 IF Z$="," THEN PRINT Z$;
   :ZL%=ZL%+1
   :GOTO 232
   :ELSE IF Z$="." AND ZD=0 THEN ZD=1
   :GOTO 228
218 IF (Z$="-" OR Z$="+") AND ZS=0 AND ZL%=0 THEN ZS=1
   :GOTO 228
220 IF Z$<>CHR$(8) THEN 224
   :ELSE IF ZL%=0 THEN 206
   :ELSE PRINT RO$;
   :IF Z1>0 THEN 222
222 A$=LEFT$(A$,LEN(A$)-1)
   :ZL%=ZL%-1
   :PRINT CU$;RO$;
   :GOTO 206
224 IF Z$=RO$ THEN PRINT STRING$(ZL%,RO$);
   :GOTO 202
   :ELSE IF Z$<>CHR$(13) THEN 206
226 PRINT STRING$(ABS(Z1)-ZL%,32);
   :GOTO 234
228 IF Z1=1 THEN IF ASC(Z$)>96 THEN Z$=CHR$(ASC(Z$)-32)
230 PRINT Z$;
   :A$=A$+Z$
   :ZL%=ZL%+1
232 IF ABS(Z1)<>1 THEN 206
234 Z1=1
236 RETURN
247 REM
248 REM             INPUT number
249 REM
250 GOSUB 310
   :Z1=0
   :GOSUB 200
   :GOSUB 300
   :RETURN
   :REM <- inkey$
260 GOSUB 310
   :Z1=-CW%
   :GOSUB 200
   :GOSUB 300
   :RETURN
   :REM <- multi inkey$
270 REM
280 REM             Text Output Routines
290 REM
```

```
300 CR%=2
   :GOSUB 404
   :CR%=0
   :RETURN
   :REM <- PRINT w/CR
302 CR%=2
   :GOSUB 402
   :CR%=0
   :RETURN
   :REM <- PRINT w/2 CRs
310 CR%=1
   :GOSUB 404
   :CR%=0
   :RETURN
   :REM <- PRINT w/o CR
320 CR%=4
   :GOSUB 404
   :CR%=0
   :RETURN
   :REM <- PRINT w/centering
330 REM
340 REM            Adjust Text to Screen
350 REM
400 GOSUB 404
   :RETURN
   :REM <- LPRINT w/CR
402 GOSUB 404
   :GOSUB 404
   :RETURN
   :REM <- LPRINT w/2 CRs
404 IF LEN(P$)<=SW% THEN 430
   :ELSE II%=SW%
   :REM <- 400
405 IF MID$(P$,II%,1)<>" " THEN 420
410 PP$=LEFT$(P$,II%)
   :PR$=RIGHT$(P$,LEN(P$)-II%)
   :IF LEN(PP$)<SW% THEN PP$=PP$+CHR$(13)
412 GOSUB 465
415 P$=PR$
   :GOTO 400
420 II%=II%-1
   :IF II%>0 THEN 405
425 IF LEN(P$)>SW% THEN II%=SW%
   :GOTO 410
430 IF CR%=1 OR LEN(P$)=SW% THEN PP$=P$
   :ELSE PP$=P$+CHR$(13)
435 GOSUB 465
440 P$=""
445 RETURN
450 REM
455 REM            Output Text
457 REM
465 IF CR%>3 THEN PP$=FNS$(PP$)
   :REM center text?
467 PRINT PP$;
   :REM Screen
470 IF (LP=1 OR LP=3) AND (CR%=0 OR CR%=4) THEN LPRINT TAB(TB%);P
    P$;
   :REM Print
475 IF LP>1 AND (CR%=0 OR CR%=4) THEN PRINT #2,PP$;
   :REM File
480 SC%=SC%+1
   :REM Increment line counter
482 IF CR%>2 THEN IF SC%=SL%-1 THEN P$=""
   :GOSUB 510
   :RETURN
   :REM CR%=3
484 IF LP=0 AND CR%=0 THEN IF SC%=SL% THEN GOSUB 500
   :RETURN
485 RETURN
488 REM
490 REM            Common Subroutines
492 REM
500 IF LP=0 THEN P$="Press "+EN$+"to continue"
   :GOSUB 250
   :PRINT CHR$(27);STRING$(40," ");CHR$(13);CHR$(27);
```

```
     :REM move up cursor
505 RETURN
510 PRINT @ 960,"";
     :P$="Procedure: <##>, <E>xit, <?>, or "+EN$+"for next screen
              "
     :REM MSDOS=?,TR4=1840
512 GOSUB 310
     :PRINT STRING$(4,RO$);
513 Z1=1
     :GOSUB 200
     :IF A$="0" THEN X$=A$
     :ELSE IF VAL(A$)=0 THEN 516
     :ELSE X$=A$
514 Z1=1
     :GOSUB 202
     :A$=X$+A$
     :U%=ABS(VAL(A$))
516 GOSUB 310
     :SC%=SL%+1
518 RETURN
520 PX$="Log(Dose)"
     :FOR I=1 TO N(J)
     :IF X(I,J)<=0 THEN P$="Log of"+STR$(X(I,J))+" not defined! Re-
         enter or edit data."
     :PX$="Error"
     :GOSUB 300
     :I=N(J)
     :GOTO 525
522 X(I,J)=LOG(X(I,J))/LOG(10)
525 NEXT I
     :RETURN
530 GOSUB 550
     :CR%=4
     :P$=SR$
     :GOSUB 400
     :P$=VR$+" - "+DA$
     :GOSUB 400
     :REM Header
532 CR%=0
     :GOSUB 400
535 RETURN
540 IF IV$="N" THEN A$=""
     :RETURN
     :ELSE P$=EN$+"to continue or <L>ist values calculated from reg
         ression line"
     :GOSUB 250
     :GOSUB 300
     :REM <- 3,4,8,9,24
545 RETURN
550 CLS
     :SC%=1
     :RETURN
     :REM Clear Screen, APPLE=HOME
555 IF CM$="" THEN CM$="DIR" ELSE CM$="DIR "+CM$
     :REM Directory
556 CMD CM$
     :RETURN
     :REM MSDOS=FILES,TR4=SYSTEM CM$
558 SAVE CM$
     :RETURN
     :REM Save CM$
560 GOSUB 550
     :LP=0
     :A$=""
     :REM Version Header
562 P$=VR$
     :GOSUB 320
566 P$=STRING$(SW%-1,"-")
     :GOSUB 320
     :ZD=FRE(Z$)
567 P$="Data space:"+STR$(JZ)+" groups @"+STR$(IZ)+" items each."
         +STR$(FRE(A))+" Bytes Free."
     :GOSUB 320
     :GOSUB 300
568 RETURN
```

```
570 GOSUB 300
   :P$="Enter new "+PX$+" to calculate "+PY$+" or "+EN$+"to conti
    nue."
   :GOSUB 300
   :REM <- 3,8,24
579 RETURN
580 P$="Do you want to show intermediate results (Y/N) "
   :GOSUB 250
   :IV$=A$
   :GOSUB 300
   :IF IV$<>"Y" AND IV$<>"N" THEN 580
589 RETURN
590 P$="Are you entering <D>ose or <L>og(dose) data"
   :GOSUB 250
   :IF A$="D" THEN PX$="Dose" ELSE IF A$="L" THEN PX$="Log(Dose)"
    ELSE 590
599 RETURN
600 FOR I=1 TO N(J)
   :XA(I)=X(I,J)
   :YA(I)=Y(I,J)
   :NEXT I
   :NN(J)=N(J)
605 RETURN
   :REM Save X,Y matrix
610 IF L>1 THEN GOSUB 51500
   :P$=UL$+UL$
   :GOSUB 400
615 RETURN
620 OPEN "O",1,"SYS4/PCS"
   :PRINT #1,A$
   :CLOSE 1
   :RETURN
   :REM set U%, MSDOS
630 OPEN "I",1,"SYS4/PCS"
   :INPUT #1,A$
   :CLOSE 1
   :RETURN
   :REM read U%
670 REM
680 REM            Output Screen Matrix
690 REM
700 JL=0
   :P$=""
   :REM <- *
705 JS=JL+1
   :IF JS>C% THEN 765
710 IF (JS+CC%-2)>C% THEN JL=C%
   :ELSE JL=JS+CC%-2
715 FOR I=0 TO R%
720 P$=P$+FNF$(P$(I,0))
725 FOR JJ=JS TO JL
730 P$=P$+FNF$(P$(I,JJ))
735 P$(I,JJ)=""
740 NEXT JJ
745 GOSUB 400
750 NEXT I
755 GOSUB 400
760 GOTO 705
765 FOR I=0 TO R%
   :P$(I,0)=""
   :NEXT I
   :R%=0
   :C%=0
770 RETURN
775 REM
780 REM            Print Menu
785 REM
800 GOSUB 560
   :REM Header
817 FT$="SYS3"+ET$+"PCS"
   :CR%=2
   :GOSUB 58900
   :REM Procedure Names
820 IF A$="" THEN U%=0
   :GOSUB 510
```

```
     :REM Input Procedure
830 IF A$="E" THEN CLS
     :CMD "S"
     :REM MSDOS,TR4=SYSTEM
832 IF A$="D" THEN 980
833 IF A$="?" OR A$="H" THEN X$="1"
     :GOSUB 940
     :GOTO 820
838 IF A$="R" THEN 960
839 IF A$="S" THEN 971
840 IF A$="V" THEN 950
841 IF A$="" THEN 800
842 REM          Get Procedure
844 IF U%>0 AND U%<=NZ THEN JL=0
     :GOSUB 58420
     :ELSE A$=""
     :GOTO 820
846 REM
848 REM          Set Common Variables
849 REM
850 JP=2
     :L=0
     :REM Default /xy data type
856 PX$="X"
     :PY$="Y"
857 XI$="X-Intercept"
     :YI$="Y-Intercept"
     :SI$="Slope"
858 IV$=""
     :RA$=""
     :RB$=""
     :REM Random access filespecs
894 REM
896 REM          Procedure Heading & Prompts
898 REM
900 LP=2
     :CLOSE 2
     :OPEN "O",2,"REPORT"+ET$+"TXT"
     :GOSUB 530
     :REM save results
904 IF U%>25 THEN 910
906 ON U% GOSUB 1000,2000,3000,4000,5000,6000,7000,8000,9000,1000
     0,11000,12000,13000,14000,15000,16000,17000,18000,19000,200
     00,21000,22000,23000,24000,25000
908 IF U%<26 THEN 912
910 ON U%-25 GOSUB 26000,27000,28000,29000,30000,31000,32000,3300
     0,34000,35000,36000,37000,38000,39000,40000,41000,42000,430
     00,44000,45000,46000,47000,48000
912 PRINT #2,CHR$(12)
     :CLOSE
     :U%=0
913 GOSUB 962
     :REM report utility
914 GOTO 8
915 REM
916 REM          Utilities
918 REM
940 LX=LP
     :LP=0
     :SR$="<?> Help (press <ESC> to abort Help and return to menu)"
     :GOSUB 530
     :REM <?>
942 FT$="HELP"+X$+ET$+"PCS"
     :CR%=0
     :GOSUB 58900
     :LP=LX
948 RETURN
950 CLOSE
     :SR$="<V>ersion Maintenance Utility"
     :GOSUB 530
     :REM <V>
952 FT$="SYS1"+ET$+"PCS"
     :RUN FT$
     :REM VERSION
954 REM
```

```
955 GOSUB 300
    :P$="Report: <P>rint,"
959 RETURN
960 SR$="PHARM/PCS <R>eport Utility"
    :GOSUB 530
    :LP=0
    :L=1
    :J=0
    :FI$(0)="REPORT"+ET$+"TXT"
    :GOSUB 52400
    :FT$=FI$(0)
961 GOSUB 955
962 IF P$="" THEN GOSUB 955
    :P$=P$+" <S>ave,"
    :SR$=""
963 P$=P$+" or <V>iew"
    :LP=0
    :GOSUB 250
    :GOSUB 310
964 IF A$="" THEN 914 ELSE IF A$="P" THEN LP=1 ELSE IF A$="S" AND
       SR$="" THEN 968
965 IF A$="?" THEN X$="5"
    :GOSUB 940
    :GOTO 962
966 IF FI$(0)="" THEN FT$="REPORT"+ET$+"TXT"
967 CLS
    :GOSUB 58900
    :IF SR$="" THEN 962 ELSE 961
968 J=0
    :L=1
    :GOSUB 300
    :GOSUB 50800
969 CM$="RENAME REPORT"+ET$+"TXT "+FI$(0)
    :CMD CM$
    :REM MSDOS,TR4
970 GOTO 914
971 SR$="<S>ave PHARM/PCS Utility"
    :GOSUB 530
    :REM <S>
972 CM$="PHARM"+ET$+"PCS"
974 P$="Save current PROGRAM configuration as '"+CM$+"' or enter
       your own filespec "
    :GOSUB 310
976 Z1=14
    :GOSUB 200
    :GOSUB 302
    :IF A$<>"" THEN CM$=A$
978 P$="Saving '"+CM$+"' ..."
    :GOSUB 300
    :GOSUB 558
    :A$=""
    :GOTO 820
979 REM
980 SR$="<D>irectory Utility"
    :GOSUB 530
    :REM <D>
984 P$="Enter directory wildcard, or press "+EN$+"for entire dire
       ctory "
    :GOSUB 310
986 Z1=14
    :GOSUB 200
    :GOSUB 302
    :CM$=A$
988 P$="Listing '"+CM$+"' directory ..."
    :GOSUB 300
    :GOSUB 555
    :A$=""
    :GOTO 820
996 REM
997 REM            Subroutines begin below
999 REM
2000 DATA " 2> Mean, Standard Deviation & Confidence Limits",0
2010 REM 03/12/86 VER 4.0
2030 GOSUB 2100
     :REM <- 27,28,30,31
```

```
2040 GOSUB 2200
     :REM Process
2050 GOSUB 2300
     :REM Output
2060 RETURN
2070 REM
2080 REM          Input
2090 REM
2100 JP=1
     :GOSUB 50050
     :REM <- 32
2120 RETURN
2130 REM
2140 REM          Process
2150 REM
2200 J=1
     :REM 2200
2205 IF N(J)<2 THEN P$="You must enter more than ONE value!"
     :GOSUB 300
     :GOTO 2030
2210 GOSUB 2660
     :J=J+1
     :IF J<=L THEN 2205 ELSE RETURN
2220 REM
2230 REM          Output
2240 REM
2300 IF IV$="N" THEN RETURN ELSE JL=0
2310 JS=JL+1
     :IF JS>L THEN RETURN
     :ELSE IF (JS+CC%-2)>L THEN JL=L
     :ELSE JL=JS+CC%-2
2320 GOSUB 51070
     :REM List filenames
2330 FOR J=JS TO JL
     :GOSUB 2800
     :NEXT J
     :GOTO 2310
2340 RETURN
2350 REM          Calculate Stats
2660 N=N(J)
     :DE=0
     :DS=0
     :SE=0
     :VA=0
     :REM <- 8,9,29,46
2670 X=0
     :SX=0
     :MX=0
     :S1=0
     :Y=0
     :SY=0
     :MY=0
     :S2=0
     :FOR I=1 TO N
     :X=X(I,J)
     :SX=SX+X
     :S1=S1+X*X
     :Y=Y(I,J)
     :SY=SY+Y
     :S2=S2+Y*Y
     :NEXT I
     :MX=SX/N
     :MY=SY/N
     :FOR I=1 TO N
     :Y=Y(I,J)
     :DS=DS+(Y-MY)*(Y-MY)
     :NEXT I
2675 IF N=1 THEN RETURN
2680 VA=DS/(N-1)
     :DE=SQR(VA)
     :SE=DE/SQR(N)
     :SX(J)=SX
     :S1(J)=S1
     :MX(J)=MX
     :SY(J)=SY
```

```
       :S2(J)=S2
       :MY(J)=MY
       :DS(J)=DS
       :VA(J)=VA
       :DE(J)=DE
       :SE(J)=SE
2690 RETURN
2697 REM
2698 REM            Min & Max
2699 REM
2700 XS=1E+32
       :XB=-1E+32
       :YS=1E+32
       :YB=-1E+32
2720 I=1
       :IB=0
2730 IF JP=1 THEN 2760
2740 IF X(I,J)<XS THEN XS=X(I,J)
2750 IF X(I,J)>XB THEN XB=X(I,J)
2760 IF Y(I,J)<YS THEN YS=Y(I,J)
2770 IF Y(I,J)>YB THEN YB=Y(I,J)
       :IB=I
2780 I=I+1
       :IF I<=N(J) THEN 2730
2792 RETURN
2797 REM
2798 REM              Output Stats
2799 REM
2800 P$=FNF$("N:")
       :REM <- 29
2810 FOR J=JS TO JL
       :P$=P$+FNP$(N(J))
       :NEXT J
       :GOSUB 400
2812 P$=FNF$("Minimum:")
       :FOR J=JS TO JL
       :GOSUB 2700
       :P$=P$+FNP$(YS)
       :NEXT J
       :GOSUB 400
2814 P$=FNF$("Mean:")
       :FOR J=JS TO JL
       :P$=P$+FNP$(MY(J))
       :NEXT J
       :GOSUB 400
2816 P$=FNF$("Maximum:")
       :FOR J=JS TO JL
       :GOSUB 2700
       :P$=P$+FNP$(YB)
       :NEXT J
       :GOSUB 400
2818 P$=FNF$("Sum:")
       :FOR J=JS TO JL
       :P$=P$+FNP$(SY(J))
       :NEXT J
       :GOSUB 400
2820 P$=FNF$("Std. Dev.:"):FOR J=JS TO JL
       :P$=P$+FNP$(DE(J))
       :NEXT J
       :GOSUB 400
       :P$=FNF$("Std. Err.:")
       :FOR J=JS TO JL
       :P$=P$+FNP$(SE(J))
       :NEXT J
       :GOSUB 400
2825 FOR J=JS TO JL
       :N=N(J)-1
       :GOSUB 2960
       :ZA(J)=TV
       :P$=FNF$("t Value:")+FNP$(ZA(J))
       :NEXT J
       :IF U%=2 THEN GOSUB 400
2830 P$=FNF$("95% C.L.:")
       :FOR J=JS TO JL
       :P$=P$+FNP$(ZA(J)*SE(J))
```

```
      :NEXT J
      :GOSUB 402
      :RETURN
2840 REM
2850 REM          Get t-value
2860 REM
2960 IF N>30 THEN TV=1.96
      :T9=2.576
      :RETURN
      :REM <- 5
2970 NV%=N
      :RA$="T95"+ET$+"PCS"
      :GOSUB 55000
      :TV=V!
2980 IF U%>5 THEN RA$="T99"+ET$+"PCS"
      :GOSUB 55000
      :T9=V!
2999 RETURN
50000 DATA "END",0
      :REM Data File Input Routines
50010 REM 07/30/86 VER 4.0
50020 REM
50030 REM          Choose Keyboard or Disk Input
50040 REM
50050 XL$=""
      :YL$=""
      :REM <- *
50060 J=1
      :N(1)=0
      :NM=0
50070 IF L=0 THEN L=JZ
50080 P$="Input: <K>eyboard, <D>isk, or <E>xit this procedure"
      :GOSUB 250
      :GOSUB 300
      :X$=A$
50082 IF INSTR("KDE?",X$)=0 THEN 50080
50086 IF X$="E" OR X$="" THEN A$=""
      :GOTO 820
      :REM Return to menu
50088 IF X$="?" THEN X$="2"
      :GOSUB 940
      :GOTO 50050
50095 IF L>1 THEN GOSUB 50140
      :REM prompt # files
50100 IF X$="D" THEN GOSUB 50500
50120 IF X$="K" THEN GOSUB 50900
      :GOSUB 50180
50130 GOSUB 300
50132 L=J-1
50134 IF L<1 THEN 914
50136 GOTO 52000
      :REM File options
50137 REM
50138 REM          data file prompt
50139 REM
50140 P$="You may enter"+STR$(L)
      :IF JP=1 THEN P$=P$+" 'Y'" ELSE IF JP=2 THEN P$=P$+" 'XY'" E
      LSE P$=P$+" 'XYZ'"
50142 P$=P$+" data files. "
50144 RETURN
50150 REM
50160 REM          Keyboard Input
50170 REM
50180 IF PX$="" AND JP<>1 THEN GOSUB 590
      :REM dose or log(dose) ?
50185 P$=P$+"Type 'END' after last file. Enter file name or "+EN$
      +"for default name
      :"
      :GOSUB 300
50190 J$=STR$(J)
      :J$=RIGHT$(J$,LEN(J$)-1)
50200 FI$(J)="FILE"+J$+ET$
50210 IF JP=1 THEN A$="Y" ELSE IF JP=2 THEN A$="XY" ELSE IF JP=3
      THEN A$="XYZ"
50218 FI$(J)=FI$(J)+A$
```

```
50220 P$="'"+FI$(J)+"' (or 'END') "
      :GOSUB 310
50230 Z1=14
      :GOSUB 200
      :GOSUB 300
      :IF A$="END" THEN 50640
50240 IF A$<>"" THEN FI$(J)=A$
50250 IF ASC(FI$(J))<65 THEN 50220
50255 LT=LP
      :LP=0
50260 IL=0
      :I=1
      :GOSUB 50340
      :GOSUB 300
      :REM input data
50265 LP=LT
50270 N(J)=I-1
      :IF N(J)=0 THEN 50640
50280 IF N(J)>NM THEN NM=N(J)
50290 J=J+1
      :IF J<=L THEN 50190
50300 RETURN
50310 REM
50320 REM          Key Data
50330 REM
50340 GOSUB 300
      :P$="You may enter up to"+STR$(IZ-N(J))
50350 IF JP=1 THEN P$=P$+" observations." ELSE IF JP=2 THEN P$=P$
      +" x,y data pairs." ELSE P$=P$+" x,y,z data sets."
50360 P$=P$+" Press "+EN$+"after the last entry."
      :GOSUB 300
50370 JS=J
      :JL=J
      :GOSUB 51070
      :REM print heading
50390 P$=FNF$("#"+STR$(I)+"
      :")+" "
      :GOSUB 310
50400 IF JP<>1 THEN Z1=-CW%+1
      :GOSUB 202
      :PRINT " ";
      :X$=A$
      :IF A$="" THEN 50450
50410 Z1=-CW%+1
      :GOSUB 202
      :PRINT " ";
      :Y$=A$
      :IF A$="" THEN 50450
50415 IF JP=3 THEN Z1=-CW%+1
      :GOSUB 202
      :PRINT " ";
      :YZ$=A$
      :IF A$="" THEN 50450
50420 GOSUB 300
50430 X(I,J)=VAL(X$)
      :Y(I,J)=VAL(Y$)
      :IF JP=3 THEN Z(I,J)=VAL(YZ$)
50440 I=I+1
      :IF I+IL<=IZ THEN 50390
50450 GOSUB 302
50460 RETURN
50470 REM
50480 REM          Disk File Input
50490 REM
50500 IF L>1 THEN P$=P$+"Press "+EN$+"after last file name."
      :GOSUB 300
50510 GOSUB 50800
      :REM enter filename
50520 IF FI$(J)="" THEN 50640
50530 IF ASC(FI$(J))<65 THEN 50510
50540 OPEN "I",1,FI$(J)
      :REM <- 60
50550 I=1
      :GOSUB 55500
      :REM data id
```

```
50560 IF EOF(1) THEN 50600
50570 IF JP<>1 THEN INPUT #1,X(I,J)
50580 INPUT #1,Y(I,J)
50585 IF JP=3 THEN INPUT #1,Z(I,J)
50590 I=I+1
      :GOTO 50560
50600 CLOSE 1
50610 N(J)=I-1
50620 IF N(J)>NM THEN NM=N(J)
50630 J=J+1
      :IF J<=L THEN 50510
50640 RETURN
50680 REM
50690 REM          Enter Filename
50700 REM
50800 FI$(J)=""
50810 PRINT "File name";
      :IF L>1 THEN PRINT J;
      :ELSE PRINT ": ";
50820 IF FI$(J)<>"" THEN PRINT FI$(J);" ";
50840 Z1=14
      :GOSUB 200
      :GOSUB 300
      :IF A$<>"" THEN FI$(J)=A$
50860 RETURN
50870 REM
50880 REM          Edit PX$, PY$, PZ$
50890 REM
50900 IF (PX$<>"X" AND PY$<>"Y") OR JP=1 THEN RETURN
50910 P$="Enter new variable name(s), or "+EN$+"for default(s)
      :"
      :GOSUB 300
50940 IF JP<>1 THEN P$="Variable X: '"+PX$+"' "
      :GOSUB 310
      :Z1=CW%-1
      :GOSUB 200
      :GOSUB 300
      :IF A$<>"" THEN PX$=A$
50950 P$="Variable Y: '"+PY$+"' "
      :GOSUB 310
      :Z1=CW%-1
      :GOSUB 200
      :GOSUB 300
      :IF A$<>"" THEN PY$=A$
50960 IF JP=3 THEN P$="Variable Z: '"+PZ$+"' "
      :GOSUB 310
      :Z1=CW%-1
      :GOSUB 200
      :GOSUB 300
      :IF A$<>"" THEN PZ$=A$
50970 RETURN
50975 REM
50980 REM          Print Raw Data
50990 REM
51000 JS=1
      :REM list data
51015 IF JP<>1 THEN JL=JS
      :GOTO 51030
51020 IF (JS+CC%-2)>L THEN JL=L
      :ELSE JL=JS+CC%-2
51030 GOSUB 51050
51040 JS=JL+1
51042 IF JS<=L THEN 51015
51045 RETURN
51050 GOSUB 51070
51060 GOTO 51200
51070 GOSUB 51510
      :REM Print Filespec
51075 REM
51080 REM          Print Variable Names
51100 REM
51120 IF JP=1 THEN 51180
      :ELSE P$=FNF$("Variable:")
51130 FOR JJ=JS TO JL
51140 P$=P$+FNF$(PX$)+FNF$(PY$)
```

```
51150 IF JP=3 THEN P$=P$+FNF$(PZ$)
51155 IF YC$<>"" THEN P$=P$+FNF$(YC$)
51160 NEXT JJ
51170 GOSUB 400
51180 FOR II=1 TO 1+JP*(JL-JS+1)
      :P$=P$+UL$
      :NEXT II
      :IF YC$<>"" THEN P$=P$+UL$
51185 GOSUB 400
51190 RETURN
51192 REM
51195 REM          Print Values
51199 REM
51200 FOR I=1 TO NM
51210 FOR J=JS TO JL
51220 GOSUB 51300
51230 NEXT J
51240 IF P$=STRING$(LEN(P$)," ") THEN P$=""
      :I=NM
      :GOTO 51270
51250 P$=FNF$("#"+STR$(I)+"
      :")+P$
51260 GOSUB 400
51270 NEXT I
51285 IF YC$<>"" THEN GOSUB 3890
51288 GOSUB 400
51290 RETURN
51300 IF I>N(J) THEN FOR II=1 TO JP
      :P$=P$+STRING$(CW%," ")
      :NEXT II
      :RETURN
51310 IF JP<>1 THEN P$=P$+FNP$(X(I,J))
51320 P$=P$+FNP$(Y(I,J))
51321 IF JP=3 THEN P$=P$+FNP$(Z(I,J))
51322 IF YC$<>"" THEN P$=P$+FNP$(M(J)*X(I,J)+B(J))
51330 RETURN
51470 REM
51480 REM          Print File Name
51490 REM
51500 IF L=1 THEN RETURN ELSE JS=J
      :JL=J
      :GOSUB 51510
      :RETURN
51510 P$=FNF$("File name:")
      :FOR JJ=JS TO JL
51512 REM IF JP=1 THEN FI$(JJ)="GROUP" ELSE FI$(JJ)="LINE"
      :REM demo
51515 REM FI$(JJ)=FI$(JJ)+RIGHT$(STR$(JJ),LEN(STR$(JJ))-1)
      :REM demo
51520 P$=P$+FNF$(FI$(JJ))
51530 IF JP<>1 THEN P$=P$+FNF$(" ")
51535 IF JP=3 THEN P$=P$+FNF$(" ")
51540 NEXT JJ
      :GOSUB 400
51550 RETURN
51970 REM
51980 REM          File Options
51990 REM
52000 P$="Data: <E>dit, <L>ist, <S>ave, or "+EN$+"to continue"
52010 GOSUB 250
      :GOSUB 300
      :SC%=SC%-1
52020 IF A$="" OR A$="C" THEN RETURN
52025 IF A$="E" THEN LT=LP
      :LP=0
      :GOSUB 52100
      :LP=LT
      :GOTO 52000
52030 ON INSTR("LPS?",A$) GOSUB 51000,56000,54000,52050
52040 GOTO 52000
52050 X$="3"
      :GOSUB 940
52060 RETURN
52070 REM
52080 REM          Choose File to Edit
```

```
52090 REM
52100 IF L=1 THEN JN=1
      :GOTO 52300
52110 P$=EN$+"to continue or edit: "
52120 FOR J=1 TO L
52130 P$=P$+"<"+RIGHT$(STR$(J),LEN(STR$(J))-1)+"> '"+FI$(J)+"'   "
52140 NEXT J
52150 GOSUB 310
52170 Z1=-2
      :GOSUB 200
      :GOSUB 302
      :IF A$="" THEN PRINT
      :RETURN
      :ELSE JN=VAL(A$)
52180 IF JN=0 THEN RETURN
52190 IF JN>L OR JN<1 THEN 52100
52200 PRINT
52270 REM
52280 REM          Edit Subcommands
52290 REM
52300 IF L>1 THEN P$="Editing '"+FI$(JN)+"'"
      :GOSUB 300
52310 P$="Edit: <C>hange, <D>elete, <I>nsert, <L>ist, or <R>ename
      "
      :GOSUB 250
      :GOSUB 300
52330 J=JN
52340 IF A$="" THEN 52370
52350 ON INSTR("CDILR?",A$) GOSUB 52600,52800,53000,51000,52400,5
      2365
52360 GOTO 52300
52365 X$="4"
      :GOSUB 940
      :REM help
52370 RETURN
52400 P$="Enter new filename or press "+EN$+"for no change
      :"
      :GOSUB 300
      :GOSUB 50810
      :GOSUB 300
      :REM change filename
52410 IF J<>0 THEN GOSUB 50910
      :GOSUB 300
      :REM change PX$,PY$
52460 RETURN
52470 REM
52480 REM          Get Input #
52490 REM
52500 IN=N(JN)
52510 P$=E$+": which entry (1 -"+STR$(IN)+") in '"+FI$(J)+"' "
      :GOSUB 310
52530 Z1=-3
      :GOSUB 200
      :GOSUB 302
      :IF A$="" THEN RETURN
      :ELSE I=VAL(A$)
52540 IF I<1 OR I>IN THEN 52510
      :ELSE RETURN
52570 REM
52580 REM          Change
52590 REM
52600 E$="Change"
      :GOSUB 52500
52610 IF A$="" THEN RETURN
52620 JS=JN
      :JL=JN
      :GOSUB 51070
52630 J=JN
      :GOSUB 51300
      :P$=FNF$("#"+STR$(I)+"
      :")+P$
      :GOSUB 300
52640 P$=FNF$("#"+STR$(I)+"
      :")+"  "
      :GOSUB 310
```

```
52650 IF JP<>1 THEN Z1=-CW%+1
      :GOSUB 202
      :IF A$<>"" THEN X(I,JN)=VAL(A$)
      :PRINT " ";
      :ELSE PRINT " ";
52660 Z1=-CW%+1
      :GOSUB 202
      :IF A$<>"" THEN Y(I,JN)=VAL(A$)
      :PRINT " ";
52665 PRINT " ";
      :IF JP=3 THEN Z1=-CW%+1
      :GOSUB 202
      :IF A$<>"" THEN Z(I,JN)=VAL(A$)
52670 PRINT
      :GOTO 52600
52770 REM
52780 REM          Delete
52790 REM
52800 E$="Delete"
      :GOSUB 52500
      :IF A$<>"" THEN GOSUB 52820
      :GOTO 52800
52810 RETURN
52820 FOR K=I TO N(JN)
52830 IF JP<>1 THEN X(K,JN)=X(K+1,JN)
52840 Y(K,JN)=Y(K+1,JN)
52845 IF JP=3 THEN Z(K,JN)=Z(K+1,JN)
52850 NEXT K
52860 N(JN)=N(JN)-1
52870 RETURN
52970 REM
52980 REM          Insert
52990 REM
53000 E$="Insert at"
      :IN=N(JN)+1
      :GOSUB 52510
53010 IF A$="" THEN RETURN
53020 J=JN
53030 IL=N(J)-I+1
53040 FOR K=0 TO IL-1
53050 IF JP<>1 THEN XA(K)=X(I+K,J)
53060 YA(K)=Y(I+K,J)
53065 IF JP=3 THEN ZA(K)=Z(I+K,J)
53070 NEXT K
53080 GOSUB 50340
      :REM keyboard input
53090 FOR K=0 TO IL-1
53100 IF JP<>1 THEN X(I+K,J)=XA(K)
53110 Y(I+K,J)=YA(K)
53115 IF JP=3 THEN Z(I+K,J)=ZA(K)
53120 NEXT K
53130 N(J)=I+IL-1
53140 IF N(J)>NM THEN NM=N(J)
53150 RETURN
53970 REM
53980 REM          Save Data Files to Disk
53990 REM
54000 FOR J=1 TO L
      :GOSUB 54050
      :NEXT J
      :GOSUB 300
54030 RETURN
54050 CLOSE 1
      :OPEN "I",1,FI$(J)
      :CLOSE 1
      :REM <- 60
54060 GOSUB 54200
54090 ON INSTR("RCS",A$) GOTO 54120,54110,54200
54100 GOTO 54060
54110 GOSUB 50800
      :GOTO 54050
54120 PRINT "Saving '";FI$(J);"' ..."
54130 OPEN "O",1,FI$(J)
54140 GOSUB 55400
      :REM save data id
```

```
54150 FOR I=1 TO N(J)
54160 IF JP=1 THEN PRINT #1,Y(I,J)
54170 IF JP=2 THEN PRINT #1,X(I,J);Y(I,J)
54175 IF JP=3 THEN PRINT #1,X(I,J);Y(I,J);Z(I,J)
54180 NEXT I
      :CLOSE 1
54190 RETURN
54200 P$="'"+FI$(J)+"' already exists!"
      :GOSUB 300
54210 P$="<R>eplace, <C>hange name, or <S>kip"
      :GOSUB 250
      :GOSUB 300
54290 RETURN
54910 REM
54920 REM         Open Random Access Files
54930 REM
54940 REM x95/PCS & x99/PCS
      : T,C,F,Q,D; A12/PCS
54950 REM Input = NV%, Output = V!
54960 REM
55000 IF ST$="0" THEN 55100 ELSE IF RA$<>"" AND RA$=RB$ THEN 5504
      0
      :REM <- 2,27,42,46
55010 CLOSE 3
55020 OPEN "R",3,RA$,4
      :REM <- 60
55030 FIELD 3,4 AS V$
55040 GET 3,NV%
      :REM <- 60
55050 V!=CVS(V$)
      :RB$=RA$
55070 RETURN
55080 REM
55090 REM         Manual Table Lookup
55095 REM
55100 IF MID$(RA$,2,1)<>"9" THEN PRINT"ERROR
      : This procedure requires the file
      : ";RA$
      :CLOSE
      :END
55110 P$="Enter '"+MID$(RA$,1,1)+"' value at "+MID$(RA$,2,2)+"% l
      evel for"+STR$(NV%)+" degrees of freedom
      :"
      :GOSUB 300
55120 GOSUB 260
      :V!=VAL(A$)
55130 RETURN
55397 REM
55398 REM         Save Data ID
55399 REM
55400 IF JP=1 THEN PRINT #1,"Y"
55410 IF JP=2 THEN PRINT #1,"XY"
55415 IF JP=3 THEN PRINT #1,"XYZ"
55420 PRINT #1,N(J)
55430 IF JP<>1 THEN PRINT #1,PX$
55440 PRINT #1,PY$
55445 IF JP=3 THEN PRINT #1,PZ$
55450 RETURN
55497 REM
55498 REM         Input Data ID
55499 REM
55500 IF EOF(1) THEN RETURN
55520 INPUT #1,X$
55522 IF INSTR(X$,"Y")=0 THEN 55580
      :REM old format data
55540 INPUT #1,N(J)
55560 IF JP<>1 THEN INPUT #1,PX$
55570 INPUT #1,PY$
55575 IF JP=3 THEN INPUT #1,PZ$
55578 RETURN
55580 IF PX$="" THEN GOSUB 590
      :REM dose or log(dose) ?
55584 IF JP=1 THEN Y(1,J)=VAL(X$)
      :I=2
      :RETURN
```

```
55588 X(1,J)=VAL(LEFT$(X$,INSTR(2,X$," ")))
      :Y(1,J)=VAL(RIGHT$(X$,LEN(X$)-1-LEN(STR$(X(1,J)))))
      :I=2
55590 RETURN
56000 RETURN
      :REM          plot routine (reserved for future use)
58000 REM
58010 REM          Read System Variables
58015 REM
58020 ET$="/"
      :REM Extension, MSDOS=.
58022 RA$="SYS0"+ET$+"PCS"
      :OPEN "I",1,RA$
      :REM <- 60
58035 INPUT #1,JZ
      :REM Number of groups/lines/files
58040 INPUT #1,IZ
      :REM Number of items/group
58055 INPUT #1,TB%
      :REM Left margin for printouts
58060 INPUT #1,SN$
      :SN$=SN$+" (04/06/86)"
      :REM Serial number
58065 CLOSE
58070 VR$="Pharmacologic Calculation System - Version 4.0"
58072 CU$=CHR$(95)
      :REM cursor character
58074 SW%=64
      :REM Screen width MSDOS,TR4=80
58076 SL%=16
      :REM Number of lines on screen MSDOS,TR4=24
58080 RO$=CHR$(24)
      :REM Cursor left, MSDOS=29
58082 DA$=LEFT$(TIME$,8)
      :REM MSDOS=(DATE$,10),TR4=(DATE$,8)
58085 NZ=48
      :  REM Maximum number of subroutines
58092 CW%=12
      :REM Data column width, MSDOS,TR4=13
58095 CC%=INT(SW%/CW%)
      :REM Maximum columns per screen
58100 PW%=(SW%-5)/11
      :REM Plot y-increment
58105 SC%=1
      :REM Screen line counter
58110 UL$=" "+STRING$(CW%-1,"-")
      :REM Column Underline
58112 EN$="<ENTER> "
      :REM MSDOS=<RETURN>
58115 BL$=CHR$(91)
      :BR$=CHR$(93)
      :REM lf & rt brackets
58117 ST$="1"
      :REM table file installation flag
      : 0=none
58120 RETURN
58125 REM
58130 REM          Other System Variables
58135 REM
58140 REM A$ = Keyboard input
58145 REM E$ = Edit function
58146 REM FI$() = Data filespecs
58150 REM I = Item index
58155 REM II,IL,IN,K = Temp item index
58160 REM J = Group/Line index
58165 REM JJ,JN = Temp group index
58166 REM JP = Data type flag
      : 1=y, 2=xy, 3=xyz
58170 REM L = Maximum groups or files index
58175 REM LP,LT = Lineprinter flags
58180 REM NM = Maximum n
58185 REM NV%,V$,V! = Random access file values
58190 REM RA$,RB$ = Random access filespecs
58195 REM U% = Procedure number
58205 REM
```

```
58400 REM            Read Subroutine Names
58410 REM
58420 RESTORE
      :SR$=""
58427 READ SR$,II
      :IF SR$="END" THEN IF U%=0 THEN RETURN
      :ELSE II=U%
      :JL=1
      :GOTO 58445
58430 SR%(VAL(SR$))=1
      :IF U%=0 THEN P$=P$+STR$(VAL(SR$))
58440 IF SR%(II)=0 THEN 58445
58442 IF U%=VAL(SR$) THEN SR$="<"+SR$
      :IF JL=2 THEN 850
      :ELSE RETURN
58444 GOTO 58427
58445 IF JL=1 THEN GOSUB 560
      :JL=2
      :REM subs merged
58450 SR$=STR$(II)
      :SR$=RIGHT$(SR$,LEN(SR$)-1)
      :IF LEN(SR$)=1 THEN SR$="0"+SR$
58452 GOSUB 630
      :REM get U%
58454 IF A$="0" THEN A$=SR$
      :GOSUB 620
      :REM save U%
58455 SR$="PCS"+SR$+ET$+"LIB"
58460 P$="Merging "+SR$+" ..."
      :GOSUB 300
58490 MERGE SR$
      :REM CHAIN MERGE SR$, 10
      :REM TR4,MSDOS
58500 GOTO 10
58870 REM
58880 REM            List Text File
58890 REM
58900 X=1
      :A$=""
      :RA$=""
      :CLOSE 1
      :OPEN "I",1,FT$
      :REM <- 60
58902 X$=LEFT$(FT$,4)
58910 IF EOF(1) THEN 58960
      :REM close
58920 LINE INPUT #1,P$
      :IF INKEY$=CHR$(27) THEN 58960
58925 IF X$="HELP" THEN GOSUB 300
      :ELSE IF X$="SYS3" THEN GOSUB 58972
      :ELSE GOSUB 400
58932 IF A$<>"" THEN 58960
58933 REM X$="SYS2"+ET$+"PCS"
      :IF FT$=X$ THEN 58940
      :REM STARTUP
58935 IF SC%<=SL% THEN 58939
58937 IF X$="HELP" THEN GOSUB 530
      :GOTO 58940
58938 IF X$="SYS3" THEN GOSUB 560
      :GOTO 58940
58939 IF SC%>SL%-2 AND LP=0 THEN IF X$="SYS3" THEN GOSUB 510
      :SC%=1
      :IF U%<>0 THEN 58960
58940 IF SC%>SL%-1 AND LP=0 THEN GOSUB 500
58950 GOTO 58910
58960 CR%=0
      :CLOSE 1
58970 RETURN
58972 IF X>NZ THEN RETURN ELSE IF SR%(X)=1 THEN MID$(P$,5)="*"
58974 CR%=3
      :X=X+1
58976 GOSUB 400
58978 RETURN
58980 REM
59970 REM
```

```
59980 REM           ERROR Trap
59990 REM
60000 PRINT
    :ER=ERR/2+1
    :REM MSDOS=ERR,TR4=ERR
60002 IF ER=9 THEN 60200
    :REM MSDOS=,TR4=7  out of memory!!
60004 IF ERL=969 THEN 60300
    :REM file exists
60010 IF ERL=50540 THEN PRINT "File Not Found."
    :RESUME 50510
60020 IF ERL=556 THEN PRINT"Error: Bad wildcard"
    :PRINT
    :RESUME 984
60025 IF ERL=58022 THEN PRINT "'";RA$;"' not available. Load prop
    er diskette and re-run."
    :CLOSE
    :END
60030 IF ERL=55020 OR ERL=55040 THEN PRINT "'";RA$;"' not availab
    le. Enter the following table value from Appendix A."
    :RESUME 55100
60040 IF ERL=58900 OR ERL=952 THEN PRINT "'";FT$;
    :GOTO 60110
60050 IF ERL=54050 THEN RESUME 54120
60060 IF ERL=58490 THEN PRINT "'";SR$;
    :GOTO 60110
60090 PRINT
    :PRINT"*** Error #";ER;" on Line #";ERL;" ***"
    :END
60100 PRINT"Please check your data and try again!"
    :GOTO 60120
60110 PRINT"' not available on this diskette."
60120 A$=""
    :CLOSE
    :RESUME 10
60200 GOSUB 300
    :P$="ERROR: OUT OF MEMORY! Data file too large or too many p
    rocedures are loaded. Select <V>ersion Maintenance Utility
    to change 'Number of items/group'. "
60210 IF N(J)>0 THEN P$=P$+"Increase to"+STR$(N(J))+" or more."
60220 GOSUB 300
    :GOTO 60120
60300 J=0
    :GOSUB 54200
    :IF A$="R" THEN CM$="KILL "+FI$(0)
    :CMD CM$
    :RESUME 969
    :REM MSDOS="SYSTEM DEL",TR4="SYSTEM REMOVE"
60310 IF A$="C" THEN RESUME 968
60320 RESUME 914
60999 END



File name: PCS01/LIB
------------------------------------------------------------------

1000 DATA" 1> Dosage & Concentration: Drug Stock Solutions",0
1010 REM 03/05/86 VER 4.0
1020 REM
1030 REM               S1 Variables
1040 REM
1050 CO=0
    :E=0
    :G=0
    :GR=0
    :IO=1
    :ML=0
    :MO=0
    :MW=0
    :O(1)=1
    :O(2)=1.8
    :O(3)=2.6
    :O(4)=3.4
```

```
      :O(5)=4.2
      :Q=0
      :VO=0
      :X=0
1060 REM
1070 REM          Input
1080 REM
1100 P$="Enter molecular weight of drug "
      :GOSUB 260
      :MW=VAL(A$)
1110 P$="Enter concentration of stock drug solution "
      :GOSUB 300
      :P$="(grams "+EN$+"mls "+EN$+")"
      :GOSUB 310
      :Z1=-CW%
      :GOSUB 200
      :GR=VAL(A$)
      :Z1=-CW%
      :GOSUB 200
      :ML=VAL(A$)
      :GOSUB 300
1120 P$="Enter desired molarity of drug sol'n "
      :GOSUB 260
      :MO=VAL(A$)
      :P$="Enter volume of sol'n desired (mls) "
      :GOSUB 260
      :VO=VAL(A$)
      :CO=GR/ML
      :X=(MO*MW*VO)/(1000*CO)
1130 IF X>VO THEN P$="DRUG STOCK IS TOO DILUTE !"
      :GOSUB 300
      :GOTO 1110 ELSE P$="Is the drug an electrolyte (Y/N) "
      :GOSUB 250
      :IF A$<>"Y" THEN 1200
1140 P$="Enter # of ions (2-5) "
      :GOSUB 250
      :IO=VAL(A$)
      :IF IO<1 OR IO>5 THEN 1140
1150 REM
1160 REM          Process
1170 REM
1200 E=32.5*O(IO)/MW
      :G=E*((MW*MO*VO)/1000)
      :Q=(.009*VO)-G
      :IF Q<0 THEN Q=0
1210 GOSUB 400
1220 REM
1230 REM          Output
1240 REM
1500 P$="Molecular weight of drug        = "+STR$(MW)
      :GOSUB 400
      :P$="Conc. of stock drug solution    = "+STR$(GR/ML)+" grams/
      ml"
      :GOSUB 400
      :P$="Desired molarity of drug sol'n  = "+STR$(MO)
1510 GOSUB 400
      :P$="Total volume of desired sol'n   = "+STR$(VO)+" ml"
      :GOSUB 400
      :GOSUB 400
      :P$="Add"+STR$(X)+" mls of drug stock and"
      :P$=P$+STR$(INT(1000*Q+.5))+" milligrams of NaCl to"
1520 GOSUB 400
      :P$=STR$(VO-X)+" mls of distilled water"
      :IF Q=0 THEN P$=P$+".  -NOT ISOTONIC-" ELSE IF Q>0 THEN P$=P$
      +" to give an isotonic solution."
      :GOSUB 400
1999 RETURN


File name: PCS03/LIB
-----------------------------------------------------------------

103 DIM M(JZ),B(JZ),XY(JZ)
    :REM PCS03/LIB
```

```
3000 DATA" 3> Linear Regression I",2
3010 REM 03/10/86 VER 4.0
3030 GOSUB 3100
     :REM Input
3040 GOSUB 3200
     :REM <- 23,29
3050 GOSUB 3800
3060 RETURN
3070 REM
3080 REM          Input
3090 REM
3100 GOSUB 50050
     :REM <- 4,5
3110 RETURN
3120 REM
3130 REM          Process
3140 REM
3200 GOSUB 2200
     :REM <- 4,20,24
3210 FOR J=1 TO L
     :GOSUB 3230
     :NEXT J
     :RETURN
3220 REM calculate regression line
3230 N=N(J)
     :REM <- 5,9,46
3240 X=0
     :SX=SX(J)
     :MX=MX(J)
     :S1=S1(J)
     :Y=0
     :SY=SY(J)
     :MY=MY(J)
     :S2=S2(J)
     :XY=0
     :M=0
     :B=0
     :FOR I=1 TO N(J)
     :X=X(I,J)
     :Y=Y(I,J)
     :XY=XY+(X*Y)
     :NEXT I
     :M=((SX*SY/N)-XY)/(((SX*SX)/N)-S1)
     :M(J)=M
     :B=MY-(M*MX)
3250 B(J)=B
     :XY(J)=XY
     :RETURN
3260 REM
3270 REM          Output
3280 REM
3800 FOR J=1 TO L
     :GOSUB 3830
     :NEXT J
     :GOSUB 3860
     :RETURN
3830 GOSUB 51500
     :IF U%<46 THEN GOSUB 400
     :REM <- 5,9,14,46
3836 P$=FNF$(PY$+" =")+" "+STR$(M(J))+" * "+PX$+" "
     :IF B(J)>0 THEN P$=P$+"+"
3838 P$=P$+STR$(B(J))
     :GOSUB 402
     :RETURN
3840 REM
3842 REM          Output Calculated Y
3844 REM
3860 YC$="Y Calculated"
     :REM <- 5,14
3870 GOSUB 540
     :IF A$="L" THEN GOSUB 51000
3880 RETURN
3890 GOSUB 570
     :REM <- 50 Calculate new values?
3900 GOSUB 260
```

```
    :IF A$="" THEN RETURN ELSE X=VAL(A$)
    :YC=M(JS)*X+B(JS)
    :P$=FNF$("")+FNP$(X)+STRING$(CW%," ")+FNP$(YC)
    :GOSUB 400
    :GOTO 3900
3999 RETURN




File name: PCS04/LIB
------------------------------------------------------------------------

4000 DATA " 4> Linear Regression II: Lines Through Origin",3
4010 REM 02/05/86 VER 4.0
4030 GOSUB 3100
    :REM Input
4040 GOSUB 3200
    :REM Process
4050 GOSUB 4100
    :REM Output
4060 RETURN
4070 REM
4080 REM        Output
4090 REM
4100 FOR J=1 TO L
    :GOSUB 51500
    :REM <- 21,24
4120 M(J)=XY(J)/S1(J)
    :B(J)=0
4130 P$=FNF$(PY$+" =")+" "+STR$(M(J))+" * "+PX$
4140 GOSUB 400
4150 NEXT J
4160 GOSUB 400
    :GOSUB 3860
4999 RETURN




File name: PCS05/LIB
------------------------------------------------------------------------

5000 DATA " 5> Analysis of the Regression Line",3
5010 REM 03/10/86 VER 4.0
5030 GOSUB 3100
    :REM Input
5040 GOSUB 5200
    :REM Process <- 15,16
5050 GOSUB 5400
    :REM Output <- 6,7
5060 RETURN
5070 REM
5080 REM        Process
5090 REM
5200 GOSUB 2200
    :REM <- 6,7,20,24
5210 FOR J=1 TO L
    :REM <- 16,18
5215 GOSUB 5220
    :NEXT J
    :RETURN
5220 GOSUB 3230
    :REM <- 8
5230 XX=0
    :SS=0
    :R=0
    :EM=0
    :EB=0
    :EX=0
5250 FOR I=1 TO N
    :X=X(I,J)
    :XX=XX+(X-MX)*(X-MX)
```

```
    :Y=Y(I,J)
    :CY=M*X+B
    :SS=SS+((Y-CY)*(Y-CY))
    :NEXT I
5270 SS(J)=SS
    :XX(J)=XX
    :R(J)=(XY-(N*MX*MY))/SQR((S1-(N*(MX*MX)))*(S2-(N*(MY*MY))))
    :S=SQR(SS/(N-2))
    :S(J)=S
    :EM(J)=S*SQR(1/XX)
    :EY(J)=S*SQR((1/N)+(MX*MX/XX))
5280 EX(J)=ABS(S/M)*SQR((1/N)+(MY/M)*(MY/M)/XX)
    :RETURN
5290 REM
5300 REM          Output
5310 REM
5400 IF U%<>5 AND IV$="" THEN GOSUB 580
    :REM intermediate results?
5405 GOSUB 400
    :FOR J=1 TO L
    :GOSUB 5410
    :NEXT J
    :IF IV$="Y" OR U%=5 THEN GOSUB 3860
5408 RETURN
5410 GOSUB 3830
    :REM <- 8
5420 N=N(J)-2
    :IF IV$="N" AND U%<>5 THEN GOSUB 2960
    :RETURN
5430 P$=FNF$("R =")+FND$(ABS(R(J)),3)
    :REM <- 15
5440 GOSUB 402
    :GOSUB 5600
    :GOSUB 400
5480 P$(2,0)=SI$+":"
    :P$(2,1)=STR$(M(J))
    :P$(2,2)=STR$(EM(J))
    :P$(2,3)=STR$(M(J)-EM(J)*TV)
    :P$(2,4)=STR$(M(J)+EM(J)*TV)
5500 P$(3,0)=YI$+":"
    :P$(3,1)=STR$(B(J))
    :P$(3,2)=STR$(EY(J))
    :P$(3,3)=STR$(B(J)-EY(J)*TV)
    :P$(3,4)=STR$(B(J)+EY(J)*TV)
5520 P$(4,0)=XI$+":"
    :X=-B(J)/M(J)
    :P$(4,1)=STR$(X)
    :P$(4,2)=STR$(EX(J))
    :P$(4,3)=STR$(X-EX(J)*TV)
    :P$(4,4)=STR$(X+EX(J)*TV)
5530 R%=4
    :C%=4
    :GOSUB 700
5540 RETURN
5550 P$(R%,0)=P1$
    :P$(R%,1)=STR$(P2)
    :P$(R%,2)=STR$(P4)
    :P$(R%,3)=STR$(P2-P3)
    :P$(R%,4)=STR$(P2+P3)
    :RETURN
    :REM <- 8,12,17
5600 GOSUB 2960
    :REM <- 8,12,17,46
5610 P$=FNF$("t (95%) =")+STR$(TV)+FNF$(STR$(N)+" d.f.")
    :GOSUB 400
5615 IF U%=6 OR U%>38 THEN P$=FNF$("t (99%) =")+STR$(T9)
    :GOSUB 400
5620 P$(0,0)="Variable"
5630 P$(0,1)="Value"
    :P$(0,2)="Std. Err."
    :P$(0,3)="Lower C.L."
    :P$(0,4)="Upper C.L."
    :FOR II=0 TO 4
    :P$(1,II)=UL$
    :NEXT II
```

```
5640 RETURN
5700 GOSUB 5600
     :REM <- 6,39,40
5705 IF U%=41 THEN RETURN
5710 P$=FNF$("t (calc) =")+FND$(ABS(T),3)
     :IF ABS(T)<TV THEN P$=P$+"   NOT " ELSE P$=P$+"    "
5720 P$=P$+"Significant "
     :IF T>T9 THEN P$=P$+"at p < 0.01" ELSE IF T>TV THEN P$=P$+"at
        p < 0.05"
5999 RETURN



File name: PCS06/LIB
---------------------------------------------------------------------

6000 DATA " 6> Parallel Lines I: Test for Parallelism",5
6010 REM 01/06/86 VER 4.0
6030 GOSUB 6100
     :REM Input
6040 GOSUB 5200
     :REM Process
6050 GOSUB 6800
     :REM Output
6060 RETURN
6090 REM
6094 REM          Input
6096 REM
6100 GOSUB 50050
6110 IF L<2 THEN P$="YOU MUST HAVE MORE THAN ONE LINE !"
     :GOSUB 300
     :GOTO 6100
6120 RETURN
6770 REM
6780 REM          Output
6790 REM
6800 GOSUB 5050
6810 FOR J=2 TO L
6830 SP=SQR(((N(1)-2)*(S(1)*S(1))+(N(J)-2)*(S(J)*S(J)))/(N(1)+N(J
     )-4))
6840 T=ABS((M(1)-M(J))/(SP*SQR((1/XX(1))+(1/XX(J)))))
6850 GOSUB 400
     :P$=""""+FI$(1)+"' vs. '"+FI$(J)+"'
     :"
     :GOSUB 400
6860 N=N(1)+N(J)-4
     :GOSUB 5700
     :GOSUB 400
6870 NEXT J
6999 RETURN



File name: PCS07/LIB
---------------------------------------------------------------------

7000 DATA " 7> Parallel Lines II: Construction of Parallel Lines"
     ,6
7010 REM 01/26/86 VER 4.0
7030 GOSUB 6100
     :REM Input
7040 GOSUB 7200
     :REM Process
7050 GOSUB 7900
     :REM Output
7060 RETURN
7062 REM
7064 REM          S7 Variable Definitions
7066 REM
7068 REM BM = Sum of weighting factors
7070 REM CM = Common slope
```

```
7072 REM TP = Sum of W * slopes
7074 REM W = Weighting factor
7080 REM
7170 REM
7180 REM          Process
7190 REM
7200 GOSUB 5200
   :REM S10 Entry
7220 FOR J=1 TO L
   :W(J)=1/(EM(J)*EM(J))
   :NEXT J
7250 TP=0
   :BM=0
   :FOR J=1 TO L
   :TP=TP+(W(J)*M(J))
   :BM=BM+W(J)
   :NEXT J
7265 CM=TP/BM
7270 RETURN
7870 REM
7880 REM          Output
7890 REM
7900 GOSUB 5050
   :REM S10 Entry v4
7910 P$="Common Slope = "+STR$(CM)
   :GOSUB 402
7920 FOR J=1 TO L
7930 JS=J
   :JL=J
   :GOSUB 51500
   :GOSUB 400
   :REM File names
7940 P$=FNF$(PY$)+" = "+STR$(CM)+" * ( "+PX$
7950 IF MX(J)<=0 THEN P$=P$+"+"
7960 P$=P$+STR$(-1*MX(J))+") +"+STR$(MY(J))
   :GOSUB 402
7970 NEXT J
7999 RETURN




File name: PCS08/LIB
---------------------------------------------------------------------

8000 DATA " 8> Graded Dose-Response",5
8010 REM 04/06/86 VER 4.0
8020 L=1
   :PY$="Response"
   :GOSUB 8100
   :REM Input
8030 GOSUB 8200
   :REM Process
8040 RETURN
8050 REM
8060 REM          Input
8070 REM
8100 PX$=""
   :GOSUB 50050
   :GOSUB 580
   :PO$=PX$
8110 RETURN
8120 REM
8130 REM          Process
8140 REM
8200 J=1
   :MA=0
   :GOSUB 600
   :REM save x,y
8210 P$="Calculation of A50 requires the knowledge of Emax.  Pres
   s <ENTER> to do a double reciprocal plot to estimate Emax O
   R enter Emax "
   :GOSUB 260
   :GOSUB 300
   :MA=VAL(A$)
```

```
8220 IF MA<>0 THEN 8240
8230 P$="Calculating double reciprocal plot..."
     :GOSUB 302
     :GOSUB 8500
     :IF MA<0 THEN RETURN
8240 P$="Log(Dose)-Response regression between 20%-80% of Emax...
     "
     :GOSUB 400
     :GOSUB 8300
8250 RETURN
8260 REM
8270 REM          Log(Dose)-Response Plot
8280 REM
8300 IF PX$="Dose" THEN GOSUB 520
     :IF PX$="Error" THEN RETURN
8310 REM          Delete data outside 20-80% Emax
8320 IF IV$="Y" THEN GOSUB 400
     :JS=1
     :JL=1
     :JP=3
     :PZ$="% Emax"
     :GOSUB 51120
     :JP=2
8325 IX=0
     :I1=IX
     :II=1
     :I=II
     :JN=I
     :P$=""
8330 IX=IX+1
     :Y=Y(II,JN)/MA
     :IF Y>.8 OR Y<.2 THEN IX$=" deleted" ELSE IX$=""
8340 IF IV$="Y" THEN P$=FNF$("#"+STR$(IX)+"
     :")+FNP$(X(II,JN))+FNP$(Y(II,JN))+FNP$(Y(II,JN)/MA*100)+IX$
     :GOSUB 400
8350 IF IX$<>"" THEN I1=I1+1
     :GOSUB 52820
     :GOTO 8330
     :REM delete
8360 II=II+1
     :IF II<=N(JN) THEN 8330
8370 IF I1<>0 THEN GOSUB 400
     :P$="Data points deleted:"+STR$(I1)
     :GOSUB 400
8390 GOSUB 8670
     :GOSUB 8700
     :M5=MA/2
     :A5=(M5-B(J))/M(J)
8400 SE=ABS(S/M(J))*SQR(1/N(J)+(A5-MX(J))*(A5-MX(J))/XX(J))
     :N=N(J)-2
8410 IF IV$="N" THEN GOSUB 5620
     :R%=2
     :ELSE R%=0
8420 P$(R%,0)="A50"
     :P2=10[ A5
     :P3=10[ (TV*SE)
8430 P$(R%,1)=STR$(P2)
     :P$(R%,2)=""
     :P$(R%,3)=STR$(P2/P3)
     :P$(R%,4)=STR$(P2*P3)
8440 R%=R%+1
     :P1$="Log(A50)"
     :P2=A5
     :P3=TV*SE
     :P4=SE
     :GOSUB 5550
     :C%=4
     :GOSUB 700
8450 RETURN
8460 REM
8470 REM          Double-Reciprocal Plot
8480 REM
8500 J=1
     :FOR I=1 TO N(J)
     :IF PX$="Log(Dose)" THEN X(I,J)=1/10[ X(I,J) ELSE X(I,J)=1/X(I
```

```
     ,J)
8510 Y(I,J)=1/YA(I)
     :NEXT I
8520 PX$="1/Dose"
     :PY$="1/Response"
     :IF IV$="Y" THEN GOSUB 51000
8530 L=1
     :GOSUB 3200
     :J=1
     :GOSUB 3830
     :J=1
     :MA=1/B(J)
     :P$="Emax estimated from double reciprocal plot = "+STR$(MA)
     :IF IV$="Y" THEN GOSUB 402 ELSE GOSUB 302
8540 IF MA>0 THEN 8560
8550 P$="Negative Emax! You should delete one or more of the low
       doses or enter an estimated Emax."
     :GOSUB 302
8560 P$="Emax options: <E>dit data, enter <N>ew estimate, or <K>e
       ep double reciprocal estimate":GOSUB 250
     :GOSUB 300
     :IF INSTR("ENK",A$)=0 OR A$="" THEN 8560
8570 IF A$="K" THEN IF MA<0 THEN 8550 ELSE 8610
8580 IF A$="E" THEN LT=LP
     :LP=0
     :GOSUB 52100
     :LP=LT
     :GOTO 8520
8590 P$="Enter new Emax estimate"
     :GOSUB 260
     :GOSUB 300
8600 IF A$<>"" THEN MA=VAL(A$)
     :ELSE GOTO 8590
8610 P$="Emax ="+STR$(MA)+" (estimated"
     :IF A$="K" THEN P$=P$+" from double reciprocal plot"
8630 P$=P$+")"
     :GOSUB 402
8640 N(1)=NN(1)
     :REM replace original data
8650 FOR I=1 TO N(J)
     :X(I,J)=XA(I)
     :Y(I,J)=YA(I)
     :NEXT I
     :PX$=PO$
     :PY$="Response"
8660 RETURN
8670 L=1
     :GOSUB 5200
     :J=1
     :RETURN
     :REMJ=1
     :GOSUB 2660
     :GOSUB 5220
     :GOSUB 5410
     :J=1
8680 RETURN
8700 GOSUB 5410
     :GOSUB 540
     :IF A$<>"L" THEN 8999
8720 P$=FNF$(PX$)+FNF$(PY$)
     :IF PX$="1/Dose" THEN P$=P$+FNF$("Dose")+FNF$("Response")
8730 GOSUB 400
     :FOR I=1 TO N(J)
     :X=X(I,J)
     :GOSUB 8800
     :NEXT I
     :GOSUB 400
     :GOSUB 570
8740 GOSUB 260
     :X=VAL(A$)
8750 IF A$<>"" THEN GOSUB 8800
     :GOTO 8740
8760 RETURN
8800 YC=M(J)*X+B(J)
     :P$=FNP$(X)+FNP$(YC)
```

```
8810 IF PX$="1/Dose" THEN P$=P$+FNP$(1/X)+FNP$(1/YC)
8820 GOSUB 400
8999 RETURN




File name: PCS09/LIB
------------------------------------------------------------------------

9000 DATA " 9> Quantal Dose-Response: Probits",5
9010 REM 02/13/86 VER 4.0
9030 JP=2
     :PY$="Response"
     :GOSUB 9100
     :REM Input
9040 GOSUB 9200
     :IF PX$="Error" THEN RETURN
     :REM Process
9050 GOSUB 9600
     :REM Output
9060 RETURN
9090 REM Converts % to Probit w/ Zelen & Severo Approximation
9100 C0=2.515517
     :C1=.802853
     :C2=.010328
     :D1=1.432788
     :D2=.189269
     :D3=.001308
     :REM <- 46
9110 PX$=""
     :GOSUB 50050
9120 RETURN
9200 J=1
9220 GOSUB 600
     :IF PX$="Dose" THEN GOSUB 520
     :IF PX$="Error" THEN RETURN
9235 PY$="Probit"
     :REM convert % to probits
9240 FOR I=1 TO N(J)
     :PC=Y(I,J)
     :GOSUB 9980
     :Y(I,J)=PR
     :NEXT I
     :REM <- 46
9290 GOSUB 2660
     :GOSUB 3230
     :GOSUB 3830
9300 RETURN
9600 J=1
9620 B=B(J)
     :M=M(J)
     :REM <- 46
9630 E1=(4.0055-B)/M
     :E8=(5.9945-B)/M
     :E5=(5-B)/M
9635 IF U%<>9 THEN 9670 ELSE GOSUB 400
9640 P$=FNF$("")+FNF$("Dose")+FNF$("Log(Dose)")
     :GOSUB 400
9642 P$=FNF$("")+UL$+UL$
     :GOSUB 400
9650 P$=FNF$("ED16 = ")+FNP$(10[E1)+FNP$(E1)
     :GOSUB 400
     :REM **
9655 P$=FNF$("ED50 = ")+FNP$(10[E5)+FNP$(E5)
     :GOSUB 400
     :REM **
9660 P$=FNF$("ED84 = ")+FNP$(10[E8)+FNP$(E8)
     :GOSUB 402
     :REM **
9670 E1=10[E1
     :E5=10[E5
     :E8=10[E8
     :REM **
```

```
9680 SF=((E8/E5)+(E5/E1))/2
     :IF IV$="Y" THEN P$="Slope Function = "+STR$(SF)
     :GOSUB 400
9690 GOSUB 540
     :IF A$<>"L" THEN RETURN
9700 P$=FNF$("Dose")+FNF$(PX$)+FNF$("% Response")+FNF$(PY$)
     :GOSUB 400
9705 FOR I=1 TO 4
     :P$=P$+UL$
     :NEXT I
     :GOSUB 400
9710 FOR I=1 TO N(J)
9712 X=X(I,J)
     :PC=YA(I)
     :GOSUB 9980
     :P$=FNP$(10[X)+FNP$(X)+FNP$(YA(I))+FNP$(PR)
     :REM **
9713 GOSUB 400
9714 NEXT I
9716 GOSUB 400
9720 P$="Press <ENTER> to continue, or calculate a new value from
     : <L>og(dose) or % <R>esponse"
     :GOSUB 250
9740 IF A$="" THEN RETURN
9750 ON INSTR("LR",A$) GOSUB 9780,9900
9760 RETURN
9780 P$="Enter Log(Dose) "
     :GOSUB 260
     :X=VAL(A$)
9790 IF A$="" THEN RETURN
9800 P$=FNP$(10[X)+FNP$(X)
     :REM **
9810 GOSUB 9840
9820 P$=P$+FNP$(PC)+FNP$(PR)
     :GOSUB 400
9830 GOTO 9780
9835 REM calculate probit from regression & convert to %
9840 P=M(J)*X+B(J)
     :REM <- 46
9850 IF P<2.6737 THEN PC=1
     :PR=P
     :RETURN
9851 IF P>7.3263 THEN PC=99
     :PR=P
     :RETURN
9852 PH=99
     :PL=1
9854 PC=(PH-PL)/2+PL
9860 GOSUB 9980
     :REM Get estimated probit
9862 IF ABS(P-PR)<0.001 THEN RETURN
9864 IF PR>P THEN PH=PC ELSE PL=PC
9866 GOTO 9854
9900 P$="Enter % Response "
     :GOSUB 260
     :PC=VAL(A$)
9910 IF A$="" THEN RETURN
9920 IF PC>=100 OR PC<=0 THEN P$="ERROR: Enter a number between 0
     and 100% ONLY."
     :GOSUB 300
     :GOTO 9900
9925 GOSUB 9980
9930 X=(PR-B(J))/M(J)
9940 P$=FNP$(10[X)+FNP$(X)+FNP$(PC)+FNP$(PR)
     :GOSUB 400
     :REM **
9950 GOTO 9900
9960 REM
9970 REM Converts % to probit using 'Zelen & Severo Approx.'
9972 REM Input = PC, Output = PR
9974 REM
9980 PP=PC/100
     :IF PP>0.5 THEN PP=1-PP
     :REM <- 46
9982 T=SQR(LOG(1/(PP*PP)))
```

```
9984 PZ=T-(C0+(C1*T)+(C2*T*T))/(1+(D1*T)+(D2*T*T)+(D3*T*T*T))
9986 IF PC<=50 THEN PR=5-PZ ELSE PR=5+PZ
9999 RETURN




File name: PCS10/LIB
-----------------------------------------------------------------------

10000 DATA "10> Relative Potency I",7
10010 REM 07/06/86 VER 4.0
10020 P$="This procedure calculates the relative potency of the f
      irst dose-response curve versus one or more additional curv
      es."
      :GOSUB 302
10030 IF U%=11 THEN P$="Calculation of confidence limits for the
      potency ratio requires an equal number of points (n>2) in e
      ach line."
      :GOSUB 302
10100 PX$=""
      :PY$="Response"
10120 GOSUB 50050
10130 IF L<2 THEN PRINT"You must enter at least 2 dose-response c
      urves!"
      :GOSUB 300
      :GOTO 10100
10140 IF PX$="Log(Dose)" THEN 10170
10150 J=1
10160 GOSUB 520
      :IF PX$="Error" THEN RETURN
10165 J=J+1
      :IF J<=L THEN 10160
10170 IF N(1)<3 THEN 10500
      :REM do 2x2 assay
10180 GOSUB 580
      :GOSUB 7200
      :GOSUB 7900
10190 S=-MY(1)/CM+MX(1)
      :GOSUB 400
10192 REM
10194 REM          Parallel Line Assay
10196 REM
10200 P$="Parallel Line Assay:"
      :GOSUB 10900
10210 FOR J=2 TO L
10220 U=-MY(J)/CM+MX(J)
10230 RP=10[(U-S)
      :IF N(1)=N(J) THEN LN=1 ELSE LN=0
10300 IF U%=10 THEN 10440
10320 N=2*N(1)-3
      :GOSUB 2960
      :T2=TV*TV*2
10350 SP=((S(1)*S(1))+(S(2)*S(2)))/2
10360 A=(CM*CM)-.25*((T2*SP)/XX(1))
      :REM 07/06/86
10370 B=(2*CM)*(MY(2)-MY(1))
10380 YD=MY(1)-MY(2)
      :C=(YD*YD)-((T2*SP)/N(1))
10390 X=-B/(2*A)
      :Y=SQR((B*B)-(4*A*C))/(2*A)
      :QL=X-Y
      :QU=X+Y
10410 LL!=MX(2)-MX(1)
      :LU!=LL!+QU
      :LL!=LL!+QL
      :PL=10[LL!
      :PU=10[LU!
10440 GOSUB 10600
10450 NEXT J
10490 RETURN
10492 REM
10494 REM          2 and 2 Assay
10496 REM
10500 P$="2 and 2 Dose Assay:"
```

```
        :LN=0
        :GOSUB 10900
10510 D1=X(1,1)
        :D2=X(2,1)
        :X=D2-D1
        :U1=Y(1,1)
        :U2=Y(2,1)
10520 FOR J=2 TO L
10530 IF D1=X(1,J) AND D2=X(2,J) THEN 10560
10540 P$="All dose-response curves must use equivalent doses!"
        :GOSUB 400
10550 J=L
        :GOTO 10590
10560 S1=Y(1,J)
        :S2=Y(2,J)
10570 U=(U2-S2+U1-S1)/2
        :S=(S2-S1+U2-U1)/(2*X)
10580 RP=10[(U/S)
        :GOSUB 10600
10590 NEXT J
10599 RETURN
10600 P$=FNF$(FI$(J))+FNP$(RP)
10610 IF LN=1 AND U%=11 THEN P$=P$+FNP$(PL)+FNP$(PU)
10620 GOSUB 400
10899 RETURN
10900 GOSUB 402
        :P$="Relative Potency of '"+FI$(1)+"' versus
        :"
        :GOSUB 402
10910 P$=FNF$("Curve")+FNF$("Pot. Ratio")
10920 IF U%=11 THEN P$=P$+FNF$("Lower")+FNF$("Upper")
10930 GOSUB 400
10940 P$=UL$+UL$
        :IF U%=11 THEN P$=P$+P$
10950 GOSUB 400
10999 RETURN




File name: PCS11/LIB
---------------------------------------------------------------------

11000 DATA "11> Relative Potency II: Statistical Analysis",10
11010 REM 11/04/85 VER 4.0
11020 GOTO 10020
11999 RETURN




File name: PCS12/LIB
---------------------------------------------------------------------

12000 DATA "12> Dissociation Constant I: Agonists",5
12010 REM 02/26/86 VER 4.0
12020 GOSUB 12100
        :REM Input
12030 GOSUB 12200
        :REM Process
12040 GOSUB 12500
        :REM Output
12050 RETURN
12100 DC=0
        :PX$=BL$+"A'"+BR$
        :PY$=BL$+"A"+BR$
        :P$="Enter equiactive dose pairs ("+PX$+","+PY$+")."
        :GOSUB 302
        :GOSUB 50050
        :PX$="1/"+PX$
        :PY$="1/"+PY$
12110 RETURN
12200 FOR J=1 TO L
        :FOR I=1 TO N(J)
```

```
      :X(I,J)=1/X(I,J)
      :Y(I,J)=1/Y(I,J)
      :REM <- 13
12210 NEXT I,J
12220 GOSUB 580
      :IF IV$="Y" THEN GOSUB 51000
12230 GOSUB 5040
12240 RETURN
12500 FOR J=1 TO L
      :GOSUB 610
      :DC=(M(J)-1)/B(J)
      :P$=FNF$("Ka =")+STR$(DC)
      :GOSUB 400
      :NEXT J
12999 RETURN
```

File name: PCS13/LIB

```
13000 DATA "13> Dissociation Constant II: Partial Agonists",12
13010 REM 02/26/86 VER 4.0
13020 GOSUB 13060
      :REM Input
13030 GOSUB 13120
      :REM Process
13040 GOSUB 13150
      :REM Output
13050 RETURN
13060 DC=0
13070 P$="Enter equiactive dose pairs ("+BL$+"Partial Agonist"+BR
      $+","+BL$+"Agonist"+BR$+") in molar units."
      :GOSUB 302
13090 PX$=BL$+"Partial"+BR$
      :PY$=BL$+"Agonist"+BR$
      :GOSUB 50050
13110 RETURN
13120 PX$="1/"+PX$
      :PY$="1/"+PY$
      :GOSUB 12200
13140 RETURN
13150 FOR J=1 TO L
      :GOSUB 610
      :P$=FNF$("Kp =")+STR$(M(J)/B(J))
      :GOSUB 400
      :NEXT J
13999 RETURN
```

File name: PCS14/LIB

```
14000 DATA "14> Dissociation Constant III: Perturbation Methods",
      5
14010 REM 02/26/86 VER 4.0
14020 GOSUB 14060
      :REM Input
14030 GOSUB 14100
      :REM Process
14040 GOSUB 14500
      :REM Output
14050 RETURN
14060 DC=0
      :PX$=BL$+"Agonist"+BR$
      :PY$="tau"
      :GOSUB 50050
14090 RETURN
14100 FOR J=1 TO L
      :FOR I=1 TO N(J)
      :Y(I,J)=1/Y(I,J)
```

```
14110 NEXT I,J
14120 PY$="1/"+PY$
      :GOSUB 580
      :IF IV$="Y" THEN GOSUB 51000
14130 SI$="k1"
      :YI$="k2"
      :U%=5
      :GOSUB 5040
14200 RETURN
14500 FOR J=1 TO L
      :GOSUB 610
      :P$=FNF$("K =")+STR$(B(J)/M(J))
      :GOSUB 400
      :NEXT J
14999 RETURN




File name: PCS15/LIB
-------------------------------------------------------------------

15000 DATA "15> pA2 Analysis I: Schild Plot",5
15010 REM 02/26/86 VER 4.0
15020 GOSUB 15060
      :REM Input
15030 GOSUB 15500
      :REM Process & Output
15050 RETURN
15060 P$="Computation of pA2 uses molar units of antagonist. You
      may enter antagonist concentrations in several ways:"
      :GOSUB 300
15070 U$(1)="Molar"
      :U$(2)="ug/ml or mg/kg"
      :U$(3)="mg/ml"
      :U$(4)="g/100ml"
15080 FOR X=1 TO 4
      :P$=P$+STR$(X)+" = "+U$(X)+","
      :NEXT X
      :GOSUB 300
15090 PRINT
      :PRINT"Enter option: ";
15100 GOSUB 200
      :PRINT
      :OP=VAL(A$)
      :IF OP<1 OR OP>4 THEN 15080
15110 IF OP>1 THEN INPUT"Enter molecular wt of antagonist ";MW
15130 PX$=BL$+"B"+BR$
      :PY$=BL$+"A'"+BR$+"/"+BL$+"A"+BR$
15140 GOSUB 300
      :GOSUB 50050
15150 IF OP=1 THEN 15260
15160 IF OP=2 THEN FA=.001 ELSE IF OP=3 THEN FA=1 ELSE IF OP=4 TH
      EN FA=10
15180 FA=FA/MW
      :P$="Doses in moles:"
      :GOSUB 400
15200 FOR J=1 TO L
      :FOR I=1 TO N(J)
15220 X(I,J)=X(I,J)*FA
      :P$=P$+FNP$(X(I,J))
15230 NEXT I
      :GOSUB 400
      :NEXT J
      :GOSUB 400
15260 PX$="-Log("+BL$+"B"+BR$+")"
      :PY$="Log(A'/A-1)"
15270 FOR J=1 TO L
      :FOR I=1 TO N(J)
15280 X(I,J)=-LOG(X(I,J))/LOG(10)
15290 Y(I,J)=LOG(Y(I,J)-1)/LOG(10)
15300 NEXT I,J
15310 GOSUB 580
      :IF IV$="Y" THEN GOSUB 51000 ELSE IV$="Y"
```

```
15320 RETURN
15500 XI$="pA2"
      :U%=5
      :GOSUB 5040
15999 RETURN




File name: PCS16/LIB
------------------------------------------------------------------

16000 DATA "16> pA2 Analysis II: Time-Dependent Method",5
16010 REM 02/26/86 VER 4.0
16020 GOSUB 16060
      :REM Input
16030 GOSUB 16120
      :REM Process
16040 GOSUB 16500
      :REM Output
16050 RETURN
16060 P$="The Time-Dependent Method requires dose ratio data to b
      e collected over several time periods for a single concentr
      ation of antagonist."
      :GOSUB 302
16070 P$="Enter concentration of antagonist in molar units"
      :GOSUB 260
      :BC=VAL(A$)
      :IF BC<=0 THEN 16070
16080 GOSUB 300
      :P$="Concentration of antagonist ="+STR$(BC)+" M"
      :GOSUB 402
16100 PX$="time"
      :PY$=BL$+"A'"+BR$+"/"+BL$+"A"+BR$
      :GOSUB 50050
16110 RETURN
16120 FOR J=1 TO L
      :FOR I=1 TO N(J)
16140 Y(I,J)=LOG(Y(I,J)-1)/LOG(10)
16150 NEXT I,J
16170 PY$="Log(A'/A-1)"
      :GOSUB 5040
16190 RETURN
16500 FOR J=1 TO L
      :GOSUB 610
      :P$=FNF$("pA2 =")+STR$(B(J)-LOG(BC)/LOG(10))
      :GOSUB 402
16600 P$="Half-life of antagonist ="+STR$(-LOG(2)/(M(J)/.434294))
      :GOSUB 402
      :NEXT J
16999 RETURN




File name: PCS17/LIB
------------------------------------------------------------------

17000 DATA "17> pA2 Analysis III: Constrained Plot",15
17010 REM 02/26/86 VER 4.0
17020 GOSUB 15060
      :REM Input
17030 GOSUB 17060
      :REM Process
17040 GOSUB 17180
      :REM Output
17050 RETURN
17060 GOSUB 2200
      :GOSUB 5210
17080 FOR J=1 TO L
      :XM=MX(J)
      :YM=MY(J)
      :SS=0
```

```
17120 FOR I=1 TO N(J)
     :X=X(I,J)
     :Y=Y(I,J)
     :SS=SS+((Y-YM)+(X-XM))*((Y-YM)+(X-XM))
     :NEXT I
17140 SE(J)=SQR(SS/(N(J)-1))/SQR(N(J))
     :NEXT J
17170 RETURN
17180 FOR J=1 TO L
     :N=N(J)-1
     :B=MX(J)+MY(J)
     :GOSUB 400
17200 P$=FNF$(PY$+" =")+" -1 x "+PX$+" +"+STR$(B)
     :GOSUB 402
     :GOSUB 5600
     :GOSUB 400
17220 R%=2
     :P1$="pA2:"
     :P2=B
     :P3=SE(J)*TV
     :P4=SE(J)
     :GOSUB 5550
     :C%=4
     :GOSUB 700
     :NEXT J
17999 RETURN




File name: PCS18/LIB
----------------------------------------------------------------------

18000 DATA "18> Enzyme Kinetics I: Michaelis-Menten Equation",12
18010 REM 02/05/86 VER 4.0
18020 GOSUB 18100
     :REM Input
18030 GOSUB 18200
     :REM Process
18040 GOSUB 18500
     :REM Output
18050 RETURN
18100 DC=0
     :PX$=BL$+"Substrate"+BR$
     :PY$="Velocity"
     :GOSUB 50050
18110 RETURN
18200 PX$="1/"+BL$+"Substrate"+BR$
     :PY$="1/Velocity"
     :GOSUB 12200
18210 RETURN
18500 FOR J=1 TO L
     :GOSUB 610
     :P$=FNF$("Vmax =")+STR$(1/B(J))
     :GOSUB 400
     :P$=FNF$("Km =")+STR$(M(J)/B(J))
     :GOSUB 402
18520 NEXT J
18999 RETURN




File name: PCS19/LIB
----------------------------------------------------------------------

19000 DATA "19> Enzyme Kinetics II: Competitive Inhibition",18
19010 REM 01/30/86 VER 4.0
19020 GOSUB 19100
     :REM Input
19030 GOSUB 19200
     :REM Process
19040 GOSUB 19500
     :REM Output
```

```
19050 RETURN
19100 PN$=""
19110 P$="You must input data for two curves. The first must be w
      ithout an inhibitor, and the second must be in the presence
      of a "
19120 P$=P$+PN$+"competitive inhibitor."
      :GOSUB 302
19130 P$="Enter concentration of inhibitor "
      :GOSUB 260
      :CI=VAL(A$)
      :GOSUB 300
19140 P$="Concentration of "+PN$+"competitive inhibitor ="+STR$(C
      I)
      :GOSUB 402
19150 L=2
      :GOSUB 18020
      :IF L<>2 THEN 19110
19160 RETURN
19200 CI=CI/(((1/B(1))*M(2)/(M(1)/B(1))-1)
19300 RETURN
19500 P$=FNF$("Ki =")+STR$(CI)
      :GOSUB 400
19999 RETURN
```

```
File name: PCS20/LIB
---------------------------------------------------------------------------

20000 DATA "20> Enzyme Kinetics III: Noncompetitive Inhibition",1
      9
20010 REM 02/05/86 VER 4.0
20020 GOSUB 20060
      :REM Input
20030 GOSUB 20100
      :REM Process
20040 GOSUB 19500
      :REM Output
20050 RETURN
20060 PN$="Non-"
20070 GOSUB 19110
      :IF L<>2 THEN 20060
20090 RETURN
20100 RATIO=((M(2)/M(1))+(B(2)/B(1)))/2
      :CI=CI/(RATIO-1)
20999 RETURN
```

```
File name: PCS21/LIB
---------------------------------------------------------------------------

21000 DATA "21> First Order Drug Decay",4
21010 REM 02/05/86 VER 4.0
21020 GOSUB 21060
      :REM Input
21030 GOSUB 21100
      :REM Process
21040 GOSUB 21200
      :REM Output
21050 RETURN
21060 P$="The first entry must be the tissue concentration or amo
      unt at time = 0."
      :GOSUB 302
21080 PX$="Time"
      :PY$="Tissue Conc."
      :GOSUB 50050
21090 RETURN
21100 FOR J=1 TO L
21110 IF X(1,J)<>0 THEN PRINT "BAD DATA, T(0) MUST = 0"
      : GOTO 21000
21120 N(J)=N(J)-1
      :T0=Y(1,J)
```

```
21150 FOR I=1 TO N(J)
      :X(I,J)=X(I+1,J)
21160 Y(I,J)=LOG(T0/Y(I+1,J))
21180 NEXT I,J
      :PY$="ln (A/A-X)"
      :GOSUB 3200
      :GOSUB 4100
21190 RETURN
21200 FOR J=1 TO L
      :SL=XY(J)/S1(J)
      :GOSUB 610
21220 P$=FNF$("K =")+STR$(SL)
      :GOSUB 400
21230 NEXT J
21999 RETURN




File name: PCS22/LIB
------------------------------------------------------------------

22000 DATA "22> Scatchard Plot",5
22010 REM 06/24/86 VER 4.0
22020 GOSUB 22060
      :REM Input
22030 GOSUB 5040
      :REM Process
22040 GOSUB 22090
      :REM Output
22050 RETURN
22060 PX$=BL$+"Bound"+BR$
      :PY$=BL$+"Bnd"+BR$+"/"+BL$+"Free"+BR$
      :GOSUB 50050
22080 RETURN
22090 GOSUB 5620
      :FOR J=1 TO L
      :GOSUB 610
22095 P$(2,0)="K :":P$(2,1)=STR$(ABS(1/M(J)))
      :P$(2,2)=""
      :P$(2,3)=STR$(1/ABS(M(J)-EM(J)*TV))
      :P$(2,4)=STR$(1/ABS(M(J)+EM(J)*TV))
22100 P$(3,0)="(P)t* :"
      :X=ABS(-B(J)/M(J))
      :P$(3,1)=STR$(X)
      :P$(3,2)=STR$(EX(J))
      :P$(3,3)=STR$(X-EX(J)*TV)
      :P$(3,4)=STR$(X+EX(J)*TV)
      :REM 06/24/86
22120 R%=3
      :C%=4
      :GOSUB 700
      :P$="* Estimated concentration of binding sites."
      :GOSUB 400
      :NEXT J
      :REM 06/24/86
22999 RETURN




File name: PCS23/LIB
------------------------------------------------------------------

23000 DATA "23> Henderson-Hasselbalch Equation",0
23010 REM 02/03/86 VER 4.0
23020 P$="Enter A for weak Acid or B for weak Base "
      :GOSUB 250
      :IN$=A$
23030 IF IN$<>"A" AND IN$<>"B" THEN 23020
23040 P$="Enter pK of drug "
      :GOSUB 260
      :PK=VAL(A$)
23050 P$="Enter pH of medium"
      :GOSUB 260
      :PH=VAL(A$)
```

```
23060 RA=10[(PH-PK)
      :GOSUB 400
23070 P$="The drug is a weak "
      :IF IN$="A" THEN P$=P$+"acid "
      :ELSE P$=P$+"base "
23080 P$=P$+"with a pK of"+STR$(PK)+"."
      :GOSUB 400
23090 P$="The pH of the medium is"+STR$(PH)+"."
      :GOSUB 400
23100 P$="The ratio of ionized to unionized drug = "
23110 IF IN$="A" THEN P$=P$+STR$(RA) ELSE P$=P$+STR$(1/RA)
23120 GOSUB 402
      :P$="Run again (Y/N) "
      :GOSUB 250
      :IF A$="Y" THEN 23020
23999 RETURN
```

File name: PCS24/LIB

```
24000 DATA "24> Exponential Growth & Decay",5
24010 REM 02/25/86 VER 4.0
24020 GOSUB 24100
      :REM Input
24030 GOSUB 24200
      :REM Process
24040 GOSUB 24500
      :REM Output
24050 RETURN
24100 PX$="time"
      :PY$="X"
      :SI$="K"
      :GOSUB 50050
24110 RETURN
24200 PY$="ln("+PY$+")"
      :FOR J=1 TO L
      :FOR I=1 TO N(J)
      :Y(I,J)=LOG(Y(I,J))
24210 NEXT I,J
      :GOSUB 580
      :IF IV$="Y" THEN GOSUB 51000
24220 IV$="Y"
      :GOSUB 5200
      :FOR J=1 TO L
      :GOSUB 5410
24230 P$(0,0)="half-life:":P$(0,1)=STR$(ABS(LOG(2)/M(J)))
      :P$(0,2)=""
      :P$(0,3)=STR$(ABS(LOG(2)/(M(J)-EM(J)*TV)))
      :P$(0,4)=STR$(ABS(LOG(2)/(M(J)+EM(J)*TV)))
      :R%=0
      :C%=4
      :GOSUB 700
      :NEXT J
24250 RETURN
24500 FOR J=1 TO L
      :GOSUB 610
      :P$=FNF$("X =")+STR$(EXP(B(J)))+" x E^ "+STR$(M(J))+" t"
      :GOSUB 402
24510 REM P$=FNF$("K =")+STR$(M(J))
      :GOSUB 400
      :P$=FNF$("A =")+STR$(EXP(B(J)))
      :GOSUB 402
24520 NEXT J
24999 RETURN
```

File name: PCS25/LIB

```
25000 DATA "25> Area Under a Curve: Trapezoidal & Simpson's Rules
      ",4
```

```
25010 REM 07/10/86 VER 4.0
25020 GOSUB 25100
      :REM Input
25030 GOSUB 25500
      :REM Process
25040 RETURN
25100 P$="For the greatest accuracy, the area under the curve sho
      uld be divided into an even number (n) of EQUALLY spaced su
      bintervals. Enter n+1 pairs of X and Y values from the curv
      e."
      :GOSUB 302
25110 P$="If the X interval width is divided into UNEQUAL subinte
      rvals, the area will be based on an approximation using the
       Trapezoidal rule.  Enter X values first."
      :GOSUB 302
      :GOSUB 50050
25120 RETURN
25500 FOR J=1 TO L
      :XI=X(2,J)-X(1,J)
      :I=3
      :REM equal or unequal?
25510 IF L>1 THEN GOSUB 51500
      :GOSUB 400
25520 IF XI<>(X(I,J)-X(I-1,J)) THEN XI=0
      :ELSE I=I+1
      :IF I<=N(J) THEN 25520
25530 N=N(J)
      :IF XI=0 THEN 25610
25540 H=(X(N,J)-X(0,J))/(N-1)
      :SY=Y(1,J)+Y(N,J)
25550 FOR I=2 TO N-1
      :SY=SY+(2*Y(I,J))
      :NEXT I
25560 AT=H*SY/2
      :SY=Y(1,J)+Y(N,J)
25570 FOR I=2 TO N-1
      :IF I/2=INT(I/2) THEN F=4 ELSE F=2
25580 SY=SY+(F*Y(I,J))
25590 NEXT I
25600 AS=H*SY/3
2561? P$="Area under "+PY$+"( "+PX$+" ) between "+PY$+"("+STR$(X(
      1,J))+" ) and "+PY$+"("+STR$(X(N,J))+" )
      :"
      :GOSUB 402
25620 IF XI=0 THEN 25670
25630 P$="Using equal subintervals:"
      :GOSUB 400
25640 P$="     Trapezoidal Rule -  Area ="+STR$(AT)
      :GOSUB 400
25650 P$="     Simpson's Rule -    Area ="+STR$(AS)
      :GOSUB 402
25660 IF XI<>0 THEN 25700
25670 GOSUB 25800
25680 P$="Approximation using unequal intervals:"
      :GOSUB 400
25690 P$="     Trapezoidal Rule -  Area ="+STR$(AA)
      :GOSUB 402
25700 NEXT J
      :RETURN
25800 AA=0
      :FOR I=2 TO N
      :AA=AA+((Y(I,J)+Y(I-1,J))*(X(I,J)-X(I-1,J))/2)
      :NEXT I
      :REM <- 29,30
25999 RETURN
```

File name: PCS26/LIB

```
26000 DATA "26> Pharmacokinetics I: Constant Infusion, 1st Order
      Elimination",3
```

```
26010 REM 02/03/86 VER 4.0
26020 GOSUB 26100
     :REM Input
26030 GOSUB 26500
     :REM Process
26040 RETURN
26100 L=1
     :PX$="Time"
     :GOSUB 26200
     :GOSUB 26280
26110 RETURN
26200 SC=1
     :SA$="Saturation concentration (Default=1) ... "
26210 KE!=0
     :KE$="Elimination rate constant (1/hr), Ke ... "
26220 T2=0
     :T2$="Elimination half-time, t1/2 ............ "
26230 RI=0
     :RI$="Infusion rate (mg/hr) ................. "
26240 VD=0
     :VD$="Apparent volume of distribution (liters) "
26250 E$="="
26260 P$="Enter values or press <ENTER> if unknown."
     :GOSUB 300
26270 RETURN
26280 P$=SA$
     :GOSUB 260
     :IF A$<>"" THEN SC=VAL(A$)
26290 P$=KE$
     :GOSUB 260
     :KE!=VAL(A$)
26300 IF KE!<>0 THEN 26330
26310 P$=T2$
     :GOSUB 260
     :T2=VAL(A$)
26320 IF T2<>0 THEN KE!=LOG(2)/T2
26330 P$=RI$
     :GOSUB 260
     :RI=VAL(A$)
26340 IF RI<>0 AND KE!<>0 THEN VD=RI/(SC*KE!)
     :RETURN
26350 P$=VD$
     :GOSUB 260
     :VD=VAL(A$)
26360 IF VD<>0 AND RI<>0 AND KE!=0 THEN KE!=RI/(SC*VD)
26370 IF KE!<>0 THEN RETURN
26380 GOSUB 300
     :P$="More information is required.  Do you want to enter pla
     sma concentrations at various time intervals (Y/N) "
     :GOSUB 250
     :IF A$="N" THEN RETURN
26390 IF SC=0 THEN P$="Saturation concentration is required."
     :GOSUB 302
     :GOTO 26280
26400 P$="Enter each concentration as a fraction of the saturatio
     n concentration,"+STR$(SC)
     :GOSUB 302
26410 GOSUB 300
     :PX$="Time"
     :PY$="Conc."
     :GOSUB 50050
26420 FOR I=1 TO N(1)
     :Y(I,1)=LOG((1-Y(I,1))/SC)
     :NEXT I
26430 ID=0
     :PY$="ln(1-C/Cmax)"
     :GOSUB 3200
     :GOSUB 4100
     :KE!=-1*M(1)
26440 RETURN
26500 GOSUB 400
     :P$="Results:"
     :GOSUB 400
26510 IF SC<>0 THEN P$=SA$+E$+STR$(SC)
     :GOSUB 400
```

```
26520 IF KE!<>0 THEN P$=KE$+E$+STR$(KE!)
      :GOSUB 400
26530 IF T2=0 AND KE!<>0 THEN T2=LOG(2)/KE!
26540 IF T2<>0 THEN P$=T2$+E$+STR$(T2)
      :GOSUB 400
26550 IF RI<>0 THEN P$=RI$+E$+STR$(RI)
      :GOSUB 400
26560 IF VD<>0 THEN P$=VD$+E$+STR$(VD)
      :GOSUB 400
26570 GOSUB 400
      :GOSUB 540
      :IF A$="L" THEN GOSUB 570 ELSE RETURN
26580 GOSUB 400
      :PY$="Conc."
      :JS=1
      :JL=1
      :GOSUB 51120
26590 GOSUB 260
      :IF A$="" THEN RETURN ELSE X=VAL(A$)
26600 YC=-1*SC*(EXP(-1*KE!*X)-1)
26610 P$=STRING$(CW%," ")+FNP$(X)+FNP$(YC)
      :GOSUB 400
      :GOTO 26590
26999 RETURN




File name: PCS27/LIB
--------------------------------------------------------------------------------

27000 DATA "27> Pharmacokinetics II: Multiple Intravenous Injecti
      ons",26
27010 REM 02/05/86 VER 4.0
27020 GOSUB 27050
      :REM Input
27030 GOSUB 27300
      :REM Process
27040 RETURN
27050 DO=0
      :DO$="Dose of drug (mg) ...................... "
27060 TI=0
      :TI$="Dosing interval (hrs) .................. "
27070 FR=0
      :FR$="Fraction remaining ..................... "
27080 ND=0
      :ND$="Number of doses ........................ "
27090 CM=0
      :CO$="Plasma concentration (mg/ml) .......... "
27100 PS=0
      :PS$="Single dose plasma concentration (mg/ml) "
27110 PC=95
      :PC$="Desired level as % of upper limit ...... "
27120 GOSUB 26200
27130 P$=KE$
      :GOSUB 260
      :KE!=VAL(A$)
27140 P$=ND$
      :GOSUB 260
      :ND=VAL(A$)
27150 P$=TI$
      :GOSUB 260
      :TI=VAL(A$)
27160 IF KE!<>0 AND TI<>0 THEN FR=EXP(-KE!*TI)
27170 P$=PC$+STR$(PC)
      :GOSUB 300
      :REM PC=VAL(A$)
      :IF PC=0 THEN 27190
27180 IF TI=0 AND ND<>0 THEN FR=EXP(LOG(1-PC/100)/ND)
27190 IF FR=0 THEN P$=FR$
      :GOSUB 260
      :FR=VAL(A$)
      :IF FR=0 THEN RETURN
27200 IF ND=0 AND PC<>0 THEN ND=INT(LOG(1-PC/100)/LOG(FR)+.5)
```

```
27210 IF TI=0 AND KE!<>0 THEN TI=-LOG(FR)/KE!
27220 IF KE!=0 AND TI<>0 THEN KE!=-LOG(FR)/TI
27230 P$=PS$
      :GOSUB 260
      :PS=VAL(A$)
27240 IF PS=0 THEN P$=DO$
      :GOSUB 260
      :DO=VAL(A$)
      :P$=VD$
      :GOSUB 260
      :VD=VAL(A$)
      :IF VD<>0 THEN PS=DO/(VD*1000)
27250 IF PS=0 THEN RETURN
27260 CU=PS*(1/(1-FR))
27270 CM=PS/-LOG(FR)
27280 CL=FR*CU
27290 RETURN
27300 GOSUB 400
      :P$= "Results:"
      :GOSUB 400
27310 IF KE!<>0 THEN P$= KE$+E$+STR$(KE!)
      :GOSUB 400
27320 IF ND<>0 THEN P$= ND$+E$+STR$(ND)
      :GOSUB 400
27330 IF TI<>0 THEN P$= TI$+E$+STR$(TI)
      :GOSUB 400
27340 IF PC<>0 THEN P$= PC$+E$+STR$(PC)
      :GOSUB 400
27350 IF PS<>0 THEN P$= PS$+E$+STR$(PS)
      :GOSUB 400
27360 IF DO<>0 THEN P$= DO$+E$+STR$(DO)
      :GOSUB 400
27370 IF VD<>0 THEN P$= VD$+E$+STR$(VD)
      :GOSUB 400
27380 IF FR<>0 THEN P$= FR$+E$+STR$(FR)
      :GOSUB 400
27390 IF CM<>0 THEN P$=CO$+":":GOSUB 400
      :P$=FNF$("Peak  "+E$)+STR$(CU)
      :GOSUB 400
      :P$=FNF$("Mean  "+E$)+STR$(CM)
      :GOSUB 400
      :P$=FNF$("Lower "+E$)+STR$(CL)
      :GOSUB 400
27999 RETURN
```

File name: PCS28/LIB

```
28000 DATA "28> Pharmacokinetics III: Volume of Distribution",5
28010 REM 02/20/86 VER 4.0
28020 GOSUB 28100
      :REM Input
28030 GOSUB 28200
      :REM Process
28040 RETURN
28100 P$="This procedure calculates the volume of distribution, V
      d, from a single i.v. bolus of a drug and values of its pla
      sma concentration, Cp, over several time periods."
      :GOSUB 302
28110 P$="Enter the drug dose (i.v. bolus, mg) "
      :GOSUB 260
      :GOSUB 300
28120 D=VAL(A$)
      :P$="Intravenous bolus dose (mg) ="+STR$(D)
      :GOSUB 402
28150 PX$="time"
      :PY$="Cp (mg/l)"
      :L=1
      :GOSUB 50050
28160 RETURN
```

```
28200 GOSUB 580
      :J=1
      :FOR I=1 TO N(J)
      :Y(I,J)=LOG(Y(I,J))
      :YA(I)=Y(I,J)
      :NEXT I
      :PY$="ln("+PY$+")"
28210 P$="Enter time at which phase 2 begins "
      :GOSUB 260
      :GOSUB 300
      :TP=VAL(A$)
      :IF TP<X(1,1) OR TP>X(N(1),1) THEN 28210
28220 ID=1
      :IF IV$="Y" THEN GOSUB 51000
28230 JN=1
      :NN=N(1)
      :IX=1
      :RX=0
28240 IF X(ID,1)=TP THEN 28250 ELSE ID=ID+1
      :GOTO 28240
28250 FOR IX=1 TO ID-1
      :I=1
      :GOSUB 52820
      :NEXT IX
      :REM delete point
28300 P$="Regression from "+PX$+" ="+STR$(X(1,1))+" to"+STR$(X(N(
      1),1))+"
      :"
      :GOSUB 5040
      :R=ABS(R(1))
28310 R=ABS(R(1))
      :P1$=FNF$("ln(Co) =")+STR$(B(1))+FNF$("Co =")+STR$(EXP(B(1))
      )+FNF$("R =")+STR$(R)
      :P2$=FNF$("Vd =")+STR$(D/EXP(B(1)))
28500 REM IF R>RX THEN RX=R
      :IX=IX+1
      :IF IX<(NN-2) THEN 28250
28600 P$=P1$
      :GOSUB 402
      :P$=P2$
      :GOSUB 400
28999 RETURN


File name: PCS29/LIB
--------------------------------------------------------------------

29000 DATA "29> Pharmacokinetics IV: Plasma Concentration-Time Da
      ta",25
29010 REM 07/10/86 VER 4.0
29020 PX$="time"
      :PY$="Cp"
      :L=1
29030 GOSUB 50050
      :REM Input
29040 GOSUB 29130
      :REM Time of peak Cp
29050 GOSUB 29210
      :REM Ke from tail of ln(Cp)-Time curve
29060 GOSUB 29340
      :REM Ka from regression of ln(Cp'-Cp) vs Time
29070 GOSUB 29430
      :REM Area of Cp-Time curve from 0 to infinity
29090 RETURN
29100 REM
29110 REM          Time of Cp
29120 REM
29130 P$="Enter amount of single oral dose given"
      :GOSUB 260
      :D=VAL(A$)
      :IF D=0 THEN 29130
29140 GOSUB 300
      :P$="Single oral dose = "+A$
      :GOSUB 402
```

```
29150 J=1
      :GOSUB 2700
      :REM find time of Cmax
29160 P$="The greatest "+PY$+" measured is"+STR$(YB)+" and occurs
      at "+PX$+" ="+STR$(X(IB,J))
      :GOSUB 402
29162 P$="How many periods after peak time do you want to begin a
      nalysis of Ke (default=1) "
      :GOSUB 260
      :GOSUB 300
      :I=1
      :IF A$<>"" THEN I=VAL(A$)
29164 IF (IB+I)>N(J) OR I<1 THEN 29162 ELSE IX=IB+I
29166 P$="Ke analysis begins at t ="+STR$(X(IX,J))
      :GOSUB 400
29170 RETURN
29180 REM
29190 REM          Ke from tail of ln(Cp)-time curve
29200 REM
29210 II=1
      :REM define curve
29220 FOR I=1 TO N(1)
      :XA(I)=X(I,1)
      :YA(I)=Y(I,1)
      :NEXT I
      :N(2)=N(1)
29230 FOR I=IX TO N(1)
      :REM start w/ 1st pt after peak
29240 X(II,1)=X(I,1)
      :Y(II,1)=LOG(Y(I,1))
      :II=II+1
29270 NEXT I
      :N(1)=II-1
      :PY$="ln("+PY$+")"
      :GOSUB 3040
29300 KE!=ABS(M(1))
      :P$=FNF$("Ke =")+" "+STR$(KE!)
      :GOSUB 402
29320 SL=EXP(B(1))
      :P$=FNF$("Cp' =")+" "+STR$(SL)+" exp("+STR$(M(1))+" "+PX$+")
      "
      :GOSUB 400
29330 RETURN
29340 FOR I=1 TO IB-1
      :X(I,1)=XA(I)
29360 CP=SL*EXP(M(1)*X(I,1))
      :REM C' = slope exp(ke*t)
29370 Y(I,1)=LOG(CP-YA(I))
29380 NEXT I
      :N(1)=IB-1
      :PY$="ln(Cp'-Cp)"
      :GOSUB 3040
29410 KA!=ABS(M(1))
      :P$=FNF$("Ka =")+" "+STR$(KA!)+FNF$("Tp =")+STR$(LOG(KE!/KA!
      )/(KE!-KA!))
      :GOSUB 402
29420 RETURN
29430 N=N(2)
      :N(1)=N(2)
      :J=1
29440 FOR I=1 TO N
      :X(I,J)=XA(I)
      :Y(I,J)=YA(I)
      :NEXT I
29460 GOSUB 25800
      :P$="A.U.C.(Trapezoidal approximation) ="+STR$(AA)
      :GOSUB 402
29480 AT=Y(N(1),1)/KE!
      :P$="A.U.C.(t ="+STR$(X(N(1),1))+" to infinity) ="+STR$(AT)
      :GOSUB 402
29500 AT=AA+AT
      :P$=FNF$("Total A.U.C.")+" = "+STR$(AT)
29520 FV=(AT*KE!)/D
      :P$=P$+FNF$("F/Vd")+" = "+STR$(FV)
      :GOSUB 402
```

```
29540 CP=(FV*D*KA!)/(KA!-KE!)
      :P$="Cp ="+STR$(CP)+" x (exp("+STR$(-KE!)+"t) - exp("+STR$(-
      KA!)+"t) )"
      :GOSUB 402
29999 RETURN




File name: PCS30/LIB
-----------------------------------------------------------------

30000 DATA "30> Pharmacokinetics V: Renal Clearance",25
30010 REM 02/05/86 VER 4.0
30020 P$="Two methods are available."
      :GOSUB 302
30030 P$="Method A requires plasma concentration of drug (mg/l),
      and amount of drug in urine (mg) over several time periods
      (hr)."
      :GOSUB 302
30040 P$="Method B requires amount of drug in urine (mg) over sev
      eral time periods (hr) and the plasma concentration of drug
       (mg/l) obtained at the midpoints of each collection interv
      al."
      :GOSUB 302
30050 P$="Enter method <A> or <B> "
      :GOSUB 250
      :GOSUB 300
      :OP$=A$
      :IF OP$<>"A" AND OP$<>"B" THEN 30050
30060 PX$="Time (hr)"
      :PY$="Cp (mg/l)"
      :PZ$="Amount (mg)"
      :JP=3
      :L=1
      :GOSUB 50050
30070 P$="Method "+OP$+"
      :"
      :GOSUB 402
30080 IF OP$="B" THEN 30500
30090 REM          method A
30100 N=N(1)
      :JP=2
      :J=1
      :GOSUB 25800
      :REM A.U.C.
30130 SY=0
      :FOR I=1 TO N(1)
      :SY=SY+Z(I,1)
      :NEXT I
30140 P$="Integral of Cp over time ="+STR$(AA)+" (mg x hr)/liter"
      :GOSUB 402
30150 P$="Total amount collected in urine ="+STR$(SY)+" mg"
      :GOSUB 402
30160 M(1)=SY/AA
      :GOTO 30700
30490 REM          method B
30500 J=1
      :X=0
      :FOR I=1 TO N(1)
30520 Y=Y(I,J)
      :Y(I,J)=Z(I,J)/(X(I,J)-X)
      :X=X(I,J)
      :X(I,J)=Y
30530 NEXT I
      :PX$=PY$
      :PY$="Rate (mg/hr)"
      :JP=2
30600 GOSUB 51000
      :GOSUB 4040
      :GOSUB 300
30700 P$="Renal clearance ="+STR$(M(1))+" liters/hr"
      :GOSUB 402
30999 RETURN
```

File name: PCS31/LIB

```
31000 DATA "31> Pharmacokinetics VI: Renal Excretion Data Followi
      ng I.V. Administration",3
31010 REM 01/14/86 VER 4.0
31020 REM DIM Z(IZ,JZ)
31030 L=1
      :JP=3
      :PX$="Time (hr)"
      :PY$="Volume (ml)"
      :PZ$="Conc.(mg/l)"
31032 P$="Enter the dose of drug administered intravenously (mg)
      "
      :GOSUB 260
      :GOSUB 300
      :D=VAL(A$)
31040 P$="Enter the collection time (hr), volume of urine collect
      ed, and the concentration of drug in the urine."
      :GOSUB 302
31100 GOSUB 50050
      :TD=0
      :TT=X(N(1),1)
31110 REM calc midpoint time & amount excreted
31120 FOR I=N(1) TO 1 STEP -1
      :X=X(I,1)-X(I-1,1)
      :X(I,1)=X(I-1,1)+(X(I,1)-X(I-1,1))/2
      :Z(I,1)=Y(I,1)*Z(I,1)/1000
      :TD=TD+Z(I,1)
      :Z(I,1)=Z(I,1)/X
      :Y(I,1)=LOG(Z(I,1))
      :NEXT I
31140 PX$="t"
      :PY$="ln(dU/dt)"
      :PZ$="dU/dt"
      :GOSUB 51000
      :REM list calculated values
31200 JP=2
      :GOSUB 3040
      :REM do linear regresssion
31300 KE!=-M(1)
      :KR!=EXP(B(1))/D
31310 P$="Dose of drug given i.v. (mg) ="+STR$(D)
      :GOSUB 402
31320 P$="Drug excreted at the end of"+STR$(TT)+" hours (mg) ="+S
      TR$(TD)
      :GOSUB 402
31330 P$="Ke ="+STR$(KE!)+FNF$("Kr =")+STR$(KR!)
      :GOSUB 402
31999 RETURN
```

File name: PCS32/LIB

```
32000 DATA "32> Pharmacokinetics VII: Multiple Dosing from Absorp
      tive Site",2
32010 REM 02/05/86 VER 4.0
32030 CL=0
      :CL$="Clearance rate (1/hr) .................. "
32040 CM=0
      :CM$="Mean limiting concentration (Cm, mg/l) .. "
32050 DO=0
      :DO$="Dose of drug (mg) ..................... "
32060 FR=1
      :FR$="Fractional absorption .................. "
32070 KA!=0
      :KA$="Absorption rate constant (1/hr), Ka ..... "
32080 KE!=0
      :KE$="Elimination rate constant (1/hr), Ke .... "
32090 TI=0
      :TI$="Dosing interval (hrs) .................. "
```

```
32100 T2=0
      :T2$="Elimination half-time, t1/2 ............ "
32110 VD=0
      :VD$="Apparent volume of distribution (l) ..... "
32200 P$="Enter the following required data (enter t1/2 or Ke):"
      :GOSUB 302
32210 P$=DO$
      :GOSUB 260
      :DO=VAL(A$)
32220 P$=TI$
      :GOSUB 260
      :TI=VAL(A$)
32230 P$=T2$
      :GOSUB 260
      :T2=VAL(A$)
32240 IF T2<>0 THEN KE!=LOG(2)/T2 ELSE P$=KE$
      :GOSUB 260
      :KE!=VAL(A$)
32250 IF KE!<>0 AND T2=0 THEN T2=LOG(2)/KE!
32260 IF KE!=0 AND T2=0 THEN 32230
32270 GOSUB 300
      :P$="Enter the following data, or press <ENTER> if value is
      unknown:"
      :GOSUB 302
32280 P$=FR$+STR$(FR)
      :GOSUB 260
      :IF A$<>"" THEN FR=VAL(A$)
32290 P$=VD$
      :GOSUB 260
      :VD=VAL(A$)
      :IF VD<>0 THEN CL=(LOG(2)*VD)/T2
32300 P$=CL$+STR$(CL)
      :GOSUB 260
      :CL=VAL(A$)
32310 IF CL=0 AND VD=0 THEN 32290
32320 P$=KA$
      :GOSUB 260
      :KA!=VAL(A$)
32330 IF CL=0 THEN CL=(LOG(2)*VD)/T2 ELSE IF VD=0 THEN VD=(CL*T2)
      /LOG(2)
32340 CA=(DO*FR)/(CL*TI)
      :IF KA!=0 THEN 32500
32360 M=(KA!*DO*FR)/(VD*(KE!-KA!))
      :G=EXP(-KE!*TI)
32400 A=M*(EXP(-KA!*TI)-G)
      :S=A/(1-G)
32405 TC=(1/(KE!-KA!))*LOG((KE!*(M-S))/(KA!*M))
32410 CM=M*(1/TI)
      :B=((1/KA!)*(1-EXP(-KA!*TI)))-((1/KE!)*(1-G))
32420 CM=CM*B+(A/(TI*KE!))
32430 CU=M*(EXP(-KA!*TC)-EXP(-KE!*TC))+(S*(EXP(-KE!*TC)))
32440 CX=((FR*DO)/(VD*TI*KE!))*(1-EXP(-KA!*TI))
32490 REM          output
32500 GOSUB 300
      :P$="Results:"
      :GOSUB 302
32510 P$=DO$+"="+STR$(DO)
      :GOSUB 400
32520 P$=TI$+"="+STR$(TI)
      :GOSUB 400
32530 P$=T2$+"="+STR$(T2)
      :GOSUB 400
32545 P$=FR$+"="+STR$(FR)
      :GOSUB 400
32550 IF KA!<>0 THEN P$=KA$+"="+STR$(KA!)
      :GOSUB 400
32555 P$=KE$+"="+STR$(KE!)
      :GOSUB 400
32560 P$=VD$+"="+STR$(VD)
      :GOSUB 400
32570 P$=CL$+"="+STR$(CL)
      :GOSUB 400
32580 TP=4.32193*T2
      :P$="Time to reach 95% of Cm (hr) ............ ="+STR$(TP)
      :GOSUB 402
```

```
32590 IF CM=0 THEN P$=CM$+"="+STR$(CA)+" approx."
      :GOSUB 400
32600 IF CM<>0 THEN P$=CM$+"="+STR$(CM)
      :GOSUB 402
32610 IF CU<>0 THEN P$="Maximum plasma concentration (Cmax, mg/1)
      ="+STR$(CU)
      :GOSUB 400
32999 RETURN



File name: PCS33/LIB
-----------------------------------------------------------------------

33000 DATA "33> Analysis of Variance I: One-way",2
33010 REM 01/07/86 VER 4.0
33020 AN$="1"
33030 GOSUB 33100
      :REM Input
33040 GOSUB 33160
      :REM Process
33050 GOSUB 33680
      :REM Output
33060 RETURN
33100 IF AN$="2" THEN GOSUB 300
      :P$="For 2-way ANOVA, each file represents a different 'trea
      tment' and entries (mean values) across all treatments repr
      esent a 'block'."
      :GOSUB 302
33105 IF IV$="" THEN GOSUB 580
33110 GOSUB 2030
      :IF AN$="1" THEN RETURN
33120 J=2
33130 IF N(J)<>N(1) THEN P$="ERROR: n's must be equal for 2-way A
      NOVA!"
      :GOSUB 302
      :GOTO 33100
33140 J=J+1
      :IF J<=L THEN 33130
33150 RETURN
33160 NG=0
      :GT=0
      :GM=0
      :TS=0
      :ST=0
      :SE=0
      :VP=0
      :VT=0
      :F=0
      :SB=0
33170 FOR J=1 TO L
33180 NG=NG+N(J)
33190 GT=GT+SY(J)
33200 ST=ST+(MY(J)*MY(J)*N(J))
33210 SE=SE+(VA(J)*(N(J)-1))
33220 NEXT J
      :IF U%=44 THEN RETURN
33230 GM=GT/NG
      :N1=L-1
      :N2=NG-L
33240 ST=ST-(GM*GM*NG)
33250 VT=ST/N1
33260 IF AN$="1" THEN 33340
33270 REM
33280 REM         2-way anova
33290 REM
33300 FOR I=1 TO N(1)
      :Y=0
      :FOR J=1 TO L
      :Y=Y+Y(I,J)
      :NEXT J
      :SB=SB+(Y*Y)
      :NEXT I
      :REM s.s.b
```

```
33310 C=GT*GT/(N(1)*L)
33320 SB=SB/L-C
      :SE=SE-SB
33330 N1=N(1)-1
      :N2=N1*(L-1)
      :VB=SB/N1
33340 VP=SE/N2
      :F=VT/VP
      :FB=VB/VP
33350 RETURN
33360 REM
33370 REM          Get F table values
33380 REM
33390 IF N1=0 OR N2=0 THEN STOP
      :REM N1=L-1
      :N2=NG-L
33400 IF N1<7 THEN 33460
33410 IF N1=7 THEN N1=6
33420 IF N1>7 AND N1<12 THEN N1=7
33430 IF N1>11 AND N1<24 THEN N1=8
33440 IF N1>23 AND N1<48 THEN N1=9
33450 IF N1>47 THEN N1=10
33460 IF N2<31 THEN 33520
33470 IF N2>30 AND N2<40 THEN N2=30
33480 IF N2>39 AND N2<60 THEN N2=31
33490 IF N2>59 AND N2<120 THEN N2=32
33500 IF N2>119 AND N2<240 THEN N2=33
33510 IF N2>239 THEN N2=34
33520 NV%=(10*(N2-1)+N1)
33530 RA$="F95"+ET$+"PCS"
      :GOSUB 55000
      :F5=V!
33540 RA$="F99"+ET$+"PCS"
      :GOSUB 55000
      :F9=V!
33550 RETURN
33560 GOSUB 33390
      :P$=FNF$("F (95%):")+FNP$(F5)+FNF$("F (99%)
      :")+FNP$(F9)
      :GOSUB 402
33570 P$="Differences between"
33580 RETURN
33590 REM
33600 REM          ANOVA header
33610 REM
33620 P$(0,0)="Source of"
      :P$(0,1)="Sum of "
      :P$(0,2)="Deg. of"
      :P$(0,3)="Mean   "
33630 P$(1,0)="Variation"
      :P$(1,1)="Squares"
      :P$(1,2)="Freedom"
      :P$(1,3)="Square"
      :P$(1,4)="F Value"
33640 FOR I=0 TO 4
      :P$(2,I)=UL$
      :NEXT I
33650 RETURN
33660 REM          Print ANOVA table
33670 REM
33680 GOSUB 33620
      :REM header
33690 P$(3,0)="Total:"
      :P$(3,1)=STR$(SE+ST+SB)
      :P$(3,2)=STR$(NG-1)
      :R%=4
33700 P$(R%,0)="Between:"
      :P$(R%,1)=STR$(ST)
      :P$(R%,2)=STR$(L-1)
      :P$(R%,3)=STR$(VT)
      :P$(R%,4)=FND$(ABS(F),2)
33710 IF AN$="1" THEN 33730 ELSE P$(R%,0)="Treatments
      :"
      :R%=R%+1
33720 P$(R%,0)="Blocks:"
```

```
        :P$(R%,1)=STR$(SB)
        :P$(R%,2)=STR$(N1)
        :P$(R%,3)=STR$(VB)
        :P$(R%,4)=FND$(ABS(FB),2)
33730 R%=R%+1
        :P$(R%,0)="Within:"
        :P$(R%,1)=STR$(SE)
        :P$(R%,2)=STR$(N2)
        :P$(R%,3)=STR$(VP)
33740 C%=4
        :GOSUB 700
33750 N1=L-1
        :GOSUB 33560
        :REM get F values
33760 IF AN$="1" THEN P$=P$+" means
        :"
        :GOSUB 33790
        :RETURN
33770 P$=P$+" treatments:"
        :GOSUB 33790
        :GOSUB 400
33780 N1=N(1)-1
        :GOSUB 33560
        :P$=P$+" blocks:"
        :F=FB
        :GOSUB 33790
        :RETURN
33790 IF F<F5 THEN P$=P$+" NOT"
33800 P$=P$+" Significant at p < 0.0"
33810 IF F>=F9 THEN P$=P$+"1" ELSE P$=P$+"5"
33820 GOSUB 402
33999 RETURN




File name: PCS34/LIB
-------------------------------------------------------------------

34000 DATA "34> Analysis of Variance II: Two-way, Single Observat
        ion",33
34010 REM 01/05/86 VER 4.0
34020 AN$="2"
34030 GOTO 33030
34999 RETURN




File name: PCS35/LIB
-------------------------------------------------------------------

35000 DATA "35> Analysis of Variance III: Two-way, with Replicati
        on",33
35010 REM 01/05/86 VER 4.0
35020 SS=0
        :L=0
        :NN=0
35030 P$="Two factor ANOVA with replications requires entry of 2
        Blocks (e.g. male & female), each with 2 or more treatments
        . Each file represents a different treatment (e.g. dose 1,
        dose 2, etc.)."
        :GOSUB 300
        :GOSUB 300
35040 P$="Enter Block A now:"
        :GOSUB 300
        :GOSUB 300
35050 GOSUB 33100
        :REM input
35060 GOSUB 33160
        :REM process
35070 IF SS=0 THEN FOR J=1 TO L
        :XA(J)=SY(J)
        :SS=SS+S2(J)
        :NEXT J
```

```
      :NX=N(1)
      :P$="Enter Block B now:"
      :GOSUB 300
      :GOSUB 300
      :GOTO 35050
35080 IF NX<>N(1) THEN P$="ERROR: n's must be equal for all treat
      ments (files) for Block A and Block B."
      :GOSUB 300
      :GOTO 35000
35090 B1=0
      :B2=0
      :TT=0
      :ST=0
      :SC=0
      :SB=0
      :SE=0
35100 NG=2*L*N(1)
      :REM total N
35110 FOR J=1 TO L
      :SS=SS+S2(J)
      :NEXT J
      :REM SStotal
35120 FOR J=1 TO L
      :T(J)=SY(J)+XA(J)
      :NEXT J
      :REM sum treatments
35130 FOR J=1 TO L
      :B1=B1+XA(J)
      :B2=B2+SY(J)
      :NEXT J
      :REM sum blocks
35140 TT=B1+B2
      :TT=TT*TT
      :REM total treatments & blocks
35150 C=TT/NG
      :REM correction
35160 SS=SS-C
      :DS=NG-1
      :REM SStotal
35170 FOR J=1 TO L
      :SC=SC+(SY(J)*SY(J))+(XA(J)*XA(J))
      :NEXT J
      :SC=(SC/N(1))-C
      :DC=2*L-1
      :REM SScells
35180 SE=SS-SC
      :DE=2*L*(N(1)-1)
      :REM SSerror
35190 FOR J=1 TO L
      :ST=ST+(T(J)*T(J))
      :NEXT J
      :ST=ST/(2*N(1))-C
      :DT=L-1
      :REM SStreatments
35200 SB=(((B1*B1)+(B2*B2))/(L*N(1)))-C
      :DB=1
      :REM SSblocks
35210 SI=SC-ST-SB
      :DI=DT
      :REM SSinteractions
35220 MT=ST/DT
      :MB=SB/DB
      :MI=SI/DI
      :ME=SE/DE
      :REM mean squares
35230 FT=MT/ME
      :FB=MB/ME
      :FI=MI/ME
      :REM F values
35240 GOSUB 33620
      :REM ANOVA header
35250 P$(3,0)="Treatments:"
      :P$(3,1)=STR$(ST)
      :P$(3,2)=STR$(DT)
      :P$(3,3)=STR$(MT)
```

```
           :P$(3,4)=STR$(FT)
           :R%=4
35260 P$(R%,0)="Blocks:"
           :P$(R%,1)=STR$(SB)
           :P$(R%,2)=STR$(DB)
           :P$(R%,3)=STR$(MB)
           :P$(R%,4)=STR$(FB)
           :R%=5
35270 P$(R%,0)="Interaction:"
           :P$(R%,1)=STR$(SI)
           :P$(R%,2)=STR$(DI)
           :P$(R%,3)=STR$(MI)
           :P$(R%,4)=STR$(FI)
           :R%=6
35280 P$(R%,0)="Error:"
           :P$(R%,1)=STR$(SE)
           :P$(R%,2)=STR$(DE)
           :P$(R%,3)=STR$(ME)
           :C%=4
           :GOSUB 700
35290 REM
35300 REM           calculate significance
35310 REM
35320 N2=DE
           :P$(0,0)="Variation"
           :P$(0,1)="F (95%)"
           :P$(0,2)="F (99%)"
           :P$(0,4)="Significance"
           :P$(1,0)=UL$
           :P$(1,1)=UL$
           :P$(1,2)=UL$
           :P$(1,4)="-------------"
35330 N1=DT
           :FV=FT
           :R%=2
           :P$(R%,0)="Treatments:"
           :GOSUB 35380
35340 N1=DB
           :FV=FB
           :R%=3
           :P$(R%,0)="Blocks:"
           :GOSUB 35380
35350 N1=DI
           :FV=FI
           :R%=4
           :P$(R%,0)="Interaction:"
           :GOSUB 35380
35360 C%=4
           :GOSUB 700
35370 RETURN
35380 IF NN<>N1 THEN GOSUB 33390
           :REM get new f values
35390 IF FV>F9 THEN SI$="p < 0.01" ELSE IF FV>F5 THEN SI$="p < 0.
      05" ELSE SI$="n.s."
35400 P$(R%,1)=STR$(F5)
           :P$(R%,2)=STR$(F9)
           :P$(R%,4)=SI$
           :NN=N1
35999 RETURN




File name: PCS36/LIB
------------------------------------------------------------------

136 DIM IX%(JZ)
   :REM PCS36/LIB
36000 DATA "36> Newman-Keuls Test",33
36010 REM 03/25/86 VER 4.0
36020 GOSUB 33020
           :REM do ANOVA
36030 REM Convert from df to y coordinate of Q array
36040 NF=NG-L
           :DX=0
```

```
      :IF NF<15 THEN ND=NF
      :GOTO 36160
36050 IF NF>120 THEN ND=23
      :GOTO 36160
36060 IF NF=120 THEN ND=22
      :GOTO 36160
36070 IF NF>59 THEN ND=21
      :DX=60
      :DZ=120
      :GOTO 36160
36080 IF NF>39 THEN ND=20
      :DX=40
      :DZ=60
      :GOTO 36160
36090 IF NF>29 THEN ND=19
      :DX=30
      :DZ=40
      :GOTO 36160
36100 IF NF>23 THEN ND=18
      :DX=24
      :DZ=30
      :GOTO 36160
36110 IF NF>19 THEN ND=17
      :DX=20
      :DZ=24
      :GOTO 36160
36120 IF NF>17 THEN ND=16
      :DX=18
      :DZ=20
      :GOTO 36160
36130 IF NF>15 THEN ND=15
      :DX=16
      :DZ=18
      :GOTO 36160
36140 IF NF>14 THEN ND=14
      :DX=14
      :DZ=16
      :GOTO 36160
36150 REM Get Q(r,df) - the Studentized range statistic
36160 RA$="Q95/PCS"
      :IF DX<>0 THEN SF=(NF-DX)/(DZ-DX)
36170 FOR I=2 TO L
      :NV%=14*(ND-1)+(I-1)
      :GOSUB 55000
      :XA(I)=V!
      :NV%=14*ND+(I-1)
      :GOSUB 55000
      :ZA(I)=V!
36180 IF DX<>0 THEN XA(I)=SF*(ZA(I)-XA(I))+XA(I)
36190 NEXT I
36200 RA$="Q99/PCS"
      :FOR I=2 TO L
      :NV%=14*(ND-1)+(I-1)
      :GOSUB 55000
      :YA(I)=V!
      :NV%=14*ND+(I-1)
      :GOSUB 55000
      :ZA(I)=V!
36210 IF DX<>0 THEN YA(I)=SF*(ZA(I)-YA(I))+YA(I)
36220 NEXT I
36230 REM
36240 REM          Print Results
36250 REM
36260 GOSUB 36300
      :GOSUB 36740
      :GOSUB 36500
      :GOSUB 36700
36270 RETURN
36280 REM          Print Q Stats
36290 REM
36300 P$(0,0)="Step (w):"
36310 FOR I=2 TO L
      :P$(0,I-1)=STR$(I)
      :NEXT I
36320 FOR I=0 TO L
```

```
        :P$(1,I)=UL$
        :NEXT I
36330 P$(2,0)="q95% ("+STR$(NF)+")
        :"
36340 FOR I=2 TO L
        :P$(2,I-1)=STR$(XA(I))
        :NEXT I
36350 P$(3,0)="q99% ("+STR$(NF)+")
        :"
36360 FOR I=2 TO L
        :P$(3,I-1)=STR$(YA(I))
        :NEXT I
36370 R%=3
        :C%=L-1
        :GOSUB 700
36380 RETURN
36390 REM
36400 REM          Comparison
36410 REM
36500 P$=FNF$("Filename")+FNF$("vs Filename")+FNF$("Difference")+
        FNF$("Std. Err.")+FNF$("q")
        :GOSUB 400
36510 FOR I=1 TO 5
        :P$=P$+UL$
        :NEXT I
        :GOSUB 400
36520 FOR J=1 TO L-1
        :FOR I=J+1 TO L
36530 X=ABS(MY(IX%(J))-MY(IX%(I)))
        :X$=STR$(X)
36540 SE=SQR((VP/2)*((1/N(IX%(J)))+(1/N(IX%(I)))))
        :Q=X/SE
36550 IF Q>=YA(I-J+1) THEN X$=X$+"**" ELSE IF Q>=XA(I-J+1) THEN X
        $=X$+"*"
36560 P$(J+2,I)=X$
36570 P$=FNF$(FI$(IX%(J)))+FNF$(FI$(IX%(I)))+FNP$(X)+FNP$(SE)+FNP
        $(Q)
        :GOSUB 400
36590 NEXT I,J
        :GOSUB 402
        :P$="Newman-Keuls Test Summary:"
        :GOSUB 402
36600 GOSUB 36680
        :R%=L+1
        :C%=L
        :GOSUB 700
36610 RETURN
36680 FOR I=1 TO L
        :P$(0,I)=FI$(IX%(I))
        :P$(I+2,0)=P$(0,I)
        :P$(1,I)=STR$(MY(IX%(I)))
        :P$(2,I)=UL$
        :NEXT I
        :P$(L+2,0)=""
        :REM <- 37,38
36690 RETURN
36700 P$="* Significant at p < 0.05"
        :GOSUB 400
36710 P$="** Significant at p < 0.01"
        :GOSUB 400
36720 RETURN
36730 REM Shell-Metzner Sort
36740 FOR I=1 TO L
        :IX%(I)=I
        :NEXT I
        :N%=L
        :M%=N%
        :REM <- 37,38
36750 M%=INT(M%/2)
        :IF M%=0 THEN RETURN
36760 K%=N%-M%
        :J%=1
36770 I%=J%
36780 LL%=I%+M%
        :IF MY(IX%(I%))>MY(IX%(LL%)) THEN 36800
```

```
36790 J%=J%+1
      :IF J%>K% THEN 36750 ELSE 36770
36800 WW%=IX%(I%)
      :IX%(I%)=IX%(LL%)
      :IX%(LL%)=WW%
      :I%=I%-M%
36810 IF I%<1 THEN 36790 ELSE 36780
36999 RETURN




File name: PCS37/LIB
--------------------------------------------------------------------

37000 DATA "37> Duncan Multiple Range Test",36
37010 REM 02/11/86 VER 4.0
37020 GOSUB 33020
      :REM do ANOVA
37030 GOSUB 37050
      :REM process
37040 RETURN
37050 NF=L*(N(1)-1)
      :N2=NF
      :IF N2<25 THEN N2=N2-2
      :GOTO 37070
37054 IF N2>25 AND N2<35 THEN N2=19
37056 IF N2>35 AND N2<45 THEN N2=20
37058 IF N2>45 AND N2<90 THEN N2=21
37062 IF N2>90 AND N2<121 THEN N2=22
37064 IF N2>120 THEN N2=23
37070 FOR I=1 TO L-1
      :IF NF=1 THEN D5!=18
      :GOTO 37080
      :ELSE IF NF=2 THEN D5!=6.08
      :GOTO 37080
37072 N1=I+1
      :IF N1>15 AND N1<25 THEN N1=11
37074 IF N1>35 AND N1<75 THEN N1=12
37076 IF N1>=75 THEN N1=12 ELSE N1=N1-1
37078 GOSUB 37900
37080 XA(I)=D5!*SQR(VP/N(1))
      :P$(2,I-1)=STR$(XA(I))
37085 X$=STR$(I+1)
      :MID$(X$,1,1)="R"
      :P$(0,I-1)=X$
      :P$(1,I-1)=UL$
37090 NEXT I
      :R%=2
      :C%=L-2
      :GOSUB 700
      :REM show Rp
37095 P$="Duncan's Multiple Range Test Summary: Differences"
      :GOSUB 402
37100 GOSUB 36740
      :REM sort means
37110 GOSUB 36680
      :REM header
37120 FOR X=1 TO L-1
      :FOR I=1 TO L-X
      :REM adjacent steps
37140 Y=ABS(MY(IX%(I))-MY(IX%(I+X)))
      :X$=STR$(Y)
37150 IF Y>XA(X) THEN X$=X$+"*"
37160 P$(I+2,I+X)=X$
37180 NEXT I,X
      :R%=L+1
      :C%=L
      :GOSUB 700
37190 P$="* Significant at p < 0.05"
      :GOSUB 400
37200 RETURN
37900 NV%=(10*(N2-1)+N1)
```

```
37910 RA$="D95"+ET$+"PCS"
      :GOSUB 55000
      :D5=V!
37920 REM RA$="D99"+ET$+"PCS"
      :GOSUB 55000
      :D9=V!
37999 RETURN
```

File name: PCS38/LIB

```
38000 DATA "38> Least Significant Difference Test",36
38010 REM 03/12/86 VER 4.0
38020 GOSUB 33020
      :REM do ANOVA
38030 GOSUB 38050
      :REM process
38040 RETURN
38050 P$="L.S.D. Test Summary:"
      :GOSUB 402
38060 N=NG-L
      :GOSUB 2960
38070 D5=TV*SQR((2*VP)/L)
      :D9=T9*SQR((2*VP)/L)
      :REM L.S.D. p < .05 & p < .01
38080 P$="L.S.D., p < 0.05 ="+STR$(D5)
      :GOSUB 400
38085 P$="L.S.D., p < 0.01 ="+STR$(D9)
      :GOSUB 402
38090 GOSUB 36740
      :REM sort means
38100 GOSUB 36680
      :REM header
38110 FOR J=1 TO L-1
      :FOR I=J+1 TO L
38120 X=ABS(MY(IX%(J))-MY(IX%(I)))
      :X$=STR$(X)
      :IF X>D9 THEN X$=X$+"**" ELSE IF X>D5 THEN X$=X$+"*"
38130 P$(J+2,I)=X$
38150 NEXT I,J
      :R%=L+1
      :C%=L
      :GOSUB 700
38160 P$="* Significant at p < 0.05"
      :GOSUB 400
38170 P$="** Significant at p < 0.01"
      :GOSUB 400
38999 RETURN
```

File name: PCS39/LIB

```
39000 DATA "39> t-Test I: Grouped Data",5
39010 REM 03/12/86 VER 4.0
39020 GOSUB 2030
      :REM Input
39030 GOSUB 39200
      :REM Process
39040 RETURN
39200 FOR J=2 TO L
      :GOSUB 39220
      :NEXT J
39210 RETURN
39220 DF=N(1)+N(J)-2
      :REM <- 41
39230 SP=((N(1)-1)*VA(1)+(N(J)-1)*VA(J))/DF
39240 DI=SQR((N(1)+N(J))/(N(1)*N(J)))
39250 T=ABS((MY(1)-MY(J))/(SQR(SP)*DI))
```

```
39260 P$= "'"+FI$(1)+"' vs. '"+FI$(J)+"'
      :  Pooled Variance ="+STR$(SP)
      :GOSUB 400
39500 N=DF
      :GOSUB 5700
      :GOSUB 400
39999 RETURN
```

File name: PCS40/LIB

```
40000 DATA "40> t-Test II: Paired Data",39
40010 REM 02/11/86 VER 4.0
40020 GOSUB 40050
      :REM Input
40030 GOSUB 40080
      :REM Process
40040 RETURN
40050 P$="Enter 2 'Y' data files, the difference will be computed
      ."
      :GOSUB 300
      :GOSUB 300
      :L=2
      :GOSUB 2100
40060 IF N(1)<>N(2) THEN P$="ERROR
      : For paired t-test, n's for each group must be equal!
      :gosub 300
      :goto 40050
40070 RETURN
40080 FOR I=1 TO N(1)
40100 Y(I,3)=Y(I,1)-Y(I,2)
40110 NEXT I
      :L=3
      :N(3)=N(2)
      :FI$(3)="Difference"
40120 GOSUB 51000
      :GOSUB 2040
40140 T=ABS(MY(3)/(DE(3)/SQR(N(3))))
40150 DF=N(3)-1
      :REM A=J
      :B=J+1
40160 GOSUB 39500
40999 RETURN
```

File name: PCS41/LIB

```
41000 DATA "41> Ratio of Means",39
41100 REM 03/12/86 VER 4.0
41200 GOSUB 580
      :GOSUB 2030
      :REM Input
41300 FOR J=2 TO L
      :GOSUB 39220
      :P$=""
      :GOSUB 400
41400 R=MY(1)/MY(J)
      :V1=SP/N(1)
      :V2=SP/N(J)
      :C=MY(J)*MY(J)
      :C=C/(C-(V2*TV*TV))
      :CL=SQR((C-1)*(C*(R*R)+(V1/V2)))
      :CU=(C*R)+CL
      :CL=(C*R)-CL
41500 IF IV$="Y" THEN P$="V1 ="+STR$(V1)+FNF$("V2 =")+STR$(V2)+FN
      F$("C =")+STR$(C)
      :GOSUB 402
```

```
41600 P$(2,0)="Ratio"
     :P$(2,1)=STR$(R)
     :P$(2,3)=STR$(CL)
     :P$(2,4)=STR$(CU)
     :P$(0,2)="95% Limits"
     :P$(1,2)=""
41700 R%=2
     :C%=4
     :GOSUB 700
     :NEXT J
41999 RETURN




File name: PCS42/LIB
------------------------------------------------------------------------

42000 DATA "42> Chi-Square Test",2
42010 REM 02/11/86 VER 4.0
42020 GOSUB 42100
     :REM Input
42030 GOSUB 42200
     :REM Process
42040 GOSUB 42500
     :REM Output
42050 RETURN
42100 P$="Each data file represents a 'Row' in the contingency ta
     ble. Since data values across all rows represent a 'Column'
      in the contingency table, n's for each file (Row) must be
      equal."
     :GOSUB 302
42110 IV$="N"
     :L=0
     :GOSUB 2030
     :X=0
42120 N=N(1)
     :FOR J=2 TO L
     :IF N(J)<>N THEN X=1
     :NEXT J
42130 IF X=0 AND L>1 THEN 42170 ELSE P$="ERROR: "
42140 IF X=1 THEN P$=P$+"Each file (Row) must have the same numbe
     r of entries. "
42150 IF N<2 OR L<2 THEN P$=P$+"You must have more than one row a
     nd/or column!"
42160 P$=P$+" Please re-enter your data!"
     :GOSUB 302
     :GOTO 42100
42170 RETURN
42200 GT=0
     :YS=0
     :FOR J=1 TO L
     :GT=GT+SY(J)
     :NEXT J
42210 FOR J=1 TO L
     :E(J)=SY(J)/GT
     :NEXT J
42220 FOR I=1 TO N(1)
     :S(I)=0
     :FOR J=1 TO L
     :S(I)=S(I)+Y(I,J)
     :NEXT J,I
42230 IF N(1)=2 THEN P$="2 x 2 contingency table (using adjusted
     chi-square)."
     :GOSUB 402
42240 P$="Expected Frequencies:"
     :GOSUB 402
42250 FOR J=1 TO L
     :P$=P$+FNF$(FI$(J))
     :NEXT J
     :P$=P$+FNF$("Totals")
     :GOSUB 400
42260 FOR J=1 TO L+1
     :P$=P$+UL$
```

```
      :NEXT J
      :GOSUB 400
42270 FOR I=1 TO NM
      :FOR J=1 TO L
42280 IF I>N(J) THEN P$=P$+FNF$("")
      :GOTO 42320
42290 E=E(J)*S(I)
      :Y=Y(I,J)
      :P$=P$+FNP$(E)
42300 IF N(1)>2 THEN X=(Y-E)*(Y-E) ELSE X=(ABS(Y-E)-.5)*(ABS(Y-E)
      -.5)
42310 YS=YS+(X/E)
42320 NEXT J
      :P$=P$+FNP$(S(I))
      :GOSUB 400
      :NEXT I
42330 RETURN
42500 GOSUB 400
      :DF=(L-1)*(N(1)-1)
42510 NV%=DF
      :RA$="C95"+ET$+"PCS"
      :GOSUB 55000
42520 P$="Chi-Square, (95%) ="+STR$(V!)+"    "+STR$(DF)+" d.f."
      :GOSUB 400
42530 P$="Chi-Square, Calc. ="+FND$(YS,3)
42540 IF YS<V! THEN P$=P$+"   Not" ELSE P$=P$+"    "
42550 P$=P$+" Significant"
      :GOSUB 400
42999 RETURN
```

File name: PCS43/LIB

```
43000 DATA "43> Proportions: Confidence Limits",2
43010 REM 11/07/85 VER 4.0
43020 GOSUB 43060
      :REM INPUT
43030 GOSUB 43090
      :REM PROCESS
43040 GOSUB 43150
      :REM OUTPUT
43050 RETURN
43060 P$="Number of subjects exhibiting the effect "
      :GOSUB 260
      :X=VAL(A$)
43070 P$="Enter the total number of subjects "
      :GOSUB 260
      :N=VAL(A$)
      :GOSUB 300
43075 IF X=0 OR N=0 THEN 43060
43080 RETURN
43090 P=X/N
      :T=1.96
      :T2=T*T
      :P1=1/(2*N)
      :P4=T2/(4*N*N)
      :P2=T2/(2*N)
43100 S1=SQR(((P+P1)*(1-P-P1))/N+P4)
43110 S2=SQR(((P-P1)*(1-P+P1))/N+P4)
43120 CL=(N/(N+T2))*(P-P1+(P2)-(T*S1))
43130 CU=(N/(N+T2))*(P+P1+(P2)+(T*S2))
43140 RETURN
43150 P$="Number of subjects showing effect ="+STR$(X)
      :GOSUB 400
43160 P$="Total number of subjects           ="+STR$(N)
      :GOSUB 400
43170 GOSUB 400
43180 P$(0,0)="Proportion"
      :P$(0,1)="95% C.L.:":P$(0,2)="Lower"
      :P$(0,3)="Upper"
```

```
43190 P$(1,0)=UL$
      :P$(1,2)=UL$
      :P$(1,3)=UL$
43200 P$(2,0)=STR$(P)
      :P$(2,2)=STR$(CL)
      :P$(2,3)=STR$(CU)
43210 R%=2
      :C%=3
      :GOSUB 700
43999 RETURN



File name: PCS44/LIB
---------------------------------------------------------------------

44000 DATA "44> Dunnett's Test",2
44010 REM 10/16/85 VER 4.0
44020 GOSUB 44050
      :REM Input
44030 GOSUB 44070
      :REM Process
44040 RETURN
44050 PX$=""
      :GOSUB 2030
44060 RETURN
44070 DF=0
      :SS=0
      :S2=0
      :T2=0
44080 FOR J=1 TO L
44090 T2=T2+(SY(J)*SY(J))/N(J)
      :DF=DF+N(J)
      :SS=SS+S2(J)
44100 NEXT J
44110 DF=DF-L
      :S2=(SS-T2)/DF
      :GOSUB 400
44120 P$="S2 ="+STR$(S2)
      :S=SQR(S2)
      :P$=P$+"        S ="+STR$(S)+"        P ="+STR$(L-1)
      :GOSUB 400
44130 PRINT "Enter A.9 Table value for";L-1;"treatments and";DF;"
      d.f. ";
      :INPUT D
44140 P$="A.9 Table value for"+STR$(L-1)+" treatments and"+STR$(D
      F)+" d.f. = "+STR$(D)
      :GOSUB 400
44150 FOR J=2 TO L
44160 GOSUB 400
      :P$= "'"+FI$(1)+"' vs. '"+FI$(J)+"'
      :"
44170 A=S*D*SQR(1/N(J)+1/N(1))
      :P$=P$+"        A ="+STR$(A)
      :GOSUB 400
44180 DI=(MY(J)-MY(1))
44190 P$="Mean of '"+FI$(J)+"' differs from the mean of '"+FI$(1)
      +"'"
      :GOSUB 400
44200 P$="by an amount between: "+STR$(DI-A)+" and"+STR$(DI+A)+".
      "
      :GOSUB 400
44210 NEXT J
44220 RETURN



File name: PCS45/LIB
---------------------------------------------------------------------

45000 DATA "45> Mann-Whitney U-Test",2
45010 REM 02/13/86 VER 4.0
```

```
45020 GOSUB 45100
      :REM Input
45030 GOSUB 45200
      :REM Process
45040 GOSUB 45500
      :REM Output
45050 RETURN
45100 P$="Enter the sample with the smallest n first."
      :GOSUB 302
45110 L=2
      :GOSUB 2100
      :IF L<>2 THEN P$="You must enter 2 groups!"
      :GOSUB 302
      :GOTO 45100
45120 RETURN
45200 FOR J=1 TO 2
      :FOR I=1 TO N(J)
      :YA(I)=Y(I,J)
      :NEXT I
45210 FOR I=1 TO N(J)
      :FOR I1=1 TO N(J)-I
      :C=YA(I1)
      :D=YA(I1+1)
      :IF C<D THEN 45230
45220 YA(I1)=D
      :YA(I1+1)=C
45230 NEXT I1,I
      :P$= "'"+FI$(J)+"' Sorted
      : "
45240 FOR I=1 TO N(J)
      :P$=P$+STR$(YA(I))
      :NEXT I
      :GOSUB 400
45250 IF J=2 THEN 45260 ELSE FOR I=1 TO N(1)
      :XA(I)=YA(I)
      :NEXT I
45260 NEXT J
      :GOSUB 400
45270 P$="Sequence of ranks (members of '"+FI$(1)+"' are indicate
      d with *)"
45280 GOSUB 400
      :X=0
      :Y=0
      :R=1
      :J=0
45290 I=0
45300 J=J+1
      :I=I+1
45310 IF J>N(1) THEN 45400 ELSE IF I>N(2) THEN 45420
45320 IF XA(J)<YA(I) THEN 45420 ELSE IF YA(I)<XA(J) THEN 45410 EL
      SE I1=2
      :M=J
45330 J1=I
      :R1=2*R+1
      :R=R+2
      :J=J+1
      :I=I+1
45340 IF J>N(1) THEN 45360 ELSE IF XA(J)<>XA(J-1) THEN 45360 ELSE
      J=J+1
45350 GOTO 45370
45360 IF I>N(2) THEN 45380 ELSE IF YA(I)<>YA(I-1) THEN 45380 ELSE
      I=I+1
45370 R1=R1+R
      :R=R+1
      :I1=I1+1
      : GOTO 45340
45380 T=(J-M)*R1/I1
      :P$=P$+STR$(T)+"*"
      :X=X+T
      :T=(I-J1)*R1/I1
      :P$=P$+STR$(T)+" "
45390 Y=Y+T
      :GOTO 45310
45400 IF I>N(2) THEN 45450
45410 Y=Y+R
```

```
           :P$=P$+STR$(R)+" "
           :I=I+1
           :GOTO 45430
  45420 X=X+R
           :P$=P$+STR$(R)+"*"
           :J=J+1
  45430 R=R+1
           :GOTO 45310
  45440 REM          calculate U
  45450 U1=N(1)*N(2)+N(1)*(N(1)+1)/2-X
  45460 U2=N(1)*N(2)+N(2)*(N(2)+1)/2-Y
           :RETURN
  45500 GOSUB 402
           :P$(0,0)="File name:"
           :P$(0,1)=FI$(1)
           :P$(0,2)=FI$(2)
           :FOR I=0 TO 2
           :P$(1,I)=UL$
           :NEXT I
  45510 P$(2,0)="N:"
           :P$(2,1)=STR$(N(1))
           :P$(2,2)=STR$(N(2))
  45520 P$(3,0)="R:"
           :P$(3,1)=STR$(X)
           :P$(3,2)=STR$(Y)
  45530 P$(4,0)="U:"
           :P$(4,1)=STR$(U1)
           :P$(4,2)=STR$(U2)
           :R%=4
           :C%=2
           :GOSUB 700
  45540 P$=FNF$("N =")
           :IF N(1)<N(2) THEN P$=P$+FNP$(N(2)) ELSE P$=P$+FNP$(N(1))
  45550 GOSUB 400
           :P$=FNF$("U =")
           :IF U1<U2 THEN P$=P$+FNP$(U1) ELSE P$=P$+FNP$(U2)
  45560 GOSUB 400
  45999 RETURN



File name: PCS46/LIB
---------------------------------------------------------------------

  146 DIM Z(IZ,JZ)
      :REM PCS46/LIB
  46000 DATA "46> Litchfield & Wilcoxon I: Confidence Limits of ED5
       0",9
  46010 REM 02/13/86 VER 4.0
  46015 IF U%=47 THEN P$="This procedure takes a quantal d-r curve
        and calculates ED16, ED50, and ED85, and associated confide
        nce limits.  You may then enter a 2nd curve to get a potenc
        y ratio with confidence limits."
           :GOSUB 302
  46018 P$="You will be entering # Responding and # in Group, not p
        ercent responding."
           :GOSUB 302
  46020 P$="Do not enter more than two 0% and two 100% points for e
        ach curve."
           :GOSUB 302
           :F1=0
  46025 L=1
           :JP=3
           :PZ$="# in Group"
           :PY$="# Responding"
           :GOSUB 9100
           : REM Input dose & percent effect
  46030 GOSUB 46095
           :REM Convert dead/n to percent
  46035 GOSUB 46130
           :REM Convert dose to log(dose)
  46040 GOSUB 46165
           :REM Convert 10-90% effects to probits
  46045 GOSUB 46210
           :REM Calc. initial regression line
```

```
46050 GOSUB 46235
      :REM Calc. probits from line & convert to %
46055 GOSUB 46270
      :REM Get corrected effects for 0% & 100%
46060 GOSUB 46320
      :REM Convert % to probit & 2nd regression line
46065 GOSUB 46355
      :REM Calculate Chi-square
46070 GOSUB 46500
      :IF A$="Y" THEN 46025
      :REM Calc. ED50 with confidence limits
46075 RETURN
46080 REM
46085 REM Input # of animals at each dose
46090 REM
46095 PY$="Response"
      :NA=0
      :FOR I=1 TO N(1)
46100 Y(I,1)=100*(Y(I,1)/Z(I,1))
46105 NA=NA+Z(I,1)
      :NEXT I
      :GOSUB 580
46110 RETURN
46115 REM
46120 REM Convert dose --> log(dose)
46125 REM
46130 J=1
46135 IF PX$="Dose" THEN GOSUB 520
46140 GOSUB 600
      :REM save x & y matrix
46145 RETURN
46150 REM
46155 REM Convert % between 10-90% to probits
46160 REM
46165 NN=N(1)
      :IN=1
      :I=1
      :PY$="Probit"
46170 IF YA(I)<10 OR YA(I)>90 THEN 46180
46175 PC=YA(I)
      :GOSUB 9980
      :X(IN,J)=XA(I)
      :Y(IN,J)=PR
      :IN=IN+1
46180 I=I+1
      :IF I<=N(J) THEN 46170
46185 IN=IN-1
      :N(1)=IN
      :P$="Observed probit   :"
      :GOSUB 46650
46190 RETURN
46195 REM
46200 REM Calc. initial regression line
46205 REM
46210 PY$="(1) Probit"
      :GOSUB 2660
      :GOSUB 3230
      :GOSUB 3830
46215 RETURN
46220 REM
46225 REM Calc. probits from line & convert to %
46230 REM
46235 P$="Probit from line : "
46240 N(J)=NN
      :FOR I=1 TO N(J)
      :X(I,J)=XA(I)
      :NEXT I
      :GOSUB 46470
46245 P$="Expected effect   :"
      :GOSUB 46650
46250 RETURN
46255 REM
46260 REM Get corrected effect for 0 & 100% points
46265 REM
46270 FOR I=1 TO N(J)
```

```
46275 IF YA(I)>0 AND YA(I)<100 THEN 46290
46280 NV%=INT(Y(I,J)+.5)
46282 IF YA(I)=0 AND NV%>49 THEN YA(I)=10.5
      :GOTO 46290
46284 IF YA(I)=100 AND NV%<51 THEN YA(I)=89.5
      :GOTO 46290
46285 RA$="A12"+ET$+"PCS"
      :GOSUB 55000
      :YA(I)=V!
46290 Y(I,J)=YA(I)
      :NEXT I
46295 P$="Obs./Corrected % :"
      :GOSUB 46650
46300 RETURN
46305 REM
46310 REM Convert % to probits & calc. 2nd regression line
46315 REM
46320 PY$="(2) Probit"
      :GOSUB 9240
      :P$="Corrected probit :"
      :GOSUB 46650
46325 P$="Corrected probit : "
      :GOSUB 46470
      :REM calc probit -> %
46330 P$="Expected effect  :"
      :GOSUB 46650
46335 RETURN
46340 REM
46345 REM Calc. Chi-square
46350 REM
46355 X2=0
      :P$= "Chi-square: "
46360 FOR I=1 TO N(J)
46365 G=YA(I)-Y(I,J)
      :G=G*G
46370 G=G/(Y(I,J)*(100-Y(I,J)))
46375 P$=P$+STR$(G)+" "
      :X2=X2+G
46380 NEXT I
46385 IF IV$="Y" THEN GOSUB 402
46400 X2=X2*(NA/N(J))
      :NV%=N(J)-2
      :RA$="C95"+ET$+"PCS"
      :GOSUB 55000
      :XT=V!
46410 GOSUB 9620
      :REM Calc. ED50 & S function
46415 NP=0
      :FOR I=1 TO N(1)
      :D=10[X(I,1)
      :IF (D>=E1 AND D<=E8) OR (D>=E8 AND D<=E1) THEN NP=NP+Z(I,1)
      :REM # between 16 & 84
46425 NEXT I
      :P$="Total number of animals used ="+STR$(NA)
      :GOSUB 400
46430 P$="Animals between ED16 & ED84  ="+STR$(NP)
      :GOSUB 402
46432 P$="Chi-Square for"+STR$(N(J)-2)+" d.f.      ="+STR$(XT)
      :GOSUB 400
46434 P$="Chi-Square, calculated      ="+STR$(X2)
      :GOSUB 402
46436 IF NP<1 THEN P$="Confidence Limits Undetermined"
      :GOSUB 402
      :RETURN
46440 IF X2<XT THEN F=SF[(2.77/SQR(NP)) ELSE N=N(J)-2
      :GOSUB 5600
      :F=SF[(1.4*TV*SQR(X2/(N*NP)))
46445 IF IV$="Y" THEN P$="Factor(ED50) ="+STR$(F)
      :GOSUB 400
46450 RETURN
46455 REM
46460 REM Calculate probit from regression line & convert to %
46465 REM
46470 FOR I=1 TO N(J)
      :X=X(I,J)
```

```
          :GOSUB 9840
          :P$=P$+STR$(P)+" "
          :Y(I,J)=PC
          :NEXT I
46475 IF IV$="Y" THEN GOSUB 402
          :ELSE P$=""
46480 RETURN
46485 REM
46490 REM Calculate Confidence Limits
        : ED16,ED50,ED84
46495 REM
46500 J=1
          :GOSUB 2700
          :XB=10[ XB
          :XS=10[ XS
          :REM get Xbig/Xsmall
46505 SF=LOG(SF)/LOG(10)
          :A=10[ (1.1*(SF*SF)/(LOG(XB/XS)/LOG(10)))
46510 K=N(1)
          :IF X2<XT THEN FS=A[ ((10*(K-1))/(K*SQR(NP)))
46515 IF X2>XT THEN FS=A[ ((5.1*TV*(K-1)*SQR(X2/(N*NP)))/K)
46520 F8=10[ ((LOG(FS)/LOG(10)*LOG(FS)/LOG(10))+(LOG(F)/LOG(10)*LO
      G(F)/LOG(10)))
46525 U8=E8*F8
      :L8!=E8/F8
      :U1=E1*F8
      :L1!=E1/F8
      :L5!=E5/F
      :U5=E5*F
46530 GOSUB 400
      :GOSUB 5620
      :P$(0,2)="95% Limits:":P$(1,2)=""
      :P$(0,0)=FI$(1)
46535 IF U%=46 THEN P$(2,0)="ED50"
      :R%=3
      :ELSE P$(2,0)="ED16"
      :P$(3,0)="ED50"
      :P$(4,0)="ED84"
      :R%=4
46540 GOSUB 46580
46545 IF F1=0 THEN F1=E5
      :F3=F
      :FI$=FI$(1)
      :ELSE F2=E5
      :F4=F
      :REM save ED50,Fed50
46550 IF U%=46 THEN P$(0,0)="Log(ED50)" ELSE P$(0,0)="Log(ED16)"
      :P$(1,0)="Log(ED50)"
      :P$(2,0)="Log(ED84)"
46555 IF U%=47 THEN E1=LOG(E1)/LOG(10)
      :L1!=LOG(L1!)/LOG(10)
      :U1=LOG(U1)/LOG(10)
46560 E5=LOG(E5)/LOG(10)
      :L5!=LOG(L5!)/LOG(10)
      :U5=LOG(U5)/LOG(10)
      :R%=1
46565 IF U%=47 THEN E8=LOG(E8)/LOG(10)
      :L8!=LOG(L8!)/LOG(10)
      :U8=LOG(U8)/LOG(10)
      :R%=2
46570 GOSUB 46580
      :GOSUB 46610
46575 RETURN
46580 IF U%=47 THEN P$(R%-2,1)=STR$(E1)
      :IF F<>0 THEN P$(R%-2,3)=STR$(L1!)
      :P$(R%-2,4)=STR$(U1)
46585 P$(R%-1,1)=STR$(E5)
      :IF F<>0 THEN P$(R%-1,3)=STR$(L5!)
      :P$(R%-1,4)=STR$(U5)
46590 IF U%=47 THEN P$(R%,1)=STR$(E8)
      :IF F<>0 THEN P$(R%,3)=STR$(L8!)
      :P$(R%,4)=STR$(U8)
46595 C%=4
      :GOSUB 700
      :REM Print screen matrix
```

```
46600 RETURN
46605 REM Potency Ratio w/ confidence limits
46610 IF U%=46 THEN RETURN ELSE IF F2=0 THEN 46635
46615 PR=F1/F2
      :F3=LOG(F3)/LOG(10)
      :F4=LOG(F4)/LOG(10)
      :FR=10[ SQR((F3*F3)+(F4*F4))
46620 P$(0,0)="Pot. Ratio:"
      :P$(0,1)=STR$(PR)
      :P$(0,3)=STR$(PR/FR)
      :P$(0,4)=STR$(PR*FR)
46625 R%=0
      :C%=4
      :GOSUB 700
46627 P$="The Potency Ratio of "+FI$+" versus "+FI$(1)+" is"
      :IF (PR/FR)<=1 THEN P$=P$+" not"
46628 P$=P$+" significant."
      :GOSUB 402
46630 REM Compare w/ another curve?
46635 P$="Do you want to compare the potency of '"+FI$+"' with an
      other quantal dose-response curve (Y/N)"
      :GOSUB 250
      :GOSUB 300
46640 RETURN
46645 REM Print Y array
46650 IF IV$="N" THEN P$=""
      :RETURN
      :ELSE P$=P$+" "
      :FOR I=1 TO N(1)
      :P$=P$+STR$(Y(I,1))+" "
      :NEXT I
      :GOSUB 402
46999 RETURN
```

File name: PCS47/LIB

```
47000 DATA "47> Litchfield & Wilcoxon II",46
47010 REM 10/17/85 VER 4.0
47020 GOTO 46000
47999 RETURN
```

File name: PCS48/LIB

```
48000 DATA "48> Differential Equations",2
48010 REM 03/04/86 VER 4.0
48012 REM CLOSE 2
      :LP=0
      :REM turn off report save
48020 GOSUB 48050
      :REM input
48030 GOSUB 48160
      :REM process
48040 RETURN
48050 L=1
      :JP=2
48060 P$="This procedure solves 1st order differential equations
      using the Runge-Kutta approximation.  You will be prompted
      for the equation, initial values, and increment in x."
      :GOSUB 302
48070 P$="For example, the equation, dY/dX = X - 2Y, must be ente
      red as:  dY/dX = X - 2*Y.  Be sure to use parenthesis when n
      eeded."
      :GOSUB 302
48080 OPEN "I",1,"SYS5/PCS"
      :LINE INPUT #1,EQ$
      :CLOSE 1
```

```
48090 EQ$=RIGHT$(EQ$,LEN(EQ$)-INSTR(EQ$,"="))
48100 P$="Equation currently in memory: dY/dX = "+EQ$
      :GOSUB 302
48110 P$="Press <ENTER> to retain this equation or enter new equa
      tion (right side only, no '=')."
      :GOSUB 302
48120 P$="       dy/dx = ? "
      :GOSUB 310
      :LINE INPUT A$
      :GOSUB 300
48130 IF A$<>"" THEN GOSUB 48270 ELSE 48150
48135 X$="SYS5/PCS"
      :P$="Merging equation ..."
      :GOSUB 300
48140 MERGE X$
48150 P$="Enter initial conditions:":GOSUB 300
      :P$=FNF$("X = ")
      :GOSUB 260
      :X0=VAL(A$)
      :P$=FNF$("Y = ")
      :GOSUB 260
      :Y0=VAL(A$)
      :P$=FNF$("Increment = ")
      :GOSUB 260
      :H=VAL(A$)
      :P$=FNF$("X max = ")
      :GOSUB 260
      :XM=VAL(A$)
      :GOSUB 302
48155 RETURN
48160 P$="Equation: dy/dx = "+EQ$:GOSUB 402
      :P$=FNF$("Xo =")+STR$(X0)
      :GOSUB 400
      :P$=FNF$("Yo =")+STR$(Y0)
      :GOSUB 400
      :P$=FNF$("Xmax =")+STR$(XM)
      :GOSUB 400
      :P$=FNF$("Increment =")+STR$(H)
      :GOSUB 402
      :P$="Press <ESC> to abort printout."
      :GOSUB 302
48165 P$=FNF$("Xi")+FNF$("Yi")
      :GOSUB 400
      :P$=UL$+UL$
      :GOSUB 400
48170 P$=FNP$(X0)+FNP$(Y0)
      :GOSUB 400
      :IF INKEY$=CHR$(27) THEN RETURN
48180 X=X0
      :Y=Y0
      :GOSUB 48500
      :A1=H*DY
48190 X=X0+H/2
      :Y=Y0+A1/2
      :GOSUB 48500
      :A2=H*DY
48200 Y=Y0+A2/2
      :GOSUB 48500
      :A3=H*DY
48210 X=X0+H
      :Y=Y0+A3
      :GOSUB 48500
      :A4=H*DY
48220 X0=X0+H
      :Y0=Y0+(A1+2*A2+2*A3+A4)/6
48230 IF X0>XM+H THEN RETURN ELSE 48170
48260 RETURN
48270 EZ$="48500 DY="+A$
48280 OPEN "O",1,"SYS5/PCS"
48290 PRINT #1,EZ$
48300 CLOSE 1
48350 RETURN
48400 REM dY/dX equation on line 48500
48500 DY= X + Y
48999 RETURN
```

PHARM/PCS Version 4

Program Registration & Diskette Ordering Information

Use this form to register your purchase of *Manual of Pharmacologic Calculations with Computer Programs. 2nd Edition* and to receive price information for PHARM/PCS on diskette. You will be notified of program updates and changes, and Springer-Verlag will inform you of new titles in pharmacology and related areas.

If you purchase PHARM/PCS on diskette you may deduct the cost of this book. Please retain your original receipt as proof of purchase. If you own an older version of PHARM/BAS (Version 1) or PHARM/PCS (Version 2 or 3) you may apply credit toward your purchase. You must return your original diskette with your order as proof of purchase.

Discounts are available for students and for quantity purchases.

Name: _____

Affiliation: _____

Address: _____

City: _____ State: _____ Zip: _____

Phone: (_____) _____

Computer: _____

Do you own a copy of the First Edition of this book? _____

Do you currently use an earlier version of PHARM/PCS? _____

You will be sent pricing information. Please indicate if you have interest in the following:

_____ Student discount.   _____ Quantity discount.

Mail this form to: MicroComputer Specialists
                   P.O. Box 40346
                   Philadelphia, PA 19106

Note: Version 4 is available (at the time of this publication) for all MS-DOS computers (IBM-PC and compatibles) and Tandy/Radio Shack TRS-80 Models. You will be notified of the availability of versions for other computers.

(Springer-Verlag New York, Inc. is not associated with MicroComputer Specialists.)

Index